AF574352

Work Worth Doing
Advances in Brain Injury Rehabilitation

Work Worth Doing
Advances in Brain Injury Rehabilitation

Edited by:
Brian T. McMahon
Linda R. Shaw

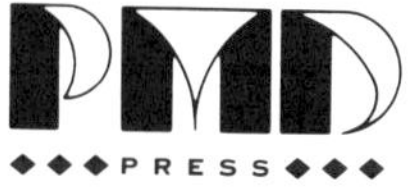

Published by
Paul M. Deutsch Press, Inc.

Editorial Staff:

Production Editor: Ann Groom
Publication Specialist: Debra Kramer

Paul M. Deutsch Press, Inc.
A Paul M. Deutsch Company
2211 Hillcrest Street
Orlando, FL 32803

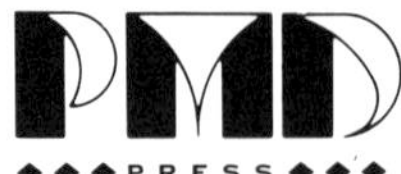

ISBN: 1-878205-19-6

Library of Congress Card Catalog Number: 91-071166

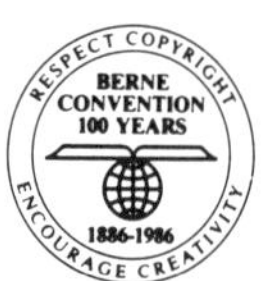

Cover designed by Groom Design

Printed in the United States of America

Dedication

This book is dedicated to the memory of Thomas J. McMahon whose life of humility, kindness, and commitment to others served as an inspiration for this work.

Far and away the best prize that life offers is the chance to work hard at work worth doing.

President Theodore Roosevelt
September 7, 1903

About the Editors

Brian T. McMahon, Ph.D., C.R.C.

Brian McMahon is Associate Professor and Director of the Rehabilitation Counselor Training Program at the University of Wisconsin – Milwaukee. He is also a certified rehabilitation counselor and consulting psychologist with offices in Milwaukee and Chicago. Dr. McMahon has authored over 40 publications regarding the vocational rehabilitation of severely disabled persons. In the 1980s, he developed and/or supervised nine head injury rehabilitation programs at five levels of care across five states. Dr. McMahon is a former board member of the American Psychological Association Division of Rehabilitation Psychology and the National Council on Rehabilitation Education. He is also past-President of the American Rehabilitation Counseling Association.

Linda R. Shaw, Ph.D., C.R.C.

Linda Shaw is an Assistant Professor in the Department of Rehabilitation Counseling, College of Health Related Professions at the University of Florida. She is a member of the Executive Council of the American Rehabilitation Counseling Association and was formerly a member of the Board of Directors of the Wisconsin Brain Trauma Association. Dr. Shaw has developed and/or managed four head injury rehabilitation programs specializing in coma management, neurobehavioral, acute, post-acute, and outpatient rehabilitation.

Contributing Authors

Deborah L. Abrams, M. Ed.
Director of Post-Acute Brain Injury Services
Sharp HealthCare
San Diego, California

Craig F. Bitter, M. S.
Behavior Specialist
New Medico Community Re-Entry Services of Ann Arbor
Ann Arbor, Michigan

Fong Chan, Ph. D.
Associate Professor, Department of Psychology
Illinois Institute of Technology
Chicago, Illinois

Lynn P. Cullity, O. T. R. - L.
Occupational Therapist
East Sandwich, Massachusetts

Patrick M. Devine, M. A.
Associate Program Director
New Medico South Bay Community Re-Entry Services
Hyannis, Massachusetts

Jack G. Dial, Ph. D.
Consulting Neuropsychologist
3-Dimensional Systems
Dallas, Texas

Charles J. Durgin, M. S.
Program Director
Community Rehabilitation Services of Annapolis
Annapolis, Maryland

Randall W. Evans, Ph. D.
Vice President, Research and Development
Learning Services Corporation
Durham, North Carolina

Robert T. Fraser, Ph. D., C. R. C.
Associate Professor
University of Washington, Department of Neurological Surgery
Seattle, Washington

Steven G. Gray, Ph. D.
Clinical Assistant Professor, Department of Rehabilitation Science
University of Texas Southwest Medical Center
Dallas, Texas

William J. Haffey, Ph. D.
Executive Director, Rehabilitation Services
Sharp HealthCare
San Diego, California

Jodi D. Jackson, O. T. R.
Program Director, Supported Living Services
Learning Services – Carolina
Durham, North Carolina

Michael L. Jones, Ph. D.
Director, Life Coach Program
Learning Services Corporation
Manassas, Virginia

Chow S. Lam, Ph. D.
Associate Professor, Department of Psychology
Illinois Institute of Technology
Chicago, Illinois

Mervin J. Langley, Ph. D.
Psychosocial Specialist
Meadowbrook of Chicago
Chicago, Illinois

Frank D. Lewis, Ph. D.
Program Administrator, Head Injury Center
St. Joseph's Rehabilitation Hospital
Augusta, Georgia

David P. Mahaffey, M. A., C. R. C.
Administrator
Meadowbrook of Chicago
Chicago, Illinois

Michelle Marmé, Ph. D.
Assistant Professor, Department of Psychology
Illinois Institute of Technology
Chicago, Illinois

Brian T. McMahon, Ph. D., C. R. C.
Associate Professor, Department of Educational Psychology
University of Wisconsin-Milwaukee
Milwaukee, Wisconsin

Peter D. Patrick, Ph. D.
Program Director
Learning Services—Shenandoah
Manassas, Virginia

Mary P. Ridgely, M. S.
Supported Employment Specialist
Department of Health and Social Services, Division of Vocational Rehabilitation
Madison, Wisconsin

Gwen Roldan, M. S.
Doctoral Candidate, Department of Psychology
Illinois Institute of Technology
Chicago, Illinois

Robert Schleser, Ph. D.
Associate Professor, Department of Psychology
Illinois Institute of Technology
Chicago, Illinois

Linda R. Shaw, Ph. D., C. R. C.
Assistant Professor, Department of Rehabilitation Counseling
University of Florida
Gainesville, Florida

Roy Tunick, Ed. D.
Professor, Department of Counseling, Rehabilitation Counseling, and Counseling Psychology
West Virginia University
Morgantown, West Virginia

J. Jepson Wulff, Ph. D.
Management Consultant
Learning Services Corporation
Montpelier, Vermont

Table of Contents

Section 1 - Management

Section 2 - Vocational Re-entry

Section 3 - Community Re-entry

Foreword

Since 1984 we have developed or managed over 12 rehabilitation programs for persons with traumatic brain injury (TBI) at five levels of care across six states. We have consulted to an equal number of programs, and have visited dozens more. The gentleman to whom this book is dedicated was obsessed with the adage, "Anything worth doing is worth doing well." In spite of the trials and tribulations, the ambiguity, and stresses of all this program development activity, we remain convinced that TBI rehabilitation is definitely work worth doing, and through this book we have endeavored to contribute something of our own to the improvement of the TBI rehabilitation practice.

During these past seven years, we have observed the dramatic, hundredfold proliferation of TBI programs nationally, and have attempted to observe, document, and replicate "best practices" wherever, whenever, and however we discovered them. Some of these are described here to provide a more solid foundation for a TBI rehabilitation industry which can grow better as well as bigger in the decade ahead.

As active educators and researchers, we witnessed the gradual evolution of TBI rehabilitation from an art to a more precise art form with some features of science. We have constantly researched our own practices and outcomes and, in collaboration with many other conscientious professionals, have endeavored to constantly refine and improve our services. Through all this, we maintained a strong allegiance to the basic philosophical principles of rehabilitation which we learned as young rehabilitation counselors many years ago. Unfortunately, divergence from these principles has sometimes occurred in recent years resulting in serious financial and image problems for the TBI industry. These are described and a course of remediation is prescribed in the first section of this book on "Management." We acknowledge that these chapters are likely to be controversial, however, we welcome any controversy that causes managers and practitioners to critically examine the important ethical and philosophical issues reviewed herein.

As rehabilitation counselors, we have a long-held professional bias toward the pre-eminence of vocational objectives and vocational restoration methods in the overall rehabilitation effort of individuals with TBI. In a society in which vocational and personal identity are co-mingled, and in which so many of our basic needs are reinforced by work activity, we have wondered aloud how we have dared for so long to regard the business of rehabilitation as complete without aggressive vocational rehabilitation. This bias is reflected in the middle section of the book entitled "Vocational Re-entry." A full seven chapters are devoted to specific strategies which are intended to maximize return-to-work outcomes for survivors of TBI. Innovative perspectives on neuropsychological and vocational evaluation, work adjustment training, and job placement methods are submitted as the cornerstones upon which a more formidable vocational rehabilitation initiative may be constructed in the future.

In the third and final section on "Community Re-entry," we have endeavored to tackle head-on those nonvocational treatment issues which represent primary impediments to long-term recovery. Persistent and sticky programming problems, such as the prevention of alcohol involvement, community skills training, home-based treatment interventions, the maintenance and generalization of treatment effects, and the sequencing of various family services, are all addressed. Not to be perceived as "miscellaneous issues," these are all matters which, if overlooked, can and will completely reverse gains which are achieved at considerable time and expense in the acute and post-acute levels of treatment. We have attempted to go beyond eloquent statements of the problem or detailed reviews of the pertinent literature to present actual methods and techniques which, if executed properly, can maximize the level of functioning and minimize the level of long-term support required of individuals with TBI.

TBI rehabilitation is work worth doing, and as such is worth doing well. We hope that the collective thinking of the 26 rehabilitationists who have contributed to this book will result in improvements in service delivery to persons with TBI and their families.

Brian T. McMahon
Linda R. Shaw

Acknowledgements

This book represents the collective wisdom, proven experience, and educated guesses of 26 dedicated rehabilitation professionals who have contributed as authors. To each we express our heartfelt appreciation for the time, energy, patience, and thorough professional preparation which have gone into each chapter. We also appreciate the scores of high-level colleagues, individuals with TBI, and their family members from whom we learned so much, and with whom we struggle shoulder-to-shoulder in our collective search for a better way. Finally, we thank our families who have nurtured our values and supported our careers as rehabilitationists.

1

Management

1

Ethics in Business Practices

Brian T. McMahon

1

Ethics in Business Practices

Brian T. McMahon

Introduction

Only a decade ago, there were but a handful of categorical post-acute traumatic brain injury (TBI) rehabilitation programs nationally. Clinical and management expertise was sparse. Facility administrators were charged with full and complete responsibility for the coordination of admissions, quality assurance, customer satisfaction, discharge planning, reimbursement, and marketing, in addition to facility operations. These were regarded as being within the proper purview of professionals and managers (most with clinical expertise themselves) who operated at the individual facility where services were actually delivered.

As with other areas of health care, however, and because of the hundredfold proliferation of TBI rehabilitation programs nationally, many TBI rehabilitation facilities have incorporated into regional and national business concerns. Due to the incorporation of rehabilitation as a business enterprise and a number of other overlapping trends, the modern-day rehabilitation setting has too often been transformed into an environment where hate, power, envy, and greed are observed in business policies, practices, and everyday operations (Mullins, 1989). According to Mullins (1989), the situation now exists:

> *...for financial concern at best, and greed at worst, to begin to rule the day....such goals as (the maintenance of quality patient care and the highest quality outcome)...must now be fulfilled in the context of cost containment and the maximizing of profit....decision making that ultimately affects direct treatment efforts takes place in a context far removed–technically and physically–from the rehabilitation setting....(by) individuals whose primary area of expertise is financial...to establish policy, objectives, and goals for an enterprise about which they know little. (pp. 741-742)*

Mullins (1989) further speculates as to how a rehabilitation industry, consumed by its focus on revenue, *could hypothetically* result in such consequences as direct overbilling, the delivery of unnecessary services, overpricing, staff dissension, burnout, mistrust of management, ethical misconduct, and jealousy. Worse yet,..."the professional who plays this game best is also the one most likely to be rewarded" (p. 742).

The purpose of this chapter is to describe how such eventualities may have moved beyond the hypothetical. Indeed, it is this author's assertion that Mullins (1989) may have understated the case. This chapter seeks to explore the ways in which organizational characteristics of select TBI rehabilitation settings relate to the nature and quality of the rehabilitation services provided. It is suggested that certain business practices (e.g., tightly centralized corporate control of selected functions) and certain treatment settings (e.g., large, residential post-acute) do, by their nature, compromise the very principles which define rehabilitation.

These features tend to cause serious conflicts of interest if not crises of conscience among ethical facility managers and professionals. They serve to distort the stated mission of the organization (typically related to the provision of quality rehabilitation services to clients); the nature of the rehabilitation services provided; and the roles, functions, and integrity of the rehabilitation professionals employed therein. State facility and discipline-specific licensing requirements, facility accreditation standards, codes of ethics of the various health-related professions, sound business practices, regard for the reputation of the organization and its employees, and even legal considerations may be compromised in the pursuit of manifest (but never publicly expressed) alternative organizational goals. Where these alternative goals exist, they typically include the blind pursuit of maximum profit, the containment of costs, the elimination of legitimate competitors, and enhanced market share.

Corporate Acquisition of Professional Rehabilitation Functions

The specific focus of this chapter is upon providers of TBI services, typically in the post-acute arena, which are very large in size, national in scope, for profit in nature, and highly centralized in terms of management power. Admittedly not all post-acute TBI service providers engage in these practices nor do all share these organizational characteristics. Among those that do, however, owners and corporate officers often feel a profound lack of control over their own business processes. This is often compounded by the rapid growth which has characterized the TBI industry in the past 10 years.

During the course of this rapid development, attention to sound human resource practices, clinical processes, and accurate management information systems lags far behind development and marketing concerns. Because local facility managers may be hired at a rapid rate, there is often little time available to establish relationships of mutual trust and respect. As growth ensues, face-to-face meetings are replaced by faxed correspondence and teleconferences. In this context, corporate owners and officers become even more reluctant to delegate to facility managers the authority which is consistent with their levels of responsibility. Caution gives way to suspicion which sometimes gives way to paranoia.

As the organization grows in size and geographic scope a number of clinical and managerial functions, once regarded as the proper purview of personnel at the facility level, begin to be subsumed by newly created corporate entities or departments. For purposes of this chapter, these functions will be limited to marketing, referral coordination, reimbursement coordination, customer satisfaction, discharge planning, legal affairs, operations management, training and development, information systems, and research.

Corporate appropriation of these functions occurs not only because of the aforementioned lack of trust which is commonplace in rapidly growing organizations, but also, in some cases, because of the failures of facility-based managers to properly discharge these responsibilities in a manner which considers both the needs of the client and the organization. While ostensibly this is the fault of the individual facility managers involved, such errors may also be attributed to their lack of orientation and training, lack of supervision, and corporate recruitment practices designed to expeditiously fill vacancies without regard to proper job temperament or experience (McMahon, Shaw, & Mahaffey, 1988).

The gradual corporate confiscation of these functions as a response to either perceived lack of corporate control or to actual local management failure temporarily ameliorates the principals (i.e., owners and corporate executives). There are, however, significant costs associated with such reorganization. For example, there are obvious financial outlays in terms of additional salaries, space, and support requirements for this new layer of bureaucracy. There is the buffering and removal of the principals even further from the actual playing field which compromises the accuracy of information exchanges in both directions. Finally, there is the aftermath of requiring universal facility cooperation with these new corporate entities regardless of an individual facility's previous record of success in managing a particular function independently. To further illustrate this process, each function is explored in terms of how its corporate acquisition may eventually distort its intended purpose, and the dynamics which cause discomfort and conflict for facility-based managers and professionals.

MARKETING ASSOCIATE

The stated purpose of the corporate Marketing Associate is to enhance the awareness of prospective consumers and referral sources regarding the services provided by the organization. In reality, the actual purpose is to increase the number of admissions to facilities, increase the client census, and increase the facility revenue. Whereas the purview and authority of Marketing Associates are variable from one provider to the next, in some "market-driven," or "consumer-driven" organizations they are near absolute. Marketing Associates are often trained and encouraged to provide assurances to prospective clients or referral sources that the organization can and will meet their expressed needs, however unreasonable these may be. Oftentimes these assurances take the form of promises regarding the provision of services which exceed the capabilities of the local facility, which is then termed "inflexible," "unresponsive," or "not cooperative" if such exaggerated claims are questioned.

A second common occurrence is the pressure exerted by Marketing Associates upon the facility managers to render immediate and positive admission decisions and to immediately generate the necessary supporting documentation to expedite admissions. No excuse for unresponsiveness is valid, whether it is rooted in budgetary restraints, priority to extant clients, concerns over client mix, current client emergencies, other reporting requirements, staff shortages, limited staff expertise, regulatory requirements, or legal considerations. Excuses rooted in expressed ethical concerns result in the immediate and enduring label of "problem employee." In such an environment, cooperation by facility managers may be measured not in terms of results, but in terms of such minutiae as the speed with which phone calls to the Marketing Associate are accepted or returned.

REFERRAL COORDINATOR

The stated purpose of the corporate Referral Coordinator is to support the facility in the facilitation and coordination of the admissions process. As there are an extraordinary number of details pursuant to an admission, particularly to residential facilities which may be in a state or region different from the client's residence, there is little question that the need exists for such a categorical occupation. Whether the Referral Coordinator should be corporate or facility-based is another question.

Many corporate referral coordinators answer dozens of questions on a daily basis about facilities which they themselves have never even visited. Referral Coordinators typically arrange for letters of medical necessity and pre-admission "plans of care" to help secure funding approval. Because insurance approval is a significant part of the Referral Coordinator's responsiblitiy, many are former insurance claim representatives with little or no background in rehabilitation.

It is the handling of insurance funding approval which best reveals the way in which the corporate Referral Coordinator's function can be compromised. Specifically, when referred clients are found not to have the necessary funding to access the services of the provider, little or no "referral" activity ensues which might connect these clients with other providers or resources. The efforts are cursory at best, and therein lies the difference between a local professional who shares the same community with financially ineligible clients vs. the corporate, business-oriented Referral Coordinator in the home office in another state.

REIMBURSEMENT COORDINATOR

The stated purpose of the corporate Reimbursement Coordinator is to identify and resolve problems with payors, monitor facility receivables, and expedite collections. This seemingly straightforward business function appears difficult to compromise. Yet one must understand the funding structure to fully appreciate how such a role might become distorted. Specifically, many post-acute TBI rehabilitation facilities have difficulty obtaining reimbursement from the most prevalent type of insurance (group accident and health) because they may not be licensed health care entities, medical necessity has often not been clearly established, and/or services may be provided by nonlicensed personnel (i.e., staff persons other than licensed/certified physical therapists, occupational therapists and assistants, speech and language pathologists, or psychologists). Approvals for these therapies are critical because all other services, while clinically necessary and required by standards in the TBI industry, are not primarily medical in nature and; thus, are not typically "covered services" in group accident and health insurance contracts. For example, these include therapeutic recreation, vocational rehabilitation, independent living, case management, health care monitoring, and family services.

Accordingly, pre-admission letters of medical necessity and "plans of care" (typically required by health insurance companies prior to funding approval), the actual post-admission treatment plans themselves, and the client schedules which result are often designed to maximize the revenue per client by *prioritizing reimbursable service needs*, which may or may not be consistent with the rehabilitation service needs as assessed by facility-based clinical professionals.

Finally, "reimbursable clinicians" are encouraged, financially and otherwise, to sign-off on the activites of nonreimbursable personnel, oftentimes paraprofessional or completely untrained personnel. These activities have varying degrees of relevance to actual client needs and treatment goals as professionally assessed, and varying degrees of relevance to the legitimate therapy being billed. Such sign-off is necessary, however, to achieve daily revenue targets which in some companies are universally prescribed by corporate managers for all clients. Moreover, such sign-off frequently occurs for activities not recommended or designed by the reimbursable therapist, or conducted by others during hours of work in which the reimbursable therapist was not present.

In some cases, it may be the actual responsibility of the corporate Reimbursement Coordinator to monitor this process and ensure that targeted revenue figures are achieved per client per day for all "fee-for-service" clientele. In some cases, FFS clients only actually receive reimbursable services, particularly in the outpatient model. Unfortunately, per diem clients may rarely receive necessary reimbursable services because their priority allocation is to FFS clients. Hence, the individuality and appropriateness of treatment programs may be severely compromised because their design is so greatly influenced by funding arrangements. There may also be considerable differences between the treatment plans as written and the treatment services which are actually delivered.

CUSTOMER SATISFACTION REPRESENTATIVE

The stated purpose of the corporate Customer Satisfaction Representative is to systematically measure and monitor the level of satisfaction with the services provided by means of periodic telephone contacts with customers. Customers may include clients, family members, referral sources, attorneys, payors, external case managers, influencers, and others, but typically are family members of currently served clients. On balance this stated purpose is maintained and the feedback received is quite helpful in problem identification, program evaluation, and service enhancement. The reliability of the data is suspect, however, when customer complaints regarding the activities of corporate entities somehow go unreported. There is very little consideration of the stress which such families are experiencing when being interviewed during such surveys (Shaw & McMahon, 1990).

Additionally, such data may be organized, compiled, and/or utilized to depict a particular facility or manager as uncooperative or unresponsive. Thus, customer satisfaction data becomes ammunition which is used to persuade, intimidate, or coerce facility management whenever conflict occurs. The Customer Satisfaction Department, when abused in this way, may become an intimidating intelligence function designed to maintain corporate control.

DISCHARGE PLANNER

Some TBI corporations have created positions entitled corporate Discharge Planners. The stated purpose of the corporate Discharge Planner is to facilitate and coordinate the discharge planning process in the best interest of the client (McKenna, 1990). Too often, however, the Discharge Planner is charged with the responsibility of policing the facility Case Managers' actions throughout the discharge planning process. Because the corporate Discharge Planners represent corporate business interests rather than clinical concerns, they may find that their actual role involves extending the length of stay by whatever legitimate or artificial means necessary; extending the funding whenever possible, regardless of clinical need for more treatment or the potential exhaustion of all available treatment funds; and maintaining the client in the facility as long as possible.

If a different level of care is clearly indicated, the new priority may become transferring the client to another facility within the corporation, whether or not this is in the best interest of that client or family. Perpetual maintenance and fostering dependency upon the corporation may be encouraged, and not always subtly. Perhaps in no other arena are the tenets of "least restrictive environment" and "de-institutionalization" more obviously violated (see Chapter 2). Good rehabilitation practice and common sense would suggest that discharge planners be locally based so that meaningful community re-entry can be facilitated by one familiar with the community in question.

Once again, the best measure of the true nature of the discharge planning function (in a rehabilitation sense) is the activity of the Discharge Planner when clients have indisputably achieved their treatment objectives and are prepared to return home. Assistance and linkages with local resources, independent from or in competition with the provider, may be minimal or nonexistent. Moreover, when clients have exhausted their funding for rehabilitation prior to the realization of treatment objectives, or when insurance approvals were discovered to be in error, the focus of the Discharge Planner may shift to immediate discharge to family with or without provisions for alternative services, with details to be arranged by the facility.

LEGAL DEPARTMENT

The stated purpose of the corporate Legal Department is, quite logically, to represent the legal interests of the organization. In reality, however, its purpose is defined by the questions and issues which it is asked to resolve, and the manner in which such questions are asked. Following up on the issue of reimbursement, for example, clinicians are often quite candid about their discomfort with prescribed billing practices. The Legal Department may be asked to provide such clinicians with a legal interpretation of the licensing code in their discipline and state, and so to ameliorate their concerns about the legality of billing practices. However, legal and ethical questions may be deliberately blurred, and a resolution of the legal issue may be presented as a solution to the ethical question.

Legal Departments may be asked to find loopholes in the facility licensing code in a particular state to determine if any legal impediment exists to the admission of behaviorally involved, chemically involved, or medically involved clients not specifically addressed in the licensing code. In this way the level of care provided and the range of clients served by that facility may be gradually broadened.

Legal Departments may be asked to review promotional materials to evaluate whether exaggerated claims constitute legal misrepresentation. Personnel actions which may involve issues of discrimination, union-busting, or disciplinary actions related to noncompliance with billing practices are also routine matters of legal review.

One can only evaluate the use or abuse of the Legal Department by looking at the issues commonly researched (examples above); the motives of executives requesting legal consultation (which may relate to relaxing admission standards, maximizing exposure, minimizing litigation and negative publicity, distorting levels of care, and maximizing revenues); and the tone of the information request (e.g., What is the least common denominator? Who might litigate against us if we pursue this course? What can we get away with?).

OPERATIONS MANAGEMENT

The stated purpose of Operations Managment is to plan, supervise, control, and direct all areas of clinical service. In reality, the actual purpose may be more accurately understood by exploring the allocation of resources for operations relative to the other entities described; the accountability of operations managers to the other entities described; and the focus of their own activities and schedules which often tend to be around (in order of priority):

a. achieving revenue targets for each facility by:

   1. achieving fee-for-service targets on each client,
   2. extending client length of stay, and
   3. minimizing unpaid leaves of absence

b. cost containment in terms of:

   1. controlling facility payroll, and
   2. controlling facility expenses

c. cooperation of facility managers with aforementioned corporate entities and the reconciliation of differences (intended to placate the latter)

The issue of minimizing unpaid client leaves of absence provides perhaps the best illustration of how post-acute programs might stray from their stated purpose. In the early years of operation in such programs, clients who so chose were routinely allowed to go on home visits with families during major holidays. One might perceive this as normalizing and therapeutic, and a good opportunity to evaluate client progress. At some point, the corporate executives become aware of significant departures from projected revenues around the holiday season. Christmas and Thanksgiving become particularly "problematic." Each facility is directed by Operations Management to form a Holiday Planning Committee to deal with this problem. Corporate directives begin to pour down. It is eventually decided that it is in the therapeutic best interest of *all TBI clients* to remain in the facility during major holidays so that "continuity of care" would be maintained.

This is a classic case of creating a false conflict by compromising one rehabilitation tenet (normalization) in the alleged interest of another (continuity of care). Families are encouraged to visit and participate in lavish holiday festivities, and toward this end no expense is spared. Free housing and, in some cases, free transportation (including airfare) are provided to visitors. Operations Managers and Discharge Planners may work day and night to review each "problem case" who might go home and for whom the insurance company did not provide a bed-hold rate (guaranteeing partial reimbursement). Interestingly, clients who *do* have pre-approved bed-hold arrangements are not reviewed. Apparently there is less concern that their continuity of care may be compromised.

The scenario continues. The Public Relations Department prepares *verbatim* statements that are to be read by each facility case manager to each family describing how it is in the clinical best interest of the client to remain in the facility during the holiday. As a last resort, the Legal Department drafts pre-admission forms that are hurriedly signed by distressed families in which they agree to be responsible for full payment to the facility if they "pull" their family member out of the facility during holidays. The management of the entire organization becomes obsessively focused on LOA days during holidays.

Another telling sign of hidden agendas which may be held by the Operations Manager is the introduction of seemingly innovative services. Examples of these services, typically not directly reimbursable in their own right in the FFS market, might include vocational rehabilitation, substance abuse counseling, case management, medical management, therapeutic recreation, and family counseling. Such services may be inserted into and withdrawn from a facility's repertoire without their clinical effectiveness ever being systematically evaluated. If these services can attract new patients, extend the length of stay of current patients, or increase revenue they are maintained and expanded. If they do not, they are downscaled or eliminated without regard to their potential to improve clinical outcomes.

For example, how can an affirmative industry approach to supported employment be abused? There is no need for clients to return home and go to work if they are provided with a job at the facility. How can an aggressive program of therapeutic recreation be abused? There is less likelihood for clients to want to return home if they cannot possibly have more fun than by staying at the facility. Extraordinary expense and management attention may be expended on such services, but if the evaluation criteria for these services are completely nonclinical, they must be suspect. Even more regrettable is that decisions, such as which clinical services to expand and which to contract, are made largely on the basis of opinions by the Marketing Department rather than either facility or Operations Management.

Operations Managers have, over time, developed "model staffing patterns" which have homogenized the TBI rehabilitation service delivery system far too early in its development. These staffing patterns are driven by extant health insurance practices which basically recognize the legitimacy of three and only three medically relevant therapies—physical, occupational, and speech therapy—which have some, but not total, relevance in a model of care which should be driven by social learning and not medicine, according to most experts (Fralish, 1988; Ylvisaker & Gobble, 1987).

When downsizing the workforce is necessary, recently rephrased as "rightsizing," nonreimbursable clinicians are the first to be let go regardless of the viability or clinical relevance of their service, or their individual performances. The model staffing pattern may also call for an inordinate proportion of nondegreed paraprofessionals who lack the required knowledge, training (pre-service or in-service), and experience to effectively intervene with TBI clients.

Operations Managers often share in the powerlessness of the facility managers. They have responsibility but little authority. Many were formerly highly regarded clinicians or clinically trained managers. They know that on a daily basis they are compromising the rehabilitation principles which they once espoused as clinicians. Many are wrought with inner conflicts. Their reputations are exploited. Many are bound by highly restrictive employment agreements. For their cooperation, they are compensated beyond their highest expectations. Because they perceive themselves as having few alternatives, they go along with the program or risk being termed "uncooperative."

TRAINING AND DEVELOPMENT, INFORMATION SYSTEMS, AND RESEARCH

The stated purposes of these departments is self-evident. The potential benefits of these functions to any organization are equally obvious, especially in a new field such as TBI rehabilitation which is still more of an art form than a science (McMahon & Fraser, 1988). But a great deal can be learned about an organization and its priorities by asking the questions in the following section.

New Guidelines for TBI Facility Evaluation

The Commission on Accreditation of Rehabilitation Facilities (CARF, 1990) has published useful guidelines to assist consumers in evaluating the quality of TBI services at a particular facility. These widely promulgated standards have been extremely useful and have served to upgrade the industry as a whole. They tend not, however, to address the areas of specific concern as outlined in this chapter. Therefore it is recommended that the following questions be put to each Program Director and each executive officer of TBI corporations which purport to be rehabilitation companies. By design, no fixed criteria nor objective measures of appropriateness are provided for the content of the responses. In all likelihood, however, rehabilitation-minded consumers will be equally interested in respondents' comfort level, clarity, and consistency of response as well as the perceived degree of truthfulness.

GENERAL QUESTIONS FOR ALL PROVIDERS

What portion/percentage of collected revenues are invested in
- clinical operations?
- corporate marketing?
- facility-based marketing?
- corporate referral coordination?
- reimbursement coordination?
- customer satisfaction surveys?
- discharge planning?
- legal affairs?
- operations management?
- clinical training?
- marketing training?
- clinical research?
- marketing research?
- information systems?

Does the actual purpose of these job classifications differ from the stated purpose?

Do the actual duties differ from those in the job description?

Do marketing, referral coordination, reimbursement coordination, customer satisfaction, or discharge planning personnel participate (directly or indirectly) in the performance appraisal of facility managers and clinicians? Why?

How do these job classifications compare with respect to compensation, authority, responsibility, job security, and overall value to the organization?

What quota and incentive systems exist and what are the criteria used for marketing associates, referral coordinators, reimbursement coordinators, discharge planners, facility managers, corporate executives, and FFS clinicians?
Are employment agreements with restrictive covenants required for employment in any of the above job classifications? Why?

MARKETING ASSOCIATES

How are Marketing Associates trained in terms of techniques for "closing?"

Are Marketing Associates encouraged and trained to make promises on behalf of the facility for
specific outcomes?
unusual services or equipment?
unusual rights or privileges?

How are Marketing Associates trained in terms of techniques for accessing referral sources?

Do Marketing Associates retain referral sources as consultants to facilities? Offer financial sharing? Offer investment opportunities?

REFERRAL COORDINATORS

Do the Referral Coordinators have any formal background or training in rehabilitation?

What has been the Referral Coordinators' direct exposure to those facilities which they represent?

Are facility managers ever asked to make admission decisions in the absense of appropriate written documentation?

What portion of prospective admissions to each facility are judged to be "clinically inappropriate" by facility management? What precise activities follow the rendering of such a decision? What pressures are brought to bear upon facility management to reverse a negative admission decision? How are such decisions reversed? To what extent are written admission criteria compromised and how often?

Are prospective admissions ever directed to a particular level of care based upon funding profile vs. clinical need?

How do Referral Coordinators' behavior differ toward prospective admissions with questionable or no known funding?

What referral assistance is provided to applicants who do not financially qualify for services?

Is the pricing for a facility's services tied to real costs?

Is the fee structure ever negotiated and under what circumstances?

Are admissions to facilities ever made without prior notification and authorization by the financial sponsor?

Does the Referral Coordinator encourage residential vs. outpatient services whenever possible?

Does the Referral Coordinator recommend one geographic location over another as clinically more relevant when the real issue is available bed space or funding?

Does the Referral Coordinator urge the family of a prospective admission to retain legal counsel or contact the state insurance commissioner when funding approval is delayed or denied?

Does the Referral Coordinator have any special arrangements with physicians for the rapid production of letters of medical necessity when required? Are these ever prepared by nonphysicians for the doctor's signature?

When a financial sponsor requires a preadmission "plan of care," are these individualized or boiler-plated? How quickly are they produced?

REIMBURSEMENT COORDINATORS

Are fixed revenue targets established for all FFS clients regardless of clinical need or the nature and degree of impairment?

Do FFS clients receive priority over per diem clients in the scheduling of reimbursable therapies? If so, do sufficient personnel exist to "reach" per diem clients with needed reimbursable services after the FFS clients have been served?

Are reimbursable therapies scheduled in preferance to nonreimbursable therapies for FFS clients regardless of clinical need?

Are treatment plans designed with the client's funding profile as a primary consideration? If so, how is this weighed against assessed clinical needs?

Are "reimbursable clinicians" encouraged or required to "sign-off" on activities

which they did not design?
which they did not supervise?
which are not therapeutic?
for which they were not present?
which are performed by untrained personnel?

Have professional, licensed clinicians ever been reprimanded or disciplined when their assessments indicated little or no impairment requiring professional attention?

What ancillary services are/are not included in the per diem rate?

Historically, what percentage of total revenues billed are for ancillary services?

CUSTOMER SATISFACTION REPRESENTATIVES

In customer satisfaction surveys, is information also requested regarding the performance of various corporate entities?

How is customer satisfaction data used in the performance appraisal of facility managers?

DISCHARGE PLANNERS

Has a quota been established regarding the maximum number of clients who may be discharged from each facility per week?

Are clients transferred to and from other facilities on the basis of funding status?

If a client or family member becomes dissatisfied, or for any other reason a "precipitous discharge" is in progress, what extraordinary measures go into effect at the corporate and facility level to dissuade the client from leaving?

What sanctions are placed upon facility managers when a "precipitous discharge" occurs?

What discharge assistance is provided to clients whose funding has abruptly and irreversibly terminated?

Is approval of the corporate Discharge Planner required to discharge a client from a facility?

What measures does the Discharge Planner take to routinely extend the length of stay as the originally contracted period of funding approval draws to a close?

How are facility-based Case Managers accountable to corporate Discharge Planners around discharge issues?

LEGAL DEPARTMENT

What questions and issues are typically referred to the legal department for research? By whom?

OPERATIONS MANAGERS

What portion of their worktime do Operations Managers spend on clinical quality assurance?

What is the role of the Operations Manager in
- minimizing unpaid leaves of absence for clients?
- monitoring FFS revenue targets?
- providing liaison between facilities and the aforementioned corporate functions?

What criteria is used for the introduction and removal of innovative services or "product lines" to particular facilities?

What nonclinical concerns go into the design of a "model staffing pattern?"

TRAINING AND DEVELOPMENT, INFORMATION SYSTEMS, AND RESEARCH

Do such departments exist? What relative resources does each have?

For whom are training programs designed and who is receiving training? Managers? Clinicians? Marketers?

What areas of information are automated? Clinical technology? Human resources? Referral? Marketing? Financial?

What questions are being researched? Clinical processes? Clinical outcome? Referral patterns? Marketing?

Conclusions and Implications

IN BUSINESS TERMS

Over a decade ago, when private sector rehabilitation was little more than a rumor, this author delineated the inherent, refractory problems which can be related directly to the prevailing, public nature of the rehabilitation service delivery system (McMahon, 1979). These problems included the corrosive effects of government funding, managerial restraints, lack of consumer choice, and limited resources. The key ingredients and advantages of private rehabilitation, on the contrary, were given as consumerism, quality control, and competition. It was predicted that with privatization, rehabilitation professionals would enjoy increased opportunity, responsibility, and exposure, an outcome orientation, and less restrained management.

The author had not anticipated that in health care alone rehabilitation would be the fastest growing field in the 1980s, due to the demographics of disability coupled with certain health care economic factors such as DRG exemption. To be sure, rehabilitation professionals experienced all the predicted benefits of this unbridled growth. Concurrently, however, management restraints upon professional practice increased as large, technocratic bureaucracies entered and applied strict business models to the operations of rehabilitation facilities.

Two established management principles speak directly to the problem of corporate aggrandizement described earlier in this chapter. The first is the Principle of Subsidiary Function, which states that:

> *It is an injustice and at the same time a grave evil and disturbance of right order to assign to a greater and higher association what lesser and subordinate organizations can do....The higher level must not absorb the functions of the lower one on the assumption that it will automatically be wiser and fulfill them more efficiently...the centre will gain in authority and effectiveness if the freedom and responsibility of the lower formations are carefully preserved....(Schumacher, 1975, pp. 244-245)*

The second, the Principle of Vindication, holds that the central authority must uphold the lower formation and defend it against reproach. This requires that both the number of criteria and points of accountability be kept very small. In the context of these two management principles, the problems of large TBI corporations which have usurped the traditional perogatives of local facility managers and clinicians become obvious. It is noted again that this does not include all TBI service providers.

It is well-known that many corporate bureaucracies use manufacturing principles because their business success is dependent upon a product with consistent quality, which in turn means a management structure which is uniform and organized (Marlett, 1986). But the utility of such corporate models is questionable when applied to endeavors requiring customization, as in rehabilitation (Woodward, 1965). Forty-three years ago, Max Weber delineated the following bureaucratic structures of large business organizations:

> 1. *A hierarchy of superordinated authority relationships.*
> 2. *Administrative rules to guide organizational tasks.*
> 3. *Decision-making procedures adhering to technical and legal rules.*
> 4. *Administrative behaviour based on the maintenance of files and records.*
> 5. *Administration as a vocation. (Marlett, 1986, p. 80)*

It is difficult for rehabilitationists who believe in individualized and personalized alternatives to do so within bureaucracies which mitigate the potential of individualization. Indeed, even the Individualized Written Rehabilitation Plan (IWRP), when applied in a bureaucratic setting, becomes translated into "management by objectives" in which professional creativity and client choices give way to paraprofessional record keeping, accountability, consistent structure, and ease of mastery (Marlett, 1986). Some have gone so far as to describe "irresolvable discrepancies" between rehabilitation organizations and industrial organizations (see Table 1).

Table 1
REHABILITATION VS. CORPORATE PRINCIPLES*

DIMENSION	CORPORATE	REHABILITATION
Manifest motive	Profit & power	Service
Beneficiaries	Owners	Disabled person
Resource base	Private capital	Public funds
Goals	Unusual/explicit	Individual/diverse
Intervention	Employee-product interactions	Staff-client interaction
Measure of performance	Quantitative	Qualitative

Reprinted from Marlett (1986).

Hummell (1977), Diamond (1984), Denhardt (1981), and others decry our dependency on corporate bureaucracies which, while meeting many of our interpersonal security needs, are displacing our social norms (as embraced in rehabilitation principles) with institutional norms such as precision, stability, control, and efficiency. Max Weber says of bureaucracies:

> *The formal characteristics of bureaucracy tend to neutralize the otherwise personal, emotional, irrational, and other often political behaviour for the bureaucracy offers job security and compensation along with a high degree of certainty of expectations and performance in return for the relinquishment of independence and autonomy of action. (Marlett, 1986, pp. 80-81)*

Kouzes and Mico (1979) use Domain Theory to further illustrate the problem. In a typical rehabilitation facility there exist three distinct domains. The Policy Domain rests with the corporate Board of Directors and is concerned with rendering policy decisions. The Service Domain rests with professional staff members who seek to control their service roles and monitor the quality of service and professional standards. The Management Domain rests with administrative persons who seek to rationalize the organization with cost efficiency and effectiveness as the measures of its success.

It is important to note that the characteristics of each domain (in terms of governing principles, measures of success, structural arrangements, and work modes) are distinct and often incongruent. This means that many rehabilitation managers fail because they attempt to dominate the system rather than recognize and support the various domain values and methods in a flexible manner.

IN REHABILITATION TERMS

It has become commonplace in the TBI industry for rehabilitationists to experience psychological dissonance, qualms of conscience, ethical conflicts, or generalized anxiety and discomfort when candidly facing issues discussed in this chapter (Mullins, 1989). Indeed the prepublication review of this material has been reported as difficult from some very accomplished professionals. Josephson (1989) points out, however, that growth will only come out of a little sense of discomfort. He writes about our "...rights orientation, which has lead to a kind of legal minimalism—as long as it's legal, it's ethical. We look for the lowest common standard of ethics" (p. 17). Although there may be disagreement over time about what is right and wrong, there is little disagreement about the root concerns of all interested parties. At the heart of the situation is the question, "How would I want to be treated if I were head-injured, the family member of a head-injured person, the referral source, or the payor?"

The answer is likely to be equally consistent, if not universal—"I want the very best, the most effective, and the most efficient rehabilitation services." For most of us this would mean that rehabilitation decisions are made by rehabilitation professionals on the basis of established rehabilitation principles.

It is typically clear to most rehabilitationists when directives are contrary to rehabilitation principles, and by extension contrary to the client's best interest. Why is it so difficult to speak out? Most rehabilitation professionals understand that advocacy is a professional responsibility for the rehabilitationist, but they somehow think that that implies advocacy in the "outside world," (i.e., the public media, the legislature, the prospective donor). Today there is a far greater need for advocacy within our own organizations, but many of us overestimate the cost of doing the right thing. We fear termination or a slower course of advancement. Worse yet, we often underestimate the cost of not doing the right thing. To be sure, there are consequences, sometimes harsh. But one who is separated from an intransigent, unethical organization for advocating for good rehabilitation practice will, in all likelihood, only miss out on the ultimate demise of that organization. Says Josephson (1989):

> *The mandate is that an ethical person ought to do more than he's required to do and less than he's allowed to do. He must exercise judgment, self-restraint, and conscience. Otherwise, we have a minimalist society where everybody's lawyering everybody else, pushing the world to the limit, and twisting the rules. We need to tell people we can do better. And if it costs us a little bit, so it costs us. It's worth it. (p. 27)*

Or stated in simpler terms, "The fact of the matter is that a good conscience is the best pillow" (Josephson, 1989, p. 20).

This chapter is not intended as a pontification or pedantic reminder about the various codes of ethics which our professional associations have developed (e.g., Commission on Rehabilitation Counselor Certification [Herlihy & Golden, 1990]). Even successful business authors are trying to redirect us toward ethical management and providing some very specific guidelines as well. Blanchard and Peale (1988) for example, suggest that we apply the "ethics check" to decisions which cause us discomfort:

> 1. *Is it legal? Will I be violating either civil law or company policy?*
> 2. *Is it balanced? Is it fair to all concerned (including competitors) in the short-term as well as the long-term? Does it promote win-win relationships?*
> 3. *How will it make me feel about myself? Will it make me proud? Would I feel good if my decision was published in the newspaper? Would I feel good if my family knew about it?. (p. 20)*

The use of such guidelines can be immensely helpful in the day-to-day decisions which confront us.

Ethical issues are clearly a matter of serious concern in rehabilitation medicine (Caplan, Callahan, & Haas, 1987). Some TBI rehabilitation providers are even publishing their own guidelines for business ethics (e.g., Learning Services Corporation, 1990). It may be that if a company is in the business of rehabilitation, and uses rehabilitation jargon to formulate its mission statement or to attract clients, then professional rehabilitationists have the right and the responsibility to hold that company true to its alleged purpose, to make sure its actions are consistent with its stated purpose. According to David Ogilve:

> *In the best institutions, promises are kept no matter what the cost in agony and overtime. (Batten, 1989, p. 14)*

It is widely known that a company's profit and future are only as strong as its corporate culture, which is founded on a statement of basic beliefs and values, a grand design, a vision, a dream. That philosophy is the broad foundation upon which policies, procedures, practices, and profit are built (Batten, 1989). If that expressed philosophy is rehabilitation, then rehabilitation principles must be taken seriously. It is the advocates' responsibility to see that this is so.

References

Batten, J. D. (1989). *Tough-minded leadership*. New York: AMACOM.

Blanchard, K., and Peale, N. V. (1988). *The power of ethical management*. New York: Fawcett Crest.

Caplan, A. L., Callahan, D., & Haas, J. (1987). *Ethical policy issues in rehabilitation medicine*. Briarcliff Manor, NY: The Hastings Center.

Commission on Accreditation of Rehabilitation Facilities (1990). *Standards manual for facilities serving people with disabilities*. Tucson, AZ: Author.

Denhardt, R. B. (1981). *In the shadow of organization*. Lawrence, KS: The Regency Press of Kansas.

Diamond, M. A. (1984). Bureaucracy as externalized self-esteem. *Administration and Society, 16*(2), 195-214.

Fralish, K. (1988). Transitional living programs. In P. Deutsch and K. Fralish (Eds.), *Innovations in head injury rehabilitation*. New York: Matthew Bender.

Herlihy, B., and Golden, L. (1990). *AACD Ethical standards casebook*. Alexandria, VA: American Association for Counseling and Development.

Hummell, R. (1977). *The bureaucratic experience*. New York: Harper and Row.

Josephson, M. (1989). Michael Josephson: Ethicist. In B. S. Flowers (Ed.), *Bill Moyers: A world of ideas*. New York: Doubleday.

Kouzes, J. M., and Mico, P. R. (1979). Domain theory: An introduction to organizational behavior in human service organizations. *The Journal of Applied Behavior Science, 15*, 449-469.

Learning Services Corporation. (1990). *Learning Services' five-part business ethics program*. Londonderry, NH: Author.

Marlett, N. J. (1986). Impact of and alternates to corporate business models in rehabilitation. In R. I. Brown (Ed.), *Management and administration of rehabilitation programs*. San Diego, CA: College-Hill Press, Inc.

McKenna, M. (1990). One step forward. *Continuing Care, 9*,(1), 8, 10, 13-14, 32.

McMahon, B. T. (1979). Private sector rehabilitation: Benefits, dangers, and implications for education. *Journal of Rehabilitation, 45*(3), 56-58.

McMahon, B. T., and Fraser, R. T. (1988). Basic issues and trends in head injury rehabilitation. In S. Rubin and N. Rubin (Eds.), *Contemporary challenges to the rehabilitation counseling profession*. Baltimore: Paul H. Brookes Publishing Company, Inc.

McMahon, B. T., Shaw, L. R., and Mahaffey, D. P. (1988). Career opportunities and professional preparation in head injury rehabilitation. *Rehabilitation Counseling Bulletin, 31*(4), 345-355.

Mullins, L. L. (1989). Hate revisited: Power, envy, and greed in the rehabilitation setting. *Archives of Physical Medicine and Rehabilitation, 70*, 740-744.

Schumacher, E. F. (1975). *Small is beautiful: Economics as if people mattered.* New York: Harper and Row.

Shaw, L. R., and McMahon, B. T. (1990). Family-staff conflict in the rehabilitation setting: Causes, consequences, and implications. *Brain Injury, 4*(1), 87-93.

Woodward, J. (1965). *Industrial organization: Theory and practice.* London: Oxford University Press.

Ylvisaker, M., and Gobble, E. M. R. (1987). *Community re-entry for head-injured adults.* Boston: College-Hill Press, Inc.

2

The Outpatient Setting: The Preferred Context for Post-acute Rehabilitation

Brian T. McMahon
Linda R. Shaw

2

The Outpatient Setting: The Preferred Context for Post-acute Rehabilitation

Brian T. McMahon
Linda R. Shaw

Introduction

The purpose of this chapter is to explore the advantages of providing post-acute TBI rehabilitation services on an outpatient basis. Residential post-acute programs were originally designed to provide transitional living services for medically stable clients with good potential for rehabilitation but whose ongoing behavioral or cognitive problems were not well-managed in the home community on an outpatient basis (Hackler & Tobis, 1983). The stated goals and treatment themes of most post-acute facilities (residential and outpatient) are reasonably consistent (i.e., to assist clients to achieve behavioral self-management, independent living status, and vocational restoration in the community).

Although these programs are often referred to as community re-entry programs, extraordinary costs, funding restrictions, geographic remoteness and, in some cases, the financial incentive to maximize lengths of stay, may serve to compromise attempts at effective community re-entry (see Chapter 1). Residential treatment centers tend to be preferred over outpatient alternatives by providers in terms of such financial issues as economies of scale, guaranteed bed and board rates, and real estate equity which may be financed for additional capital and/or depreciated for income tax purposes. Because of the financial benefits of residential over outpatient services, there has been a tendency by providers to sell the concept of the residential treatment center as a clinical necessity. This is accomplished by emphasizing the complexity of TBI symptomatology or the need for strict environmental controls in addressing the behavioral sequelae of head injury.

To be sure, there are often valid clinical bases for recommending residential over outpatient settings (McMahon & Fraser, 1988). As clients are discharged earlier and earlier from acute settings, some medical and physical restoration issues go unresolved. When these are coupled with lingering cognitive impairments, situations do exist in which clients represent a safety risk to themselves or others in the community. This does not mean, however, that all clients with behavioral symptoms require residential treatment. The management of nonviolent behavioral impairments is not necessarily beyond the capabilities of quality, categorical TBI outpatient programs. Depending upon the clinical manifestations of the client and the capabilities of the outpatient program, cognitive and behavioral impairments may be regarded as routine programming issues.

Many post-acute clients' behavior problems are matters of perseveration or disinhibition, not aggressiveness or assaultiveness. Whether organically or psychologically rooted, the treatment regimen (i.e., proper counseling, behavior analysis applications, controlled medications [when appropriate], and time) is identical whether provided in an inpatient or outpatient setting.

Furthermore, one might argue that given sufficient family support and instruction, the consequences for behavior experienced in the home community are far more effective than the simulated or contrived consequences of the residential setting. Certainly generalization is improved when the programming environment and target environment are the same (see Chapter 13). It is the authors' assertion that the "behavior involvement" argument for *mandatory and universal* residential services is often exaggerated because it better suits the business needs of the provider.

Outpatient Programming Advantages

THE FINANCIAL SPONSOR

There are several major reasons why the outpatient setting is the preferred context for TBI rehabilitation. The first advantage is to the financial sponsor. Outpatient programs are operated at a lower overhead and the primary expense is for clinical personnel. Thus, rate comparisons from provider to provider more accurately reflect the true costs of treatment. Monitoring capability is improved, because most outpatient programs are typically in major metropolitan areas near the insurance companies' offices. Improved monitoring facilitates the flexible structuring of funding arrangements (either per diem or fee-for-service) and the fading of services and associated costs as clients show improvement.

Urbanization also improves the number of vocational and educational opportunities available in the community to expedite placement. Public services (e.g., transportation, training centers, and schools) and sources of supplemental funding (e.g., state vocational rehabilitation, medical assistance, and veterans assistance monies) can be more readily accessed.

THE TBI SERVICE PROVIDER

From the provider's perspective, overhead costs are reduced because expenditures for security, housekeeping, meals, maintenance, and the like are minimized. Reimbursement tends to be more likely as most outpatient programs are licensed health care entities, either certified Comprehensive Outpatient Rehabilitation Facilities (CORF) or divisions of licensed hospitals. In contrast to most residential programs, which are typically in ex-urban or rural settings, most outpatient programs are in suburban or urban settings. Urbanization improves the recruitment of qualified clinicians, support personnel, consultants, and students. It also facilitates continuing education, collaborative research with universities, and access to media for public relations and advocacy. Finally, the outpatient setting provides greater access to clients who require a part-time program or highly selective, specialty services, such as short-term evaluation or re-evaluation, pediatric, minor head injury, work adjustment, substance abuse, or family counseling.

QUALITY OF CARE

From the perspective of improving the quality of client services, the face validity and generalizability of all services are enhanced. Continuity and communications with all interested parties are improved by proximity to referral sources, family members, third party case managers, payors, attorneys, and the like. Because shift work is minimized, there is more time for proper staffing of clients, staff training, and interdisciplinary team building activities. Clients can be scheduled with greater flexibility to accommodate work and school. Follow-up with the client is now possible as services are rescheduled, modified, or faded gradually to allow supports during and after the client's vocational or educational re-entry. According to Moore and Plovnik (1989):

> *A day treatment program is designed to integrate the individual into the daily life of the community and the family in such a way as to normalize activities and support the development of relationships which can and may continue to exist following the head injury. In day treatment, it is possible for the person with head injury to maintain positive family and community relationships while relating to a peer group and receive specialized rehabilitation services for overcoming residuals of the traumatic head injury. (pp. 5-31)*

Many costly and burdensome functions which may be perceived as necessities in the residential treatment settings operated by large corporations (see Chapter 1) can be minimized, or in some cases, obviated by utilization of an outpatient service. The discharge planning process is simplified because outpatient services exist at the end of the continuum of services (i.e., clients are already "placed" in their own homes). Length of stay issues are less controversial and the ability of payors to be more accessible and involved in monitoring quality of care may result in more careful attention to achieving timely discharges. Because point-in-time absolute discharges are rare, services are gradually faded away. As most customer complaints are about life support services (i.e., visitation, meals, housekeeping, and security) which are not provided at an outpatient facility, sound facility case management replaces the need for a categorical Customer Satisfaction Representative (Winter & Keith, 1988). The straightforward nature of licensing reduces the involvement of the Legal Department. The routine nature of funding approval reduces the complexity of the role of the Reimbursement Coordinator. Finally, while the reduced need for these various corporate functions may not alter the need for corporate supervision, it certainly alters its focus by permitting attention to the treatment-related issues.

Consistency with Rehabilitation Principles

Perhaps the most pressing question, given the above, is, "Which setting – residential or outpatient – is more conducive to rehabilitation?" The specific focus here is upon how decisions are made in the corporate, residential post-acute system vs. the outpatient facility. Some maintain that if, in the administration of a rehabilitation facility, decisions are made primarily upon the basis of rehabilitation principles, profitability and business success will follow. Plato stated that "...virtue does not come from money, but money comes from virtue...." (Josephson,

1989). Less dated and highly experienced business persons, such as IBM's F. Buck Rogers, agree that the surest route to business failure is to lose sight of the product (Rogers, 1987).

Rehabilitation is well-defined and articulated in terms of basic philosophical tenets, five of which will be explored here in light of the previous discussion. These tenets are continuity of care, normalization, criterion of ultimate functioning, social role valorization, and dignity of risk.

CONTINUITY OF CARE

The goal of continuity of treatment in rehabilitation, articulated by Jaques (1970), Wright (1980), and others, may be compromised depending upon the levels of programming available in a particular community. Most TBI facilities provide services at only one level of care — acute, post-acute residential, outpatient, supervised living, or home health (McMahon & Fraser, 1988). The vast majority of TBI facilities are of the acute care variety, and are either housed in hospital or skilled nursing environments. There are approximately seven times the number of categorical acute TBI programs as all other levels combined. This appears logical because in the early stages of recovery most, if not all, clients require the medical and restorative services which comprise the pervasive treatment themes in acute rehabilitation settings.

It is also true, however, that most TBI clients will require services beyond the acute level of care. This makes continuity difficult, if not impossible, to achieve in the local community given the paucity and uneven distribution of post-acute programs. This appears to place the TBI client at a distinct disadvantage. Some providers have responded by developing a full continuum, network, or "system" which offers services at all levels of care. With many such providers, however, there exists an assumption that each client will require all levels in a fairly rigid, pre-designed sequence. Moreover, continuity becomes defined as continuous services within the same company or system regardless of client relocation, preference, or individual circumstance.

This differs from the concept of continuity of care within the same community, which might involve cross-referrals to competitors. Even within the system of a single corporation, each facility has obvious areas of programming which are excellent and others which are weak. Still, clients may be matched to programs within the system on the basis of funding profiles, beds available, corporate needs, or geographic proximity rather than a matching of individual client needs (as professionally assessed) with a facility's special strengths. Such systems are recruititory and behave in ways intended to maintain the client within the system as long as possible, ideally resulting in an indefinite length of stay in supervised living or sustained development programs.

In the spirit of good rehabilitation and proper continuity, the facility whose services are specific to a particular level of care (level *X*) would naturally refer inappropriate clients or those who can no longer benefit from treatment at level *X* to other appropriate providers. This occurs rarely and reluctantly in the real life of predominantly residential systems in which staffing patterns, debt services, budgets, salaries, and bonuses are all tied to census objectives.

NORMALIZATION

Normalization was defined by Wolfensberger as:

> *The use of means which are culturally normative to offer a person life conditions at least as good as the average citizen and to as much as possible enhance or support personal behaviors, appearances, status, and reputation to the greatest degree possible at any given time for each individual according to his or her development needs. (Pancsofar & Blackwell, 1986, p. 6)*

Although unlikely, it is plausible that Nirjie might have been referring to residential TBI programs when he wrote:

> *Normalization means...living in normal housing in a normal neighborhood. Not in a large facility of 20, 50, or 100...and not isolated from the rest of the community. (Pancsofar & Blackwell, 1986, pp. 7-8)*

The same might be said of McCord when he described normalization as:

> *...an abused term when merely renaming cottages and rearranging furniture is the extent of adherence to a Normalization philosophy. (Pancsofar & Blackwell, 1986, p. 8)*

However, if services are functional and applied, outpatient programming is inherently normalized because of the home community setting in which it takes place.

THE CRITERION OF ULTIMATE FUNCTIONING

This term refers to:

> *...the ever-changing, expanding, localized, and personalized cluster of factors that each person must possess in order to function as productively and independently as possible in socially, vocationally, and domestically integrated community environments. (Pancsofar & Blackwell, p. 9)*

Because residential programs are, in fact, institutions, there is a tendency to sacrifice individualized treatment approaches which maximize client independence for approaches which maximize the smooth, efficient operation of the institution. In TBI residential programs, for example, it is not unusual to observe such client activities as computer-assisted cognitive retraining, sit-down meals served by waitresses, medications administered by staff when clients are capable of self-administration, the prescription of childish arts/crafts/games, the staging of elaborate "fun programs" to keep clients amused and content to stay in the institution, and the lack of provisions for privacy with visiting spouses. One may evaluate such activities according to the Criterion of Ultimate Functioning by asking such questions as:

> *Why should we engage in this activity?*
> *Is this activity necessary to prepare residents to ultimately function in complex heterogeneous community settings?*
> *Will this activity impede, restrict, or reduce the probability that residents will ultimately function in community settings?*
> *Are the skills, materials, tasks, and criteria of concern similar to those encountered in adult life?*
> *(Pancsofar & Blackwell, 1986)*

Because family visitation, facility-based meals and recreation, medication administration, and the like, are often moot issues in outpatient programming, compliance with the Criterion of Ultimate Functioning is less problematic. According to Moore and Plovnik (1989):

> *Discharge to the home is often accompanied by the emergence of family conflicts, financial problems and abandonment by friends and family. This can result in social isolation and alienation, social inappropriateness, impaired judgment and vocational failure. These life adjustment struggles cannot be simulated in an inpatient setting, and therefore cannot be successfully remediated in that setting. (pp. 5-32)*

SOCIAL ROLE VALORIZATION

This term was coined by Wolfensberger (1983) to describe a broadening of the concept of Normalization. Condeluci and Gretz-Lasky (1987) describe Social Role Valorization as:

> *...the process of bringing value to the social role that disabled individuals have in the community by (1) providing culturally normative, age-appropriate activities and training methods; e.g., by conducting community re-entry programs in real community settings rather than isolated, artificial settings; and (2) working to change societal perceptions and attitudes about the ability of head-injured individuals; e.g., by conducting community education programs about head injury. (p. 50)*

This concept extends beyond normalization to include the need to prevent devaluation and to promote the human worth and dignity of persons with TBI to the public at large. Condeluci and Gretz-Lasky (1987) pose several questions for treatment programs to help prevent the devaluation of individuals with TBI by the society in which they must function. These questions include:

> *How does the independent living program design increase the possibilities for head injured persons to present themselves in a normative fashion?*
>
> *Is the program site physically integrated in the community?*
>
> *Are considerations made concerning program size and the saturation level of the community?*
>
> *Is the physical structure designed to allow for and encourage social interaction and contact with the public so that learning and training can also occur in a nonstructured setting? (pp. 51-53)*

Generally, answers to these questions are more likely to be affirmative in reference to outpatient programs and settings, thus promoting a positive image of their clients as individuals worthy of respect and dignity.

DIGNITY OF RISK

This term is well-articulated by Perske:

> *You are a human being and so you have the right to live as other humans live, even to the point where we will not take all dangers of human life from you. [There is] human dignity in risk and there can be a dehumanizing indignity in safety. (Pancsofar & Blackwell, 1986, p. 12)*

Given today's litigious society, the safety risks which TBI clients present, and the liability associated with their proper management, it is difficult to embrace this concept in a residential program. Still, for reasons mentioned earlier, the level of acuity among clients admitted for post-acute rehabilitation is increasing, and along with it the level of risk. As the number of untoward incidents increase, the number of risk management policies and restrictive regulations intended to minimize such incidents proliferates. Both Dignity of Risk and Normalization are compromised.

How does the residential facility administrator allow for select recreational pursuits (e.g., horseback riding), provide training in skilled occupations (e.g., welding), maximize community mobility and access (e.g., driving instruction), or teach responsible socialization (e.g., dealing with bars and social drinking) without increasing the risk of reinjury and without opening the door to liability and damages of such magnitude as to close down an entire operation?

Effective risk management practices are expensive, and by their nature they restrict the range of choices, opportunities, and activities available in a residential program to such an extent that life becomes artificial and contrived. Group activities have to be modified for the safety of the one client at risk. Safety policies and procedures tend to proliferate, especially protocols for elopement, suicide prevention, accident, medical emergency, aggression, assault, and fire. The design and enforcement of such practices may require inordinate amounts of supervision and detract from the proper focus of facility management (i.e., rehabilitation services). Enforcement becomes costly, and insuring against major incidents more costly still. One can talk *ad nauseum* about the balance of dignity of risk with liability concerns, but when the safety of staff and clients is the facility's legal responsibility, most issues tend to be decided on the side of caution.

In the outpatient setting, most decisions regarding these issues are made by the client and family, with professionals providing input, suggestions, and advice based upon current assessments. As the liability for such matters rests elsewhere, managers can be more mindful of the Dignity of Risk and design treatment plans accordingly, and their focus can be upon rehabilitation activity.

A Question of Size

In most instances, outpatient programming brings with it an inherently limited geographic scope which tends, in turn, to limit the ultimate size of the program. This fact is not well-received by those providers whose roots are in large-scale, residential programming in which "economies of scale" can be realized. There exists in business an irresistible trend for units to become ever bigger even though small units may be highly prosperous and provide society with most of the really fruitful new developments.

In TBI rehabilitation, what scale is appropriate? Schumacher (1975) provides one answer which is that the correct scale depends upon what we are trying to accomplish. He also adds that, "...for every activity there is a certain appropriate scale, and the more active and intimate the activity, the smaller the number of people that can take part...." (p. 66). Considering the inherently "active and intimate" nature of TBI rehabilitation, one might reasonably conclude that while the ideal scale (that which maximizes both freedom and order) of a TBI program is not definitively known, it is likely much smaller than some residential facilities which now program over 100 TBI clients on a single site.

Is TBI rehabilitation a matter of goods, services, or people? Many providers regard it as a matter of service. To this author, however, TBI rehabilitation is clearly a matter of people, and there are few human endeavors which are as personal in nature. Schumacher states, "...people can be themselves only in small, comprehensible groups" (p. 75). It is the authors' experience that above an active daily census of 30 clients per site, regardless of the degree of decentralization of the facility or the caliber of its personnel, there is an inevitable, progressive decline in the quality of care.

Interagency Task Force Recommendations

While some of the issues discussed here are deliberately philosophical, the reader is asked to consider the recommendation of the Federal Interagency Task Force on Head Injury, which heard weeks of public hearings and reviewed other scientific input. The Interagency Head Injury Task Force Final Report (U.S. Department of Health and Human Services, 1989) contains the following among its sound recommendations:

> *...emphasizing outpatient rather that inpatient services for noncritical care and rely on outpatient services at the local level. (p. 16)*

Regrettably, this blanket recommendation follows an acknowledgement in the same report that most outpatient rehabilitation services lack organization and coordination. Specifically, most outpatient rehabilitation services are hospital-based and are not organized into disability-specific programs. Those that are often do not address the unique service needs of the head-injured individual in a categorical fashion. Nonetheless, for the reasons cited within this chapter, the authors join the Interagency Task Force in recommending the expeditious development of high quality, categorical outpatient alternatives for TBI programming to promote the resumption of TBI rehabilitation activity consistent with basic rehabilitation philosophy and principles.

References

Condeluci, A., & Gretz-Lasky, S. (1987). Social role valorization: A Model for community re-entry. *Journal of Head Trauma Rehabilitation, 2*(1), 49-56.

Hackler, E., & Tobis, J. (1983). Reintegration into the community. In M. Rosenthal (Ed.), *Rehabilitation of the head injured adult*. Philadelphia: F. A. Davis.

Jaques, M. E. (1970). *Rehabilitation counseling: Scope and services*. Boston: Houghton-Mifflin Company.

Josephson, M. (1989). Michael Josephson: Ethicist. In B.S. Flowers (Ed.), *Bill Moyers: A world of ideas*. New York: Doubleday.

McMahon, B. T., & Fraser, R. T. (1988). Basic issues and trends in head injury rehabilitation. In S. Rubin and N. Rubin (Eds.), *Contemporary challenges to the rehabilitation counseling profession*. Baltimore: Paul H. Brookes Publishing Company, Inc.

Moore, M. K., & Plovnik, N. (1989). Post-acute programs. In P. Deutsch and K. Fralish (Eds.), *Innovations in head injury rehabilitation*. New York: Matthew Bender.

Pancsofar, E., & Blackwell, R. (1986). *A user's guide to community re-entry for the severely handicapped*. Albany, NY: State University of New York Press.

Rogers, F. B. (1986). *The IBM way: Insights into the world's most successful marketing organization*. New York: Harper & Row.

Schumacher, E. F. (1975). *Small is beautiful: Economics as if people mattered*. New York: Harper and Row, Publishers.

U.S. Department of Health and Human Services. (1989). *Interagency head injury task force report*. Washington, D.C.: Author.

Winter, P. L., & Keith, R. A. (1988). A model of outpatient satisfaction in rehabilitation. *Rehabilitation Psychology, 33*(3), 131-142.

Wolfensberger, W. (1983). Social role valorization: A proposed new term for the principle of normalization. *Mental Retardation, 21*, 234-239.

Wright, G. N. (1980). *Total rehabilitation*. Boston: Little, Brown and Company.

2

Vocational Re-entry

3

Neuropsychological Evaluation: A Functional and Behavioral Approach

Jack G. Dial
Fong Chan
Roy Tunick
Steven G. Gray
Michelle Marmé

3

Neuropsychological Evaluation: A Functional and Behavioral Approach

Jack G. Dial
Fong Chan
Roy Tunick
Steven G. Gray
Michelle Marmé

Introduction

The increasing survival rate of traumatically brain-injured (TBI) individuals has placed significant demands on rehabilitation professionals responsible for the accurate assessment and subsequent treatment needs of this population. The accurate assessment/evaluation of the individual with this single event, nonprogressive condition, has been viewed as having an increasingly important role in the development of rehabilitative strategies that maximize the return of independent functioning (Norton, 1985). More specifically, the role of neuropsychological

Funds for the preparation of this chapter were provided in part by a Rehabilitation Services Administration Experimental and Innovative Training Grant (#H129T00022) and a contract (#RIRC255551IIT) from the Midwest Regional Head Injury Center for Rehabilitation and Prevention.

assessment appears to have earned a very important place in the rehabilitation of these individuals. Because there are no known medical cures for TBI, it becomes especially important that neuropsychological assessment be utilized to accurately identify a TBI client's dysfunction as well as residual functioning ability to effectively diagnose, plan, implement, and evaluate his or her rehabilitation program.

Historically, assessment concerns for this population have been focused on diagnostic criteria to identify the existence of brain dysfunction. More recent neuropsychological evaluation strategies have been directed toward the identification of deficits associated with specific brain damage, as well as remaining strengths and abilities. The goal of this latter approach is geared toward the development of remediation, accommodation, and/or compensation strategies that can be employed within a rehabilitation setting.

The emphasis on treatment/rehabilitation has replaced the limited role of clinical diagnosis as the primary purpose of a neuropsychological evaluation with the TBI population. Therefore, an integrated approach geared toward the identification of both the condition of the brain and the subsequent extrapolation of residual functional abilities has emerged. This chapter provides a theoretical foundation for the chapters on rehabilitation techniques which follow, and include information on neuroanatomy, neuropathology, and neuropsychological evaluations, and their roles in the rehabilitation of persons with TBI.

Trends in Neuropsychology

Neuropsychology has traditionally focused on two major concerns: precise localization of brain lesions responsible for specific behavioral and medical disorders; and the analysis of brain-behavior relationships in an attempt to understand the brain as the principal organ of behavior. These concerns, though complementary, have involved separate activities and interests among neuroscientists and clinicians. In contrast, relatively little has been accomplished, until recently, in the application of neuropsychological principles to the fields of vocational rehabilitation and education of individuals with TBI (Luria, 1970; McCarron & Dial, 1986).

Clinical neuropsychologists have largely emphasized localization of lesions in the hopes of developing noninvasive techniques for early diagnosis of brain disorders. In contrast, research-oriented neuroscientists have been concerned with various aspects of localization, but in the context of understanding the normal structure and function of the brain. The former have emphasized clinical instrumentation, deductive data interpretation, and pragmatic techniques of diagnosis and treatment;

while the latter have emphasized laboratory instrumentation, animal research, inductive data interpretation, and theory building (Filskov & Boll, 1981).

Recently, the interests of clinicians and researchers have converged to form a positive coalition from which many advances in the understanding of brain-behavior relationships, brain disorders, and rehabilitation approaches have been generated. The present coalition has, in part, emerged as a result of major contributions from the neurosciences, physics, medicine, psychology, and rehabilitation. These contributions include: the development and validation of noninvasive behavioral techniques for differential diagnosis of cortical brain disorders; the corresponding development of low risk and/or minimally invasive radiologic techniques for localizing brain lesions; the formulation of neurobehavioral theory which integrates many previously contradictory findings; the application of empirical findings to the rehabilitation of individuals with TBI; and the expansion of traditional vocational and educational services to neurologically impaired persons (Lassen, Ingvar, & Skinhoj, 1978; Luria, 1970; New, Scott, Schnur, Davis, & Traveras, 1974). To fully understand the implications of these developments on the rehabilitation of individuals with TBI, it is necessary to review the present status of neuropsychological theory, the functional implications of brain pathology, and approaches to neuropsychological evaluation.

The Functional Organization of the Brain

The traditional model of cerebral organization portrays a dichotomous brain with structural and functional differentiation between the right and left hemisphere. The left hemisphere dominates for language in most individuals (90 to 95%) and is described as the center of analytical and verbally oriented thought. It is considered the center for the acquisition, production, comprehension, ideation, and expression of language. The left hemisphere tends to predominate in processing and analyzing information from the environment that is presented in a sequential order, requires language encoding or decoding, or requires the use of mathematical operations (Geschwind, 1979).

In contrast, the right cerebral hemisphere is described as a simultaneous synthesizer which integrates nonverbal, visuospatial information. It predominates in the tactile-kinesthetic recognition of shapes, forms, and spatial configurations; the perception of direction and perspective; the reproduction of geometric images; and the appreciation of musical melody (Gazzaniga, 1967; Geschwind, 1979; Kimura, 1973;

Witelson, 1974; Woods & Teuber, 1973). Accordingly, the neuropsychological assessment of persons with TBI should include tests of both verbal and spatial functioning.

The traditional model of cerebral organization implies considerable lateralization of function, cerebral dominance for specific functions, and a rather isomorphic relationship between brain structure and complex behavior. Although the simplicity of this model is appealing, recent neuropsychological and physiological research evidence presents a more complicated picture. Gazzaniga (1979), for example, reevaluated his earlier work in the face of current findings and suggested that the cerebral hemispheres may differ as much in their response mode as in their capacity to mediate or process different kinds of data. His work suggests that cerebral dominance for a particular function or task may depend on several variables simultaneously, including the content of the information to be processed (i.e., verbal or visuospatial); the method of stimulus presentation (e.g., verbal, visual); the most efficient method of data analysis for the task (i.e., analytical or synthetic); and the response mode required to perform the task (e.g., verbal, manual). Therefore, the interpretation of results from neuropsychological tests must consider stimulus and response variables in addition to the special content of the task at hand.

This picture is further complicated when considering the effects of gender on the structure and function of the higher cortical centers. Though comparatively little research has been conducted in this area, various studies have suggested functional differences between males and females in cerebral organization. Norms and interpretation procedures of neuropsychological instruments must, therefore, account for possible differences in gender.

LURIA'S FUNCTIONAL SYSTEMS THEORY

The integration of isomorphic and holistic theories of cerebral organization may be conceptualized utilizing the Functional Systems Theory (Luria, 1966, 1970, 1973, 1976). Luria suggested that the brain is composed of functional systems which mediate all behavior. Each functional system involves more than one structural element (cell assembly or cylinder); however, there is a finite number of elements in each system. Functional systems are analogous to chains in that each element (or cell assembly) is involved in some way in the mediation of the behavior for which the system is responsible. Therefore, if one element (link in the chain) is damaged, the system cannot function in its most efficient or effective way. Elements may be (and usually are) involved in more than one functional system. In other words, there is multiple participation of elements among various functional systems. The extent to which behaviors mediated by different functional systems correlate may define the degree to which multiple participation of the neural substrata would be observed.

Damage to a specific region of the brain would, therefore, produce differential effects in terms of observed behaviors. Highly correlated behaviors may be most universally affected; however, many systems would be affected in some way by the same lesion. Conversely, a given behavioral act may be affected differentially by lesions in different areas of the brain or cerebral hemispheres. According to Luria, an evaluation of neurological function would, by necessity, require an assessment of a wide variety of functions involving an equally wide variety of specific tasks incrementally building toward the "clinical picture" (inductionistic approach). Conversely, a factor analytic (reductionistic) approach to interpretation would be most fruitful in both diagnosis and in developing an understanding of brain-behavior relationships. Therefore, it is impossible to develop a "single test" to detect brain damage ("organicity") or, for that matter, to develop an accurate "screening battery" — so often attempted in psychology for purely economic reasons.

According to Luria, the development of functional systems depends on genetic, hormonal, and environmental influences. Classical conditioning was also thought to influence the organization of these systems. Luria described the structural organization of the brain in terms of three units or blocks.

The first unit (Unit I) is comprised of the reticular formation, diencephalon, and limbic systems. It has extensive afferent and efferent communications with the entire brain (via thalamus and cingulate gyrus among other connections), but particularly with the frontal lobes via the medial forebrain bundle. Generally, this unit is functionally organized to mediate arousal (keeping the brain awake); filtering information that can and cannot reach the brain (selective attention, modulation); and filtering functions learned. Unit I also has specific functional systems for: (a) maintaining the metabolic processes (internal economy-homeostasis); (b) monitoring outside stimuli (e.g., alertness, mobilization, investigation, habituation, and modulating function); and (c) decoding Reticular Activating System connections from Unit III (frontal lobes) (e.g., consciousness influenced by frontal lobes to maintain activity levels sufficient to carry out complex behavioral plans, and to maintain cortical and emotional tone). It also participates in memory and learning via attentional states, filtering of stimuli, and stimulus rehearsal (hippocampus). In addition, this area probably contributes to retrieval of information from memory stores (mammillary bodies). Major lesions in the Unit I area could result in death, while minor lesions could cause Korsakoff's Syndrome (i.e., memory deficits, confabulation) and other deficits in concentration and attention.

Unit II consists of the sensory cortex and is divided into three areas responsible for detection (primary area), recognition (secondary area), and association (tertiary area) of somesthetic, auditory, and visual stimuli. The primary detection area for auditory stimuli is located in the temporal lobes (Heschl's gyrus). For visual stimuli, it is located in the calcarine cortex of the medial occipital lobes, and for somatosensory stimuli the postcentral gyrus (anterior parietal lobes). The primary detection areas for somatosensory stimuli are relatively isomorphic with respect to the representation of body areas in the cortex. The face and hands are represented in the lateral and supralateral areas, legs more superiorly, and genitalia are represented medially. The postcentral gyrus also contains many large Betz cells associated with the motor system located in the adjacent precentral gyrus. It should be noted that the motor cortex also contains an equally large number of sensory cells. Therefore, the sensorimotor cortex is considered an intermediary structure between Units II and III. Moreover, both sensory and motor functions are represented contralaterally in the cortex; hence, damage to the left hemisphere affects the right side of the body and vice versa.

In addition to being responsible for the cortical detection, recognition, and association (integration) of all sensory information, Unit II is involved in modality specific memory function and cross-modal transfer of information. As such, it is a gross understatement to view Unit II merely as the "sensory analyzer" since the memory storage and information transfer functions permit extremely complex processing of information. The right temporoparietal and parieto-occipital structures of Unit II also contribute to complex functional systems which mediate attention to and perception of space (especially to the left space), prosody of language, and the processing of complex visual-spatial information such as recognition of faces (actually, a bilateral activity including the basilar temporal lobes). Unit II left hemisphere structures are involved in processing complex verbal-cognitive and language-related information as well as certain spatial tasks, such as vertical-horizontal orientation. Finally, Unit II is interconnected with Unit I and Unit III via major and minor communicating fibers. These interconnections provide a complex feedback system among the brain's major structural areas.

Unit III is located in the frontal lobes and is divided into three subareas responsible for mediating general functional systems. The primary area is responsible for the cortical level innervation of the neuromusculature necessary for preprogrammed "voluntary" motor responses ("purposeful behavior"). The secondary area (premotor area) is located anterior to the primary motor cortex and is involved in the sequencing of motor movements necessary to carry out behavioral programs. The tertiary area is involved in the most complex aspects of planning, evaluating, and verifying the completion of behavioral programs. This area is located in the anteromedial and anterobasilar aspects of the frontal lobes bilaterally and is also intimately involved in the mediation (particularly of learned socialized aspects) of emotional behavior (in concert with limbic drive states of Unit I). Unit III has reciprocal interactions with Unit I and is capable of attenuating and modulating activational or drive states via "conscious control." It also interprets highly complex aspects of the environment, thereby serving as the neural mechanism by which various psychological variables may affect the biophysiology of the organism.

The functional organization of the various units and their associated systems follows a developmental progression. For example, Unit I is functionally organized for mediating arousal and modulation of incoming sensory stimuli by 12 months post-conception, but continues to increase its efficiency and effectiveness throughout early childhood. Until Unit I has sufficiently organized, the infant remains "stimulus bound." Areas of Units II and III functionally organize at different times and rates with the most complex systems of Unit III continuing their functional organization into early adulthood. For example, Yakolev and LeCours (1967) measured the physical size of white matter in various areas of the brain and found a correspondence between size and age (in general, the older the person the larger the size of the major parietal and frontal association areas). In fact, the size of the frontal association areas continues to increase until about age 40. After that point, the size of these areas begins to decrease.

The Functional Systems Theory proposed by Luria appears to provide an integrated approach from which various issues regarding cerebral organization, lateralization, and gender may be investigated. Previous models of cerebral dominance and lateralization have been unable to explain exceptions to their predictions or provide a means by which divergent findings may be integrated into a single model. For example, complex correlations between structure and function have been observed without apparent cause-effect relationships. An individual may be "unusual" in one respect (i.e., left-preferred handedness), but conform to the "expected" in other aspects (left hemisphere dominance for language and right hemisphere dominance for visuospatial functions). Furthermore, abnormality in structure is not clearly related to functional ability or disability; in some instances, one may observe a significant amount of tissue loss on magnetic resonance imaging (MRI) or computerized axial tomography (CAT) scan without an "apparent" behavioral deficit, particularly in unilateral lesions of the anterior frontal lobes (Hardyck, Petrinovich, & Goldman, 1976).

In the authors' opinion, the Functional Systems Theory would appear to be the most comprehensive model from which to conceptualize the development of neuropsychological tests and to guide their interpretation. Luria's personal assessment techniques, however, were qualitative in nature, involving little quantification of data. He relied primarily on extensive observation over long periods of time and on informal techniques often involving himself as the "test stimulus." As a result, his procedures were virtually impossible to replicate even by some of his better students.

Nevertheless, the Functional Systems Theory may be extremely helpful in understanding the behavioral or functional implications of brain damage and dysfunction frequently associated with traumatic brain injury. The theory provides a guideline for predicting the behavioral consequences of craniocerebral trauma, in general, and serves as an interpretative system that may be applied to virtually any neuropsychological assessment data.

A basic understanding of neuroanatomy and the neuropathology of head injury is also necessary to fully appreciate the behavioral consequences observed in individual cases. The following section describes the general types of head injuries and the probable behavioral consequences which may occur.

Patterns of TBI and their Behavioral Consequences

In general, head injury or craniocerebral trauma may be divided into two major categories: closed-head and penetrating injuries. In the former, laceration of scalp and even skull fracture may occur, but the meninges (coverings of the brain) remain intact. Penetrating injuries involve direct insult to brain tissue by outside objects, such as missiles (e.g., gunshot wounds) or projectiles (e.g., falling steel reinforcing rod on a construction site). Many objects can penetrate the skull and meninges to cause brain damage and subsequent disruption of functional systems which mediate behavior.

Traditionally, penetrating wounds have been considered less devastating neuropsychologically than closed-head injuries, in that, the area of damage was restricted to the course of the penetrating object. Therefore, if a projectile entered and lodged in the right parietal lobe, damage would be restricted to its path and the resulting behavioral dysfunction would be defined by the damage to functional systems supported by right parietal structures. Behaviorally, the person would be at risk for the following problems: a loss in the ability to tactually recognize common objects presented to the left hand; spatial disorientation or confusion (e.g., difficulty finding one's car in a parking lot); difficulty orienting to a new work environment (e.g., becoming easily lost); a loss or depreciation for left space (e.g., resulting in accidents such as fender benders and difficulty in parallel parking); increased use of verbal skills to compensate for spatial disabilities; impulsivity; constriction in time concept (e.g., shows up early for appointments); and less facility in motor activities which require visuospatial and kinetic feedback (e.g., precise placements, particularly of the left hand and arm).

In contrast, closed-head injuries have been considered to be potentially even more devastating, particularly in instances of high velocity moving vehicle accidents (MVAs). To some extent these traditional views still hold true. However, with the advent of more powerful armaments in the streets (e.g., machine guns, assault rifles), many penetrating injuries can be as or more devastating than high velocity closed-head injuries. Furthermore, when the meninges are compromised by penetrating wounds, there is a significant risk for infection and abscess of brain tissue, which is not a typical complication in closed-head injuries.

A final concern in penetrating as well as in closed-head injuries, is the potential development of seizure disorders. As normal glial scarring begins to form around the damaged area of the brain, the physiology of surviving cells in the vicinity of the damage may be adversely affected. Lower thresholds for neuronal firing may be observed, resulting in a hyperexcitability of these cells. This condition may be observed as "abnormal EEG readings" in many cases. If the level of excitability of these cells affects other cells with which they communicate in such a way as to result in a "cascade effect," a seizure will be evidenced clinically. The nature of the seizure will depend on which "functional systems" are affected and the duration of that effect. For example, if the seizure is limited to the motor system, a "Jacksonian-Motor seizure" could occur.

In contrast to penetrating wounds, closed-head injuries involve other dynamics and behavioral consequences. In general, closed-head injuries may be subdivided into three categories or types: coup ("blow"); contrecoup ("counterblow"); and coup-contrecoup injuries, (although in many instances there is no clear clinical distinction among these as they present in a given case). In traditional neuropathology, coup injuries usually involve a moving object (of limited mass) striking the nonmoving head; for example, a person is struck by a high-teed drive at the golf course. The resulting blow to the head may (or may not) cause skull fracture and contusion (bruising) to the underlying brain tissue at the impact site. A minor blow may simply result in concussion (jarring of the brain) with sublethal cell injury or "dysfunction." Following a relatively brief time, normal brain function returns and the person is asymptomatic. However, if the blow results in a brain contusion, the behavior mediated by these damaged cells will be compromised. The specific behavioral consequences will reflect the impaired functional system located at the impact site.

One may recall from Luria's Theory, however, that functional systems are not rigidly localized. For example, a functional system involved in mediating a complex behavioral act, such as reading, may involve neurons and connecting processes in quite diverse areas of the brain. If the coup impact site contains cells involved in mediating one aspect of reading, then this act will be compromised in a particular way. A lesion located in a different area of the brain may also affect "reading," but in a qualitatively different way. Since multiple participation of the same cells in a given area underpins the mediation of different functional systems, damage to a single area usually involves the compromise of more than one behavior. As an example, should a coup injury occur to the left parietal lobe, one may observe a variety of behavioral consequences, such as: a disruption in reading, math processing and writing, with a particular breakdown in vertical-horizontal discrimination and graphic expression (*b's* may seen or written as *p's* and *31* may appear to be *13*); a diminished capacity to discriminate common objects by active touch senses may occur on the right side of the body; the person may demonstrate right-left confusion on self and others; and size discrimination may be mildly impaired.

Coup injuries may also result in other pathological conditions which affect brain structure, function, and behavior. For example, a blow to the head may result in tearing of the outside covering of the brain (dura mater) and branches of the meningeal arterials which supply blood to this tissue. The resulting accumulation of blood (epidural hematoma) may compress the underlying brain tissue and cause behavioral dysfunction. In the worst case scenario, sufficient blood may accumulate and ultimately force the brain to herniate from the base of the skull (foramenum magnum). The resulting mass effect lesion, particularly to the brain stem, may cause death. Fortunately, in coup injuries these hematomas are usually diagnosed before major injury occurs and are evacuated surgically. In other instances, the presence of skull fracture may actually permit a natural exit point for compressed blood. As with other types of head injury, seizure disorders can also occur and may further compromise behavioral functioning.

Contrecoup lesions, in contrast, involve damage to brain tissue at the opposite side of the head from the point of impact. This type of head injury may occur from a low velocity fall (head in motion), particularly when the back of the head, or occiput, is the impact point. In these cases, the smooth, rounded area of the occiput may protect the brain with little, if any, damage occurring at the impact site. The physical head-in-motion energy, however, may be transmitted through the essentially fluid brain with a resulting contusion in the anterobasilar frontal region or to the anterotemporal lobes medially. The base of frontal lobes anteriorly is superior to a bony region inside the skull above the nasal area. Movement of the brain inside the skull may bruise or even lacerate frontal lobes above this region. Likewise, the rather rigid outer coverings of the brain in the anterior temporal region may concentrate force in such a way as to bruise the anteromedial temporal lobes.

In other words, contrecoup lesions tend to occur opposite the point of impact, but certain regions are relatively more susceptible than others. As with other types of head injury, the behavioral consequences are associated with the underlying brain structures that may be damaged. Tearing of the dura sinuses may also occur and result in an accumulation of venous blood between the dura mater and arachnoid (middle meningeal layer). A fairly large subdural hematoma may result, giving rise to a potential mass effect lesion as described above. Seizure disorder may, likewise, result as scar tissue forms around the damaged area.

The third major type of head injury involves a high velocity head-in-motion incident. The coup-contrecoup lesion results when the head is moving rapidly through space and impacts a nonmoving object, such as the steering wheel or windshield of a car. Moving vehicle accidents (automobile and motorcycle) are the most common causes of this type of brain injury.

The coup-contrecoup lesion is not only the most commonly occurring situation, it is also has the most devastating effects on behavioral functioning. As the term implies, the coup-contrecoup injury results in brain damage to the impact site and the areas opposite the point of impact. In fact, the contrecoup area, opposite the impact site, often is considerably more bruised than the actual impact point. For similar reasons, as indicated above, the basilar frontal lobes and the medial temporal areas tend to receive the most damage. However, brain damage is often not restricted to these particular coup-contrecoup regions. Physical energy from the blow site tends to radiate in expanding ripples or waves throughout the brain. The momentum of this energy stretches the cell processes in such a way as to actually shear axons (sending units) throughout the brain. Since the head is essentially oval-shaped, any high velocity impact tends to cause a slight rotation around a central axis. For a brief moment, the brain remains stationary as the cranial vault rotates. This swirl of "shock waves" stretches and ultimately shears the axonal processes from their cell bodies. This pattern of damage occurs throughout the brain resulting in diffuse dysfunction and/or cell death in areas quite remote from the actual impact site or the contrecoup areas of damage. The behavioral consequences of such damage are profound.

Since the usual impact point in MVAs involves coup damage to the basilar frontal lobes and medial temporal lobes bilaterally, personality changes, loss of initiative and motivation, motor deficits, and poor judgement typically result. In addition, emotional/behavioral dyscontrol and memory deficits may arise from the temporal damage. More importantly, the widespread diffuse brain damage resulting from axonal shearing compromises many functional systems and is often more debilitating than the frontotemporal damage. In addition to these problems, mass effect lesions and seizure disorders may also occur.

In summary, various general types of craniocerebral trauma may all result in broad patterns of damage and associated neuropsychological dysfunction. Many different functional systems will likely be affected in a given case. Although attempts are often made to "characterize" specific behavioral consequences of TBI, each individual case differs significantly. Hence, it is necessary to consider critical issues related to the individual which may affect the presentation of behavioral consequences such as chronicity, age of onset, amount and nature of tissue damage, and location of the lesion. Therefore, it is necessary to conduct a comprehensive neuropsychological (and vocational evaluation) to identify each individual's relative strengths and deficits which may impact upon the person's ability to return to work and live independently. The following section describes major approaches and assessment technologies used in neuropsychological evaluation.

Neuropsychological Evaluation

There are a variety of approaches to neuropsychological evaluation. In general, they may be divided into two distinct groups: the "process or clinical approach" and the "battery or standardized test approach." This section summarizes the major issues, biases, and professional predispositions which interact in determining which approach one might elect to use when evaluating a person with TBI. The clinical (or process) approach to neuropsychological assessment is often conceptualized as qualitative (theoretical, flexible, informal) while the battery approach is considered quantitative (actuarial, standardized, formal). Professionals who use a process approach typically identify strongly with this position and see this as mutually exclusive from the quantitative, actuarial, or standardized approach to assessment.

THE PROCESS OR CLINICAL APPROACH

Armed with a theoretical knowledge of brain-behavior relationships, patient history, and presenting complaint, the process-oriented evaluator believes that one can make clinical or diagnostic judgements solely by interacting with the client. The importance of designing on-the-spot techniques to test the neurological system under study is emphasized (Christensen, 1984). Changes in procedures based on the presenting complaint are justified. This position is advocated by most neurologists and a minority of clinical neuropsychologists (Katzman, 1989; Pryse-Phillips & Murray, 1986).

The process approach is something like troubleshooting the wiring system of an automobile. The owner complains that the headlights do not work. During the interview with the mechanic, the owner states that he hit a tree the previous day. The mechanic immediately chooses to use the bulb tester (as opposed to the battery tester). If negative results are obtained, the mechanic then uses an ohmmeter, and so on. In other words, the mechanic responds to the specific problem as reported, and systematically rules out the probable causes. The mechanic's "approach" relies on theoretical knowledge of how the electrical system is constructed and how it functions (e.g., where the separate components are located and what "pathways" exist between the components).

Advocates of the process approach tend to subscribe to "antilocationist" theories such as Luria's Functional Systems theory (Adams & Victor, 1981). They claim, for example, that the battery approach is atheoretical and provides minimally useful, quantitative measurement of special attributes such as intellectual functioning. According to this position, most psychological tests incorporated into these batteries simply measure the same aspects of general ability and functioning.

Historically, the process approach has rejected attempts to develop a single "impairment index" (using such tests as the WAIS) to define brain damage. Christensen (1984) supports this position by arguing that the brain is not a homogeneous mass. They state that Luria's Functional Systems theory clearly indicates that lesions in different systems lead to qualitative differences in behavior. Consequently, qualitative assessment approaches are required to localize lesions.

Still, many attempts have been made to develop an "impairment index" from standardized tests. Anastasi (1986) describes a lengthy history of such attempts predating World War II. Today, it is clear that a single "index" would have little diagnostic value for localizing lesions or prescribing treatment. On the other hand, useful indices of diffuse, left and right hemisphere "dysfunction" or "damage" have been developed for various tests (Russell, 1984). Furthermore, such profiles of test scores may be useful for predicting vocational and independent living outcomes and for defining general rehabilitation efforts (McCarron & Dial, 1986).

Instead of viewing theory and empiricism in opposition to one another, a consolidation of these positions may be more productive. Indeed, it is the fervent dream of many scientist-practitioners to develop a theory; operationalize it by "tests"; and to have the "tests" produce results that correspond to the theory's predictions. To the scientist-practitioner, therefore, all debates of the merits of a theoretical approach versus an actuarial approach are really intellectual folly. What we often see as "theoretical" arguments supporting one method over another are reflections of the differing needs and goals of researchers versus practitioners. Therefore, so called "theoretical differences in approaches" are often simply representations of individual preferences.

The person who relies on the informal or qualitative approach must also have some notion of normal variance in behavior. Therefore, the process evaluator relies primarily on "head norms," regardless of whether their assessment techniques have been developed theoretically or not. Most proponents of the informal methods have themselves become very "standardized" in their approach to evaluation. By giving basically the same "informal examination" to every patient (in exactly the same way, defining errors they associate with different disorders), they have become standardized instruments normed on their patient population.

Flexibility in the approach to assessment is an important issue related to whether the evaluator should give every patient a broad spectrum screen, or whether it is more appropriate to use one's judgement and select tests that focus upon the suspected deficits. If the presenting complaint is forgetfulness, is it important to check fine and gross motor skills? The advocates of the process approach use the patient's presenting complaint(s) and history to narrow their selection of assessment techniques to address certain problems. However, to some extent, this appears to be an artificial argument.

In fact, those who use standardized batteries are conducting broad spectrum screening examinations. Developers of these test batteries have to make decisions as to what can practically be included or not. Those who give a standardized, broad spectrum battery make this decision upon completion of the core battery. They may or may not add additional tests depending upon whether the referral question has been adequately answered by the initial battery. In practice, there is not a single battery of practical length that can test every possible neurosystem in a given patient. However, some of the most commonly used batteries provide an excellent foundation from which many neuropsychological issues surrounding TBI can be resolved. The following section describes some of these batteries.

THE BATTERY OR STANDARDIZED TEST APPROACH

Historically, many behavioral instruments have been used as measures in neuropsychological research and in clinical practice. Some instruments have attempted to measure one or more of the global higher functions in man, such as perception, memory, learning, cognition, language, affect, and/or complex sensorimotor functions. From the various behavioral operations included in the tests, inferences regarding the integrity of underlying brain structures (and their dynamic physiology) have been drawn. The general assumption has been that abnormal brain structure and/or physiology is responsible for abnormal deviations in behavior and, conversely, abnormal deviations in behavior (in the absence of so-called nonorganic explanations) imply brain pathology or, at least, "brain difference."

The clinical neuropsychologist has been expected to incorporate case history information with the client's behavioral profile (derived from a variety of standardized neuropsychological tests and behavioral observations) and to formulate diagnostic hypotheses. Subsequently, treatment strategies or further diagnostics have been recommended on the basis of these tentative diagnoses (Golden, 1981; Lezak, 1976).

The effectiveness and/or usefulness of a neuropsychological instrument (or battery) depends on a number of critical factors: the degree to which these instruments meet acceptable psychometric standards (i.e., standard procedures of administration and scoring); appropriate normative or criteria references; sufficiently high reliability; and most important, the degree to which the instruments measure the constructs that they purport to assess (validity). In addition to the usual psychometric criteria, instruments used in clinical neuropsychology should ideally demonstrate two other qualities: (a) performance on the measures should have a direct relationship between changes or alterations in brain functioning; and (b) a functional relationship between performance on the instrument and the appropriateness of a particular approach to treatment, rehabilitation, and/or education should be evidenced. Beyond these fundamental qualities, it would be desirable that neuropsychological tests correlate to functional outcomes in education and rehabilitation (e.g., success in a particular academic endeavor or occupation). Unfortunately, few batteries (much less specific instruments) meet the latter criteria (McCarron & Dial, 1986).

The Halstead-Reitan Neuropsychological Testing Battery (HRNTB)

One of the most widely researched neuropsychological test batteries was developed for use with adults by Halstead (1947) and later revised and extended for use with adults and children by Reitan (1969) and Reitan and Davison (1974). The original battery included 27 tests of which 10 were used to derive an "impairment index." Reitan later dropped three of the original 10 tests and supplemented the remaining seven with additional measures. The revised battery for adults included the: **Category Test** (a measure of concept formation); **Tactual Performance Test** (a measure of various sensorimotor functions); **Tactile Form Perception Test** (a measure of spatial organization and kinesthesis); **Seashore Rhythm Test** (a measure of sustained attention and nonverbal auditory discrimination); **Speech Sounds Perception Test** (a measure of attention and verbal-auditory-visual discrimination); and the **Finger Oscillation Test** (a measure of finger tapping speed). The resulting **Halstead-Reitan Battery** (HRNTB) generated an index of possible brain damage, the "Impairment Index," as well as other specific data useful in differential diagnosis of location, chronicity, and the nature of the suspected lesion.

The HRNTB has generally been supplemented with various measures of intelligence, achievement, sensory perception, sensorimotor functions and/or emotional-personality inventories. Commonly used tests of intelligence have included the **Wechsler-Bellevue Intelligence Scale** (Wechsler, 1944), the **Wechsler Adult Intelligence Scales** (WAIS) (Wechsler, 1955), and more recently, the revised WAIS (WAIS-R) (Wechsler, 1981). The **Wide Range Achievement Test** (Jastak & Jastak, 1965) and the **Minnesota Multiphasic Personality Inventory** (MMPI) (Hathaway & McKinley, 1967) have been frequently incorporated into the battery as measures of achievement and emotional-personality factors, respectively. The assessment of perceptual and sensorimotor functions has often been augmented by the **Trail Making Test** for Adults (also considered to have a cognitive component) (Reitan, 1958), grip strength using a hand dynamometer, tactile finger recognition, finger-tip number writing, and tactile coin recognition. Certain speech, language and visual-constructional abilities have ordinarily been evaluated using the **Aphasia Screening Test** (Wheeler & Reitan, 1962).

The children's version of the HRNTB includes many of the same instruments used in the adult battery with special procedural adaptations and different norms; such as the **Category Test**, **Tactual Performance Test**, and **Finger Tapping Test** (Finger Oscillation Test). The children's battery may also include the **Marching Test** (a measure of gross skeletal-muscular function); **Color Form Test** (a measure of organizational ability, flexibility in thinking and visual-motor integration); **Progressive Figures Test** (a more complex test measuring similar constructs as the Color Form Test); **Target Test** (a measure related to the reception and expression of visual-spatial relationships); and the **Individual Performance Test** (a group of tasks that assess visual-spatial relationships) (Filskov & Boll, 1981; Reitan & Davison, 1974).

A plethora of studies using a variety of statistical techniques have documented the validity of the Halstead-Reitan Battery for assessing neuropsychological functioning of different neurological, psychiatric, and normal populations (Filskov & Goldstein, 1974; Klonoff, Fibiger, & Hutton, 1970; Mathews, Shaw, & Klove, 1966; Schreiber, Goldman, Kleinman, Goldfader, & Snow, 1976; Reitan, 1955; Vega & Parsons, 1971). For example, Wheeler, Burke, and Reitan (1963), using discriminant analysis technique, found the HRNTB variables to be extremely accurate (94% "hit rate") in predicting the actual group membership (no cerebral damage, left cerebral damage, right cerebral damage, and diffuse cerebral damage) of 140 research subjects. Other studies contrasting various brain-damaged with nonbrain-damaged groups have also reported less, but consistently high "hit rates" of about 70 to 80% (Matthews et al., 1966; Wheeler & Reitan, 1963). There is no doubt that the HRNTB is very useful for localizing lesions in adults and children (Boll, 1974; Reitan & Davison, 1974).

However, little research is available related to the validity of the HRNTB in predicting vocational rehabilitation outcomes (e.g., rehabilitation treatment, vocational training, and job placement) of TBI clients (Ben-Yishay, Diller, Gordon, & Gerstman, 1978; Diller, 1976; Filskov & Boll, 1981; Golden, 1981). Interestingly, Golden (1981) contributes more than three-fourths of a text entitled *Diagnosis and Rehabilitation in Clinical Neuropsychology* to basic principles of neuropsychology and traditional diagnostics with the HRNTB. Only two chapters are devoted to principles of rehabilitation, and neither elucidates the relationship between localization of lesions and treatment planning. Many other texts in neuropsychology which purport to deal with rehabilitation and treatment issues, in fact, are restatements of the same issue of "localization of lesions." One must question whether localization per se, is a meaningful end product of an expensive, time-consuming (4 to 6 hours) evaluation. This issue would seem particularly controversial considering the advent of improved, high-resolution computer axial tomography; positron emission tomography; single photon emission computer-enhanced tomography; magnetic resonance imaging; thermography; and minimal risk radioisotopic labeling procedures to monitor regional blood flow in the brain (Lassen, Ingvar, & Skinhoj, 1978).

The Luria-Nebraska Battery (LNNB)

In more recent years, Golden (1981) introduced the Luria-Nebraska Neuropsychological Battery (LNNB) as an assessment technology for differential diagnosis and treatment planning. The battery, as its name implies, has attempted to incorporate aspects of Luria's (1966, 1970, 1973) Functional Systems Theory in the selection of assessment tasks.

An earlier contribution to quantification of Luria's approach (at least of stimulus items) was made by Christensen (1975). Golden (1981) modified some of these procedures, added others, and later reduced the number of items based on initial pilot studies to a total of 269 items divided into 11 sections. Further modification and elaboration of the procedures have continued to be made by Golden and others. This assessment procedure takes approximately two to two and one-half hours and may be administered in a variety of settings, including hospital rooms (a virtual impossibility for the HRNTB even in its present-day form). The test sections of the LNNB include: motor functions, rhythm scale (acousticomotor), tactile scale (higher cutaneous and kinesthetic functions), visual (spatial) scale, receptive speech, expressive speech, writing, reading, arithmetic, memory, and intellectual processes scale. The raw scores from each section are plotted on a graphic profile and converted to T-scores. T-scores which exceed the "critical level" (adjusted for educational level) are considered pathological. Additional scales are derived from critical items included in the other sections; for example, pathognomonic (32 most discriminating items), right and left hemisphere scales (combinations of unilateral items from the tactile and motor sections), elevation scale, impairment scale, etc.

In the initial validation study by Golden, Hammeke, and Purisch (1978), the 30 most sensitive items (of 269) accurately placed 100% of the subjects (50 brain-damaged, 50 nonbrain-damaged) into the appropriate categories. The 14 test sections (including pathognomonic, right, and left hemisphere indicators) achieved an overall hit rate of 93%. An 88% overall hit rate was also observed between brain-damaged and schizophrenic controls. Many studies documenting the validity of the LNNB for specific localization have subsequently been published. The instrument would appear to be equally valid (as the HRNTB) in most respects for identifying and localizing brain lesions.

Luria's Functional Systems Theory, on which the LNNB is based, provides direction for hypothesis formulation and testing related to brain-behavior relationships, as well as a conceptual model by which treatment and rehabilitation strategies may be developed. The theoretical base, standardized profile, relatively shorter administration time, and ease of administration in the hospital setting would appear to be definite advantages of the LNNB as contrasted with the HRNTB. However, the LNNB also has several significant limitations. For example, the tactile scale often does not reflect the degree of impairment which actually exists. The motor scale is relatively insensitive to static, chronic anterior, and basilar frontal lesions, even when extensive tissue loss is evident radiologically (see Chapter 4). Finally, the LNNB requires the examiner to make critical judgements of the subject's behavior to rate certain items, thus necessitating considerable training and experience on the part of the examiner. In contrast, the standardization of the HRNTB (as well as other batteries) permits less extensively trained technical staff to administer and score the various tests, thus permitting the neuropsychologist to perform other more complex interpretative, report preparation and treatment functions.

One of the most important applications of a neuropsychological evaluation is the generation of practical recommendations for rehabilitation or education intervention. It is clear from Golden's work that he fully intends for the LNNB to serve as both a diagnostic and programming tool (Golden, 1981). Unfortunately, the LNNB has not totally achieved this goal. Though impressive results have been published concerning the system's diagnostic validity, like the HRNTB, only limited empirical data are available which document the relationship between the LNNB and various rehabilitation and/or educational outcomes. No data are available which suggest a valid and efficacious mechanism for selecting appropriate rehabilitation, training, or treatment goals on the basis of an individual client's profile.

McCarron-Dial System (MDS)

While the HRNTB and the LNNB were originally developed by psychologists in the field of neuropsychology, the MDS has its origin in the vocational rehabilitation field. The MDS, a neuropsychologically-based assessment battery, was originally developed as a vocational evaluation tool with a focus on assessing the work potential and vocational competency of people with neuropsychological disabilities including TBI (Dial, McCarron, & Henke, 1978). Recently, the MDS has been validated as a neuropsychological assessment battery (Dial & Chan, 1987; Dial, Chan, & Norton, 1990). As such, the authors believe that the MDS may have some advantages over other neuropsychological batteries in dealing with return-to-work issues.

The MDS is generally acknowledged as a well-developed and studied system for use in vocational evaluation (Botterbusch, 1983). It was found to be highly predictive of independent living and vocational placement outcomes of people with neuropsychological disabilities. The MDS is also useful for conceptualizing individualized rehabilitation programming and identifying treatment/training strategies for this client group (Dial, Chan, & Norton, 1990; McCarron & Dial, 1986). Recent research also suggests that the MDS is equally useful as a diagnostic and programming tool in neuropsychological evaluation. As a result, the MDS has been incorporated into many rehabilitation, public school, and clinical settings to assess educational and vocational potential of people with neuropsychological disabilities (Botterbusch, 1983).

The neuropsychological model of the MDS incorporates traditional views of brain functions as well as Luria's Functional Systems Theory (Luria, 1970). A multifactor approach to data gathering was viewed by McCarron and Dial as essential in the evaluation of higher cortical functions. In the MDS evaluation model, three neuropsychological factors were identified as important in predicting work and independent living functioning. The MDS was developed to operationalize the evaluation model and measure these factors:

Verbal-Spatial-Cognitive (VSC) Factor: This factor reflects the individual's ability to think abstractly, conceptualize, use language, and perform operations involving numbers, language, and/or visual-spatial symbols. The primary MDS measures for this factor include the

Wechsler Adult Intelligence Scale-Revised (WAIS-R) (Wechsler, 1981) and the **Peabody Picture Vocabulary Test-Revised** (PPVT-R) (Dunn & Dunn, 1981). However, supplemental data from other psychological tests, as well as behavioral observations, may also be utilized.

Sensorimotor (SM) Factor: This factor relates to the individual's ability to receive information through various senses, to integrate sensory information across modalities, to associate new information with previous experience, and to make an appropriate adaptive motor response to the particular sensation or group of sensations. The MDS measures of this factor include the **Bender Visual Motor Gestalt Test** (BVMGT) (Bender, 1938), the **Haptic Visual Discrimination Test** (HVDT) (McCarron & Dial, 1986), and the **McCarron Assessment of Neuromuscular Development** (MAND) (McCarron, 1982). As previously mentioned, supplemental data may also be included in any given case.

Emotional-Coping (EC) Factor: This factor includes information related to the person's characteristic responses to stress, general personality development, emotional-behavioral functioning, and adaptive behavior. Adaptive behavior is defined as the individual's knowledge and skills related to activities of daily living, personal-social adjustment, and work adjustment. The EC factor is measured by a combination of the **Emotional Behavioral Checklist** (EBC) (McCarron & Dial, 1986), **Observational Emotional Inventory - Revised** (OEI-R) (McCarron & Dial, 1986), the **Dial Behavioral Rating Scale** (DBRS) (Dial, 1973), the **Street Survival Skills Questionnaire** (SSSQ) (Linkenhoker & McCarron, 1980), and the **Survey of Functional Adaptive Behaviors** (SFAB) (Dial, Mezger, Massey, Carter, & McCarron, 1986). Additional data may also be incorporated from traditional clinical instruments such as the MMPI or from case history and behavioral observations.

A number of research studies have established the criterion-related validity of the MDS. For example, results from the original validation study revealed high multiple correlations (R = .90 and .70, respectively) between the MDS factors and outcome measures of work behavior and productivity. Subsequent validation studies by different researchers also reported similar results (Carsrud, Carsrud, Dodd, Thompson, & Gray, 1981; Dial, Freemon, McCarron, & Swearingen, 1979; Dial & Swearingen, 1976; Packard, Henke, & McCollum, 1976).

Predictive validity of the MDS to functional living levels was demonstrated in several studies (Linkenhoker & McCarron, 1980; Blackwell, Dial, Chan, & McCollum 1985; Mathews, 1981; Dial, Chan, Carter, Parker, & Pomeroy 1985). These studies revealed high, significant multiple correlations between MDS factors and the level of functional autonomy attained by mentally retarded adults and emotionally disturbed adolescents.

Additional studies have described the relationship of MDS variables to the successful application of modeling procedures in treatment

(Bodenhamer, 1980), use of MDS data for programming motor intervention strategies (McCarron, 1978), and the application of the MDS for personal-social adjustment training (McCarron, Kern, & Wolf, 1979) and workshop production (Presnall, 1979; Sigelman, Morris, & Danley, 1979).

The MDS has also been validated for use with a range of disability population including the psychiatrically disabled (Fortune & Eldredge, 1982); normal and mentally retarded blind adults (adapted instrumentation) (Dial & Henke, 1981; McCarron & Dial, 1976); deaf adults and children (McCarron & Ludlow, 1982); spinal cord-injured (McCarron & Clement, 1980); closed head-injured (McCarron & Clement, 1980); and learning disabled adolescents and adults (McCarron, Bihm, Jablanca, & Valente, 1984; Texas Rehabilitation Commission, 1979). In each of the investigations, the MDS (or its specific components) have been found applicable to the clinical or vocational evaluation of the various disability groups studied.

Finally, the MDS has recently been validated for use as a neuropsychological battery. For example, Dial, Chan, and Norton (1990) investigated the effects of brain damage on MDS measures of verbal-spatial-cognitive (VSC) and sensorimotor (SM) functioning. Ninety-two brain-damaged adults and 30 normal controls were subjects of this study. The groups did not significantly differ on the variables of age, educational level, racial composition, handedness, or sexual composition. The multiple discriminant analysis results indicated that 93% of the brain-damaged and normal control groups were accurately classified by a combination of MDS, VSC, and SM measures and a 74% accuracy in classifying the right, left, and diffuse brain-damaged subgroups was also reported. Earlier, Dial and Chan (1985) and McCarron and Dial (1984) also investigated the effects of brain damage on VSC and SM measures with 141 brain-damaged adults and a comparison group of 42 psychiatric patients. Results of the discriminate analysis indicated that 90% of the combined brain-damaged group and psychiatric control group subjects were accurately classified by a combination of the MDS, VSC, and SM, measures. Significant differences between the left, right, and diffuse brain-damaged groups were observed on a number of specific MDS measures. The mean performance of the posterior brain-damaged group also differed significantly in contrast to the anterior brain-damaged group on sensorimotor measures.

Considering the research findings to date, the MDS would appear to have several advantages for use as a battery in both neuropsychological and vocational evaluation. As a neuropsychological assessment tool, the MDS can provide the same kind of diagnostic information such as the type, location, and severity of neurological impairment just like the HRNTB and the LNNB. The MDS, HRNTB, and LNNB can also provide information about specific behavioral (physical, cognitive, as well as psychosocial) strengths or weaknesses for the individual TBI client over and above what their diagnostic category may communicate. This diagnostic and treatment information is very important to the rehabilitation professionals in considering treatment and training approaches for TBI clients. However, from a vocational rehabilitation perspective, the MDS would appear to have some advantages over other neuropsychological batteries by providing data that are directly interpreted functional vocational terms.

McCarron and Dial (1986) have operationally defined work and independent living potential into different placement levels. A systematic approach for predicting these placement levels and associated treatment/training models for each level are described in the MDS manual. Specifically, seven levels of vocational functioning and five residential living levels are defined by McCarron and Dial (1986):

VOCATIONAL FUNCTIONING LEVELS

1. **Daycare** - Basic self-help skills are emphasized in programming at this level; little, if any real work activity is possible.

2. **Work Activity** - Rudimentary work activities are possible at this level; the activity of work is used as a medium for education and training.

3. **Low Extended Sheltered Workshop** - Personal/social and work adjustment are emphasized in programming at this level; elementary sorting and/or assembly tasks are used for training and/or extended employment.

4. **High Extended Sheltered Workshop** - Adjustment services for sheltered employment or in preparation for special community employment are emphasized in programming at this level; numerous sorting, assembly, and light manufacturing tasks are used for training and/or extended employment.

5. **Transitional** (Sheltered Workshop to Community Employment) - Work behavior and job readiness skills necessary for community employment are emphasized at this level; vocational exploration and job training activities are also undertaken.

6. **Skilled** - Occupational exploration, skills training, and/or apprenticeship placement are emphasized at this level; with experience and training, individuals may advance to the technical/professional level.

7. **Professional/Technical** - Career development and vocational placement planning activities are emphasized at this level; individuals may enter formal technical or academic programs in preparation for specific professions.

RESIDENTIAL FUNCTIONING LEVELS

1. **Institutional** - Twenty-four-hour care and supervision are emphasized at this level; little functional autonomy is provided the residents.

2. **Intermediate Care** - Most activities of daily living are supervised at this level; residents may be involved in work activities programs during the day.

3. **Group Home** - General supervision is provided in matters of daily living, such as meals, laundry, purchasing, etc.; residents may be employed in sheltered workshops or in community employment settings; some social activities may be conducted independently by the resident.

4. **Halfway House** (Semi-independent Living) - Monitoring by counselors is provided; residents may be responsible for most matters of living; they are generally employed in community settings or in work training centers (sheltered workshops).

5. **Community Living** - Autonomous living in the community with only occasional (normal) need for assistance from others.

Specific prediction formulas are generated from extensive empirical research using the MDS variables as predictors and the operationally defined vocational and residential functioning levels as criterion variables. A structured guideline is provided by MDS for interpreting the predicted vocational and residential functioning levels according to the client's performance on different MDS factors.

A model of developmental prerequisites for work competency was also developed by McCarron and Dial to describe the relative importance of each MDS factor at different levels of vocational functioning. For example, at the work activity level, the most significant factor for interpretation and rehabilitation planning is the sensorimotor factor; second in importance is the emotional-coping factor; and finally, the verbal-spatial-cognitive factor. Therefore, the identified sensorimotor deficits should either be remediated or accommodated as an initial program priority, followed by programming efforts for deficits in other functional areas. Further, the theory suggests that the achievement of higher levels of vocational competency is not probable unless the specific deficits are systematically addressed in order of relative significance. At each progressively higher level of vocational competency, the MDS factor for predicting and describing vocational functioning shifts in order of relative significance.

To facilitate the use of the MDS process of predicting vocational behavior, identifying strengths and deficits, and recommending treatment/training strategies, the process has been automated by computer software. A computer-based job-matching system was also developed by MDS to match the residual employability profile of a client to appropriate jobs in the world of work. In addition, vocational and independent living training curriculum are available for MDS rehabilitation programming.

Summary

The purpose of this chapter is to provide the readers with a general overview of the theory, history, and research literature in neuropsychology. A conceptual formulation of neuropsychological evaluation in rehabilitation and its role in the identification of deficits and assets of individuals with TBI was presented. Additionally, the importance of doing a comprehensive evaluation encompassing the often-neglected vocational area in rehabilitation planning was discussed. A model for integrating evaluation data was described. Specifically, the authors believe that the integration of isomorphic and holistic theories of cerebral organization may be best conceptualized by considering the Functional Systems Theory (Luria, 1970, 1973, 1976). Luria suggested that the brain is composed of functional systems which mediate all behavior. Each functional system involves more than one structural element, but there is a finite number of elements in each system. Functional systems are analogous to chains in that each cell (or cell assembly) is involved in some way in the mediation of the behavior for which the system is responsible. Structures are involved in more than one functional system. In other words, there is multiple participation of elements among various functional systems. The Functional Systems Theory would appear to be the most comprehensive model from which to conceptualize the development of neuropsychological tests and to guide their interpretation.

A number of neuropsychological tests and batteries have been developed to assess higher cortical functions. Some, such as the HRNTB, are empirically based and do not subscribe to any particular theory. Others, such as the LNNB, have attempted to operationalize Luria's theory and "clinical assessment techniques." Both the HRNTB and LNNB have demonstrated validity for localizing brain lesions in the clinical setting. However, none of the traditional clinical batteries have systematic methods for translating an individual's evaluation profile to an effective rehabilitation plan, particularly when "return-to-work" issues are important.

In contrast to other neuropsychological batteries, the development of the MDS initially focused on the establishment of empirical relationships between neuropsychological profiles and functional outcomes (i.e., work, living, learning, and social-personal adjustment criteria). Research has validated the MDS with regard to its practical utility in formulating treatment plans, predicting program outcomes, and suggesting appropriate vocational or residential placement. The McCarron-Dial System (MDS) is one of the most extensively studied vocational evaluation systems (Botterbusch, 1983). In addition, research aimed at establishing diagnostic validity of the MDS as a neuropsychologicl assessment battery has begun to emerge in the literature. As a practical rehabilitation assessment and programming tool, the MDS would, therefore, appear to have some advantages over other traditional neuropsychological assessment batteries in clinical settings. Finally, to further illustrate the use of neuropsychological evaluation in head injury rehabilitation, a case study highlighting many of the issues related to neuropsychological evaluation, rehabilitation, and return-to-work will be presented in the next chapter.

References

Adams, R. D., & Victor, M. (1981). *Principles of neurology.* New York: McGraw-Hill.

Anastasi, A. (1986). *Psychological testing* (5th ed.). New York: Macmillan.

Ben-Yishay, Y., Diller, L., Gordon, W., & Gerstman, L. (1978). *Working approaches to remediation of cognitive deficits in brain damage.* New York: Institute of Rehabilitation Medicine.

Bender, L. A. (1938). *A visual motor gestalt test and its clinical use.* New York: American Orthopsychiatric Association.

Blackwell, S., Dial, J., Chan, F., & McCollum, P. (1985). Discriminating functional levels of independent living: A neuropsychological evaluation of mentally retarded adults. *Rehabilitation Counseling Bulletin, 29,* 42-52.

Bodenhamer, E. (1980). Assessing client ability to benefit from modeling procedures. *Vocational Evaluation and Work Adjustment Bulletin, 12,* 129-132.

Boll, T. J. (1974). Behavioral correlates of cerebral damage in children aged 9-14. In R. M. Reitan & L. A. Davison (Eds.), *Clinical neuropsychology: Current status and applications* (pp. 91-120). Washington, DC: Winston and Sons.

Botterbusch, K. (1983). *A comparison of commercial vocational evaluation system.* Menomonie, WI: Materials Development Center, University of Wisconsin-Stout.

Carsrud, A., Carsrud, K., Dodd, B., Thompson, M., & Gray, W. (1981). Predicting vocational aptitude of mentally retarded persons: A comparison of assessment systems. *American Journal of Mental Deficiency, 86,* 275-280.

Christensen, A. (1984). The Luria method of examination of the brain-impaired patient. In P. Logue and J. Schear (Eds.), *Clinical neuropsychology - A multidisciplinary approach* (pp. 5-28). Springfield, IL: Charles C. Thomas.

Christensen, A. L. (1975). *Luria's neuropsychological investigation.* New York: Spectrum.

Dial, J. G. (1973). *Behavioral rating scale.* Dallas, TX: McCarron-Dial Systems.

Dial, J. G., & Chan, F. (1985). The McCarron-Dial System as a neuropsychological assessment battery in rehabilitation (Abstract). *Clinical Neuropsychology, 7,* 62-63.

Dial, J. G., & Chan, F. (1987). Diagnostic validity of the McCarron-Dial System in neuropsychological rehabilitation assessment. *International Journal of Rehabilitation Research, 10*(2), 151-158.

Dial, J. G., & Henke, R. (1981). *User's guide to the Computer Assessment Program (CAP) and the Occupational Exploration System (OES).* Dallas, TX: McCarron-Dial Systems.

Dial, J. G., & Swearingen, S. (1976). The prediction of sheltered workshop performance: Special applications of the McCarron-Dial Work Evaluation System. *Vocational Evaluation and Work Adjustment Bulletin, 9,* 24-33.

Dial, J. G., Chan, F., & Norton, C. (1990). Neuropsychological assessment of brain damage: Discriminative validity of the McCarron-Dial System. *Brain Injury, 4*, 239-246.

Dial, J. G., Chan, F., Parker, H. J., Carter, S. H., & Pomeroy, V. (1985). SSSQ predictors of independent living skills: A criterion-related validation study. *Vocational Evaluation and Work Adjustment Bulletin, 18*, 141-146.

Dial, J. G., Freemon, L., McCarron, L., & Swearingon, S. (1979). Predictive validation of the McCarron-Dial Evaluation System. *Vocational Evaluation and Work Adjustment Bulletin, 12*, 11-18.

Dial, J. G., McCarron, L., & Henke, R. (1978). *A review of the McCarron-Dial Evaluation System*. Unpublished manuscript, McCarron-Dial Systems, Dallas.

Dial, J. G., Mezger, C., Massey, T., Carter, S., & McCarron, L. (1986). *Survey of Functional Adaptive Behaviors*. Dallas, TX: McCarron-Dial Systems.

Diller, L. (1976). A model for cognitive retraining in rehabilitation. *The Clinical Psychologist, 9*, 24-33.

Dunn, L., & Dunn, L. (1981). *Peabody Picture Vocabulary Test-Revised Manual*. Circle Pines, MN: American Guidance Service.

Filskov, S. B., & Boll, T. J. (Eds.) (1981). *Handbook of clinical neuropsychology*. New York: John Wiley & Sons.

Filskov, S. B., & Goldstein, S. G. (1974). Diagnostic validity of the Halstead-Reitan Neuropsychological Battery. *Journal of Consulting and Clinical Psychology, 42*, 383-388.

Fortune, J., & Eldredge, G. (1982). Predictive validation of the McCarron-Dial System for psychiatrically disabled sheltered workshop workers. *Vocational Evaluation and Work Adjustment Bulletin, 15*, 136-141.

Gazzaniga, M. S. (1967). The split brain in man. *Scientific American, 217*(2), 24-29.

Gazzaniga, M. S. (December, 1979). *Brain mechanisms underlying conscious experience*. A presentation at the University of Health Science Center at Dallas.

Geschwind, N. (1979). Specializations of the human brain. *Scientific American, 241*, 180-199.

Giller, V. L., Dial, J. G., & Chan, F. (1986). The Street Survival Skills Questionnaire: A correlational study. *American Journal of Mental Deficiency, 91*(1), 67-71.

Golden, C. J. (1981). *Diagnosis and rehabilitation in clinical neuropsychology* (2nd ed.). Springfield, IL: Charles C. Thomas.

Golden, C. J., Hammeke, T., & Purisch, A. (1978). A diagnostic validity study of the Luria Neuropsychological Battery. *Journal of Consulting and Clinical Psychology, 46*, 1258-1265.

Halstead, W. C. (1947). *Brain and intelligence: A quantitative study of the frontal lobes*. Chicago: University of Chicago Press.

Hardyck, C., Petrinovich, L., & Goldman, R. (1976). Left-handedness and cognitive deficits. *Cortex, 12,* 266-279.

Hathaway, S. R., & McKinley, J. C. (1967). *Minnesota Multiphasic Personality Inventory manual.* New York: The Psychological Corporation.

Jastak, J. F., & Jastak, S. R. (1965). *The Wide Range Achievement Test. Manual of instructions.* Wilmington, DE: Guidance Associates.

Katzman, R. (1989). Delirium and dementia. In L. P. Rowland (Ed.), *Merritt's textbook of neurology* (pp. 3-9). Philadephia: Lea and Febiger.

Kimura, D. (1973). The asymmetry of the human brain. *Scientific American, 228*(3), 70-78.

Klonoff, H., Fibiger, C. H., & Hutton, G. H. (1970). Neuropsychological patterns in chronic schizophrenia. *Journal of Nervous and Mental Disease, 150,* 291-300.

Lassen, N. A., Ingvar, D. H., & Skinhoj, E. (1978). Brain function and blood flow. *Scientific American, 239*(4), 62-71.

Lezak, M.D. (1976). *Neuropsychological assessment.* New York: Oxford University Press.

Linkenhoker, D., & McCarron, L. (1980). *Adaptive behavior: The Street Survival Skills Questionnaire.* Dallas, TX: Common Market Press.

Luria, A. R. (1966). *Higher cortical functions in man.* New York: Basic Books.

Luria, A. R. (1970). The functional organization of the brain. *Scientific American, 222*(3), 66-78.

Luria, A. R. (1973). *The working brain.* New York: Basic Books.

Luria, A. R. (1976). *The neuropsychology of memory.* Washington, DC: Winston and Sons.

Mathews, C. G., Shaw, D. J., & Klove, H. (1966). Psychological test performances in neurologic and "pseudo-neurologic" subjects. *Cortex, 2,* 244-253.

Mathews, D. (1981). *A construct validity study of the Street Survival Skills Questionaire with emotionally disturbed children.* Unpublished master's thesis. Stephen F. Austin State University, Nacogdoches, TX.

McCarron, L. (1978). A strategy for the development of motor training activities. In L. Beutler & R. Green (Eds.), *Special problems in child and adolescent behavior.* Westport, CT: Technomic Publishing Co.

McCarron, L. (1982). *McCarron Assessment of Neuromuscular Development.* Dallas, TX: Common Market Press.

McCarron, L., & Clement, C. (1980). *Progress report 1980.* Lubbock, TX: Research and Training Center in Mental Retardation, Texas Tech University.

McCarron, L., & Dial, J. G. (1976). *McCarron-Dial Work Evaluation System: Evaluation of the mentally retarded—A systematic approach.* Dallas, TX: Common Market Press.

McCarron, L., & Dial, J. G. (1984). The development of the McCarron-Dial System. *Texas Psychologist, 36*, 8-12.

McCarron, L., & Dial, J. G. (1986). *McCarron-Dial Evaluation System: A systematic approach to vocational, educational, and neuropsychological assessment.* Dallas, TX: McCarron-Dial System.

McCarron, L., & Ludlow, G. (1982). Specificity and redundancy in vocational evaluation procedures: Factor analysis of manual dexterity skills. *Vocational Evaluation and Work Adjustment Bulletin, 15*, 49-62.

McCarron, L., Bihm, E., Jablanca, J., & Valente, E. (1984). *Vocational rehabilitation for the learning disabled: A comprehensive community based model for service delivery.* Edinburg, TX: Pan American University.

McCarron, L., Kern, W., & Wolf, S. (1979). Use of leisure time activities for work adjustment training. *Mental Retardation, 17*(1), 13-16.

New, P. F. J., Scott, W. R., Schnur, J. A., Davis, K. R., & Traveras, J. M. (1974). Computerized axial tomography with the EMI scanner. *Radiology, 11*, 109-123.

Norton, C. L. (1985). *Assessment of brain damage: Discriminative validity of a neuropsychological key approach with the McCarron-Dial System.* Unpublished doctoral dissertation. University of North Texas, Denton.

Packard, R., Henke, R., & McCollum, P. (1976). A concurrent validation of the McCarron-Dial Work Evaluation System as a pre-admission screening battery. *Vocational Evaluation and Work Adjustment Bulletin, 9*, 25-32.

Presnall, D. (February, 1979). The relationship of manual dexterity and skill acquisition factors to workshop productivity. *Education and Training of the Mentally Retarded*, 11-16.

Pryse-Phillips, W., & Murray, T. J. (1986). *Essential neurology.* New York: Medical Examination Publishing Co.

Reitan, R. M. (1955). An investigation of the validity of Halstead's measures of biological intelligence. *Archives of Neurology and Psychiatry, 73*, 28-35.

Reitan, R. M. (1958). Validity of the Trail Making Test as an indicator of organic brain damage. *Perceptual and Motor Skills, 8*, 271-276.

Reitan, R. M. (1969). *Manual for administration of neuropsychological test batteries for adults and children.* Privately published by the author, Indianapolis, 1969.

Reitan, R. M., & Davison, L. A. (1974). *Clinical neuropsychology: Current status and applications.* Washington, D.C.: Winston and Sons.

Russell, E. W. (1984). Theory and development of pattern analysis methods related to the Halstead-Reitan Battery. In P. Logue and J. Schear (Eds.), *Clinical neuropsychology - A multidisciplinary approach* (pp. 50-98). Springfield, IL: Charles C. Thomas.

Schreiber, D. J., Goldman, H., Kleinman, K. M., Goldfader, P. R., & Snow, M. Y. (1976). The relationship between independent neuropsychological and neurological detection and localization of cerebral impairment. *Journal of Nervous and Mental Diseases, 162*, 360-365.

Sigelman, C., Morris, B., & Danley, W. (1979). An evaluation of vocationally-related performance among low IQ clients. *Vocational Evaluation and Work Adjustment Bulletin, 12*, 22-26.

Texas Rehabilitation Commission (1979). *Vocational rehabilitation process for specific learning disabilities*. Austin, TX: author.

Vega, A., & Parsons, O. A. (1971). Lateralized brain damage and differential psychological effects: Reply to Dr. Woo-Sam. *Perceptual and Motor Skills, 33*, 269-270.

Wechsler, D. (1944). *The measurement of adult intelligence* (3rd ed.). Baltimore, MD: Williams and Wilkins.

Wechsler, D. (1955). *Manual for the Wechsler Adult Intelligence Scales*. New York: The Psychological Corporation.

Wechsler, D. (1981). *Manual for the Wechsler Adult Intelligence Scales - Revised (WAIS-R)*. New York: The Psychological Corporation.

Wheeler, L., & Reitan, R. M. (1962). The presence and laterality of brain damage predicted from responses to a short aphasia screening test. *Perceptual and Motor Skills, 15*, 783-799.

Wheeler, L., & Reitan, R. M. (1963). Discriminant functions applied to the problem of predicting brain damage from behavioral tests: A cross validation study. *Perceptual and Motor Skills, 16*, 681-701.

Wheeler, L., Burke, C. J., & Reitan, R. M. (1963). An application of discriminant functions to the problem of predicting brain damage using behavioral variables. *Perceptual and Motor Skills, 16*, 417-440.

Witelson, S. F. (1974). Hemispheric specialization for linguistic and nonlinguistic tactual perception using a dichotomous stimulation technique. *Cortex, 10*, 3-17.

Woods, B. T., & Teuber, H. L. (1973). Early onset of complementary specialization of cerebral hemispheres in man. *Transactions of the American Neurological Association, 98*, 59-63.

Yakolev, P. I., & LeCours, A. R. (1967). *The myelogenetic cycles of regional maturation of the brain*. Paper presented at the Regional Development of the Brain Symposium. Oxford: Blackwell.

4

Neuropsychological Evaluation, Rehabilitation, and Return-to-Work: A Case Study

Jack G. Dial
Fong Chan
Steven G. Gray
Roy Tunick
Gwen Roldan

4

Neuropsychological Evaluation, Rehabilitation, and Return-to-Work: A Case Study

Jack G. Dial
Fong Chan
Steven G. Gray
Roy Tunick
Gwen Roldan

Introduction

Understanding the strengths, limitations, and needs of a person with traumatic brain injury requires a comprehensive evaluation and integration of information from a variety of professional disciplines including neuropsychology and vocational evaluation. If the primary issue in a given case relates to the individual's potential for returning to work, a

---

Funds for the preparation of this chapter were provided in part by a Rehabilitation Services Administration Experimental and Innovative Training Grant (#H129T00022) and a contract (#RIRC255551IIT) from the Midwest Regional Head Injury Center for Rehabilitation and Prevention.

comprehensive assessment of higher cortical functions, functional strengths and limitations, and vocational potential is needed.

A neuropsychological evaluation may have a "vocational orientation," a "clinical orientation," or both. In the present context, a "vocationally oriented" neuropsychological evaluation differs from traditional clinical evaluation in several respects. The vocationally oriented evaluation focuses on functional abilities and limitations which may impede activities of daily living or work. Primary diagnostic information, though important, is interpreted and communicated in the report with reference to functional and behavioral outcomes, rather than as a simple restatement of the location of structural brain damage. The vocationally oriented evaluation tends to be conducted in the mid- to late-chronic period following the brain damage incident (e.g., two to six years following injury). The vocationally oriented report focuses on accommodations to residual impairment (as well as needed vocational rehabilitation services), rather than remediation, per se – although inclusion of recommendations involving remediation strategies may, certainly, be important in a given case. The vocationally oriented neuropsychological evaluation also provides an excellent vehicle for integrating information from a variety of sources (e.g., medical, social, educational).

In contrast, the clinically oriented neuropsychological evaluation is typically conducted earlier in the recovery process. It focuses on defining dysfunction associated with the structural lesion and often attempts to make statements concerning cognitive or perceptual remediation and/or the need for particular physical medicine/rehabilitation services (speech-language, occupational and/or physical therapy). Moreover, it does not typically provide information regarding predicted vocational or independent living outcomes. Although both orientations contribute important information related to the rehabilitation process, the clinical evaluation may be more helpful in monitoring patient progress in the earlier stages of medical recovery, while the vocationally oriented neuropsychological evaluation may be more relevant to vocational rehabilitation and return-to-work.

The vocational evaluation, in contrast, may serve to integrate findings from a variety of assessments including the neuropsychological evaluation. However, some of the same issues mentioned above may apply to the vocational evaluation of persons with traumatic brain injury as well. For example, the evaluation should be conducted relatively later rather than earlier in the recovery process and it should focus on expected outcomes, accommodations to disability, and functional strengths and limitations. Although there is usually overlap between the neuropsychological and vocational evaluations, each contributes a different facet to the body of information necessary for effective rehabilitation outcomes and return-to-work. For example, the vocational evaluator may observe "relatively normal" IQ scores reported in a traditional psychological evaluation, or observe average performance on the "General and Verbal factors" of the General Aptitude Test Battery (GATB) and erroneously conclude that the person may benefit from further academic training at the college level. The neuropsychological evaluation may help to resolve this issue (saving valuable time and money) by determining whether the traditional IQ results in this example indicate the person's ability to learn new material or whether the results simply reflect premorbid knowledge, information, or problem solving ability. In this instance, the location of the lesion, its chronicity, and the specific deficit pattern on neuropsychological tests may be a better predictor of new learning ability than the functional assessment performed by the vocational evaluator or the psychological assessment performed by the traditional clinical psychologist.

Conversely, the vocational evaluation may clarify functional abilities and accommodation strategies for maximizing performance in specific jobs; while the traditional clinical evaluation of emotional-personality functioning may better describe adjustment to disability and premorbid personality issues that may affect compliance to the rehabilitation program.

In some instances, the integration of information from various sources may occur in the context of the neuropsychological evaluation. The following section presents the report of Susan Tucker (a fictitious name). Mrs. Tucker sustained a head injury as a result of a moving vehicle accident. Due to the special nature of the case (resulting visual impairment and an impending legal action), a variety of neuropsychological and vocational assessments were performed. Susan's visual functioning level is "no light perception in the right eye and 20/60 in the left eye - nasal field only." Functionally, she can read regular print in the left nasal field, can read a computer display screen, and has vision-dependent mobility. However, Susan's reading speed is slow, she cannot distinguish certain colors, and she has reported difficulty discriminating visual detail.

Given this information, the evaluator must consider the possible interaction between visual functioning level and performance on visually oriented neuropsychological or vocational assessments. Accordingly, a special battery of instruments developed specifically for the blind (Comprehensive Vocational Evaluation System [CVES]) was administered in addition to the standard versions of tests from the Halstead-Reitan, Luria Nebraska, and McCarron-Dial batteries. Traditional measures of emotional-personality functioning, such as the MMPI, and vocational interests assessments, such as the Vocational Preference Inventory (VPI), were administered. The process of evaluation also included the gathering of extensive historical information and behavioral observation during testing and interview. Both Mrs. Tucker and her husband were interviewed, as well as attorneys involved in the case.

The Case of Susan Tucker

Medical records indicate that Mrs. Tucker sustained severe head injuries from a motor vehicle accident (MVA) occurring on March 5, 1986. Reportedly, her injuries included "a depressed bifrontal skull fracture, a right temporal fracture, numerous paranasal fractures, and a right

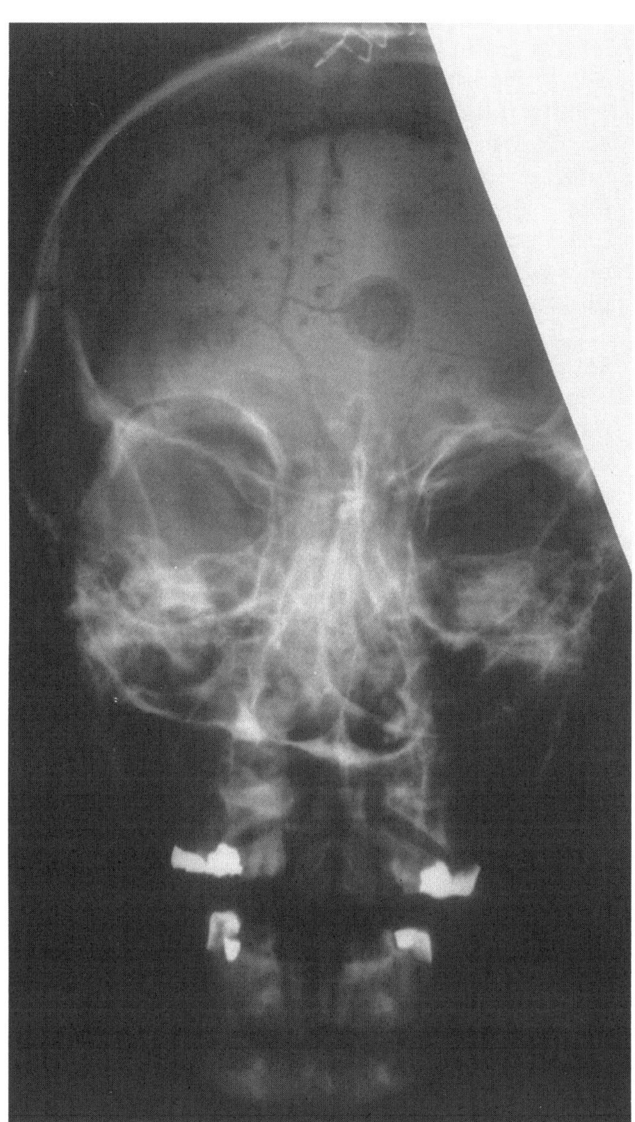

Plate A. X-ray of skull fracture.

orbital floor fracture." A large intracerebral hematoma of the left frontal lobe and an epidural hematoma of the right temporal lobe were noted. Surgery was performed to evacuate the hematomas and to repair the depressed skull fractures. Within a month there was evidence of "right third nerve paresis, optic atrophy on the right, and optic atrophy in a bow-tie distribution on the left." A resulting visual impairment was noted. The extent of Mrs. Tucker's injuries can be seen in Plates A and B. Plate A clearly illustrates the multiple skull and paranasal fractures, while Plate B defines an area of extensive left frontal damage, the left intracerebral hematoma, edema, and shifting of the midline to the right. The plates have been reversed from their usual radiographic orientation so that left structures are pictured on the left and right structures on the right.

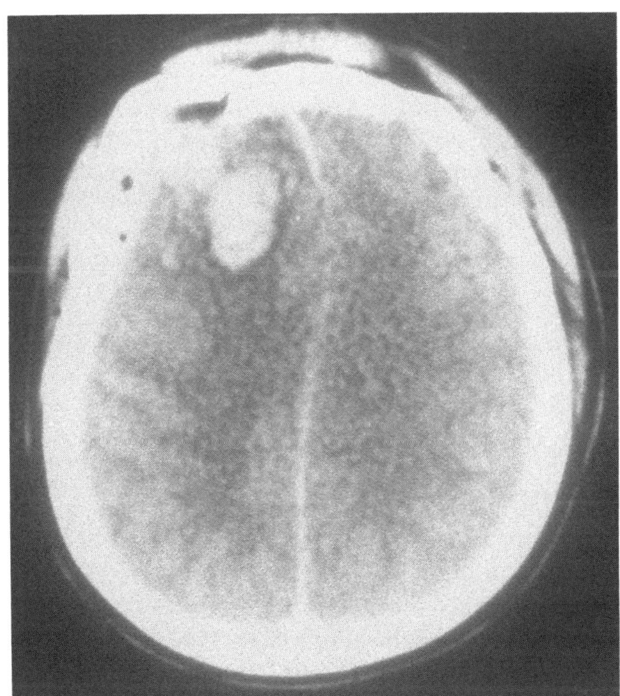

Plate B. CT showing left frontal lesion and shifting of the midline to the right.

Reason for Referral

Mrs. Tucker was referred for a comprehensive neuropsychological and vocational evaluation to determine the presence and/or extent of higher cortical dysfunction that may be associated with the reported MVA and subsequent medical findings. Specifically, verbal-spatial cognitive, sensorimotor, and emotional-coping functions were evaluated to determine whether there have been changes from estimates of her premorbid status; to assess functional strengths and limitations related to general educational and/or vocational levels; and to suggest possible avenues for remediation and/or accommodation of any observed deficits.

Tests Administered

The following tests and procedures were administered in addition to an extensive review of records and behavioral observations. The formal tests and procedures are listed under the "McCarron-Dial System" (MDS) factor structure. Note that instruments not usually associated with the MDS battery may, nevertheless, be organized under the MDS factor structure. Furthermore, some tests and procedures, such as Trails A and B from the Halstead-Reitan Battery, are listed under the Motor factor, but could as easily have been characterized as sensory or cognitive in nature.

VERBAL-SPATIAL COGNITIVE FACTOR

Wechsler Adult Intelligence Scale-Revised (WAIS-R)
Cognitive Test for the Blind (CTB)
Booklet Category Test (BCT)
Wide Range Achievement Test-Revised (WRAT-R)

SENSORY FACTOR

Bender Visual-Motor Gestalt Test (BVMGT)
Haptic Visual Discrimination Test (HVDT)
Haptic Sensory Discrimination Test (HSDT)
Seashore Rhythm Test (SRT)

MOTOR FACTOR

McCarron Assessment of Neuromuscular Development (MAND)
Finger Oscillation Test (FOT)
Trails A and B

EMOTIONAL/BEHAVIORAL FUNCTIONS

Emotional-Behavioral Checklist (EBC)
Observational Emotional Inventory-Revised (OEI-R)
Minnesota Multiphasic Personality Inventory (MMPI)

COPING/ADAPTIVE BEHAVIOR FACTOR

Survey of Functional Adaptive Behaviors (SFAB)

OTHER

Luria-Nebraska Neuropsychological Battery (LNNB)
Informal Clinical Neuropsychological Procedures
Diagnostic Interview

Background Information and Behavioral Observations

Susan is a thirty-seven-year, five-month-old female presently living with her husband, John, in a metropolitan area of the Southwest. Susan was cooperative during the interview and appeared to present a valid history. However, she has no direct memory of the automobile accident, the events immediately prior to the accident, or her hospital stay. She recalls having to work until closing (9 p.m.) the evening of the accident and awakening at her mother's house sometime after her release from the hospital. She states, "I was at my parents' house...asleep...I woke-up and thought I was in a dark room...I heard my mother's voice and tried to get up...instead, I banged my head into something." Susan's report is consistent with her injuries as described in the medical records and indicates the presence of both retrograde and anterograde amnesia during the early period of her recovery, despite the observation that she was occasionally "conscious" and "talked" during her hospital stay.

Commentary

> Retrograde and anterograde amnesia is a common finding in head injury cases. The trauma resulting in concussion (jarring), contusion (bruising), and/or laceration of brain tissue may affect functional neurological systems throughout the brain in addition to the primary lesion sites. Experiences just prior to the accident may not have undergone sufficient "rehearsal" by Unit I systems (mamillary bodies, hippocampus, fornix, etc.) to insure longer term storage in Unit II (temporal, parietal, and occipital lobes). As a result of trauma to these systems, the memory trace is lost (retrograde amnesia). The damage or sublethal dysfunction of these systems caused by the trauma may render them temporarily (or permanently) less functional; therefore, experiences encountered afterward (e.g., in the hospital) may be reacted to from a sensorimotor, perceptual, or cognitive perspective, but may not be remembered (anterograde amnesia). As the brain "heals" (swelling subsides, sublethally injured cells repair themselves) or alternate systems are invoked, memory/rehearsal functions are restored. In the interim, considerable patience is required of staff and family. The patient may need external cues, restatement, or other accommodations to function optimally.

Susan's major problems since the accident are reported by her in order as follows: 1) weight gain and change in appearance. Prior to the accident, her weight was reported to be 100 lbs. Her present weight is 149 lbs. Her hair was long prior to the accident and subsequent surgery and a change in Susan's facial appearance was noted by her husband; 2) relationship with husband has changed. ("My husband has been loyal, but not physically attracted to me since the accident.") John stated, "I still love her, but maybe for sympathetic reasons, rather than as before."; 3) blindness in the right eye, significant visual impairment. Susan can only see the color red in the left eye; 4) transportation problems; 5) financial problems. ("I was new on the job and did not have medical insurance yet...we had bought a house and my salary was to pay for the mortgage...I have not been able to find suitable [remunerative] employment yet."); 6) social isolation. ("...no close friends now...not like before..."); and 7) "recent memory" problems.

Commentary

It is extremely important to listen to the patient. The order in which they describe their problems, limitations, or complaints may identify what they perceive as the most significant or relevant issues for them. Too often, professional staff, family, or others "decide" what the person's "problems" are and proceed to address them accordingly.

Family History

Susan has been married for 15 years. This is her first and only marriage. There are no children from the marriage. Susan states that they desired children, but she was unable to conceive for medical reasons. Both of Susan's parents are living, but her father has been chronically ill. Susan reports that he had half of his stomach removed a few months ago. Susan states that there was much tension between her parents when she was growing-up and that this was a considerable stressor for her. She was the oldest child and was given much of the caretaking responsibility for her younger brother. This led to a lot of resentment and opposition directed toward her parents. Susan felt that since she was given adult responsibilities, she should be treated like an adult. Her frustration and anger led to attention-seeking behavior (e.g., skipping school) and eventually to what appears, historically, to be depression. At approximately age 15, these feelings led to a "suicide gesture." She took what remained in a bottle of her mother's tranquilizers at home while her parents were there. Susan saw a psychologist off and on after this event until she was about 18. She states, however, that "things remained about the same at home." Susan eventually dropped out of school at age 18 when she had saved enough money from part-time jobs.

Commentary

It is extremely important to obtain a thorough history for every patient with brain injury. The individual's premorbid personality development, intelligence, coping mechanisms, support systems, etc., contribute to the prediction of overall rehabilitation outcome including potential for work and independent living. Historical information may also define other problems unrelated to the head injury per se, but affecting recovery. Luria placed considerable emphasis on history in addition to his clinical findings. In formulating his Functional Systems Theory, Luria stated that the number of different ways a person has learned a particular task would define the extent to which alternate systems may be present and able to subserve behavior when primary systems were damaged. A thorough case history can provide insight into the depth of the patient's past.

Physical/Medical Information

Susan reports no illnesses other than sinus problems (congestion) at the present time. She states that the sinus problems are a result of various skull fractures sustained in the MVA (3-5-86) and takes over-the-counter medication for this problem. The sinus problem does, however, affect her sleep. She states that she wakes up two to three times a night with the feeling that she cannot breathe, but then falls back to sleep. Susan reports that her hearing is good. She has a good appetite and gets some exercise walking on a treadmill. She is overweight for her height (5'2" - 149 lbs.) and this is a concern for her. She states that the weight gain was the result of her accident (MVA).

Since the accident, Susan states that her appetite has changed to include a craving for sweets/desserts. Susan reports a history of cervical cancer in her twenties with a resulting hysterectomy at age 25. Prior injuries include a fracture of the right arm/wrist in two places as a teenager, but no complications or problems resulted from this. Susan reports that her infertility led to depression and abuse of alcohol in her mid-twenties. She sought treatment and counseling from local community resources. No residual problems associated with these events are reported. Details of Susan's injuries associated with the MVA of March 5, 1986 have been previously described in this report.

Social/Interpersonal Relationships

Susan reports no hobbies, special activities, or membership in social organizations at this time. She is, however, an active church member. Susan states that prior to the MVA she had numerous friends, particularly while attending a local university. Since the accident, Susan has been socially isolated except for casual friends at church. She states that she has always gotten along with people, but since the accident the extended period of recovery and mobility problems have interrupted many social contacts. It is also likely that other factors have affected Susan's social/interpersonal relationships since the accident (e.g., difficulties of others in accepting physical or personality changes in Susan and Susan's own perception of self in relation to others). This is most evident in the changes in her marital relationship as reported both by Susan and her husband. Both see a decline in intimacy and difficulties in adjusting to both physical and "psychological/personality" changes. John's reactions to physical changes have already been mentioned. However, he also reports that Susan seems less motivated than before; shows less initiative to do things; has a significant loss in short-term/recent memory in contrast to premorbid abilities; and that, in fact, she is a "different person" in many ways than before.

Emotional/Behavioral History

Susan describes her present emotional feelings as "anxious about my husband's continuing love and about the future...." Prior to the accident, Susan states that many things were coming together in her life. She had recovered from a long-term depression that had led to problems with alcohol. She had completed work toward her degree in psychology at a local university. She and her husband had moved into a new home and she had started a new job. Susan perceives the accident as a significant setback in her life. It has altered her physically and has affected certain cognitive abilities; it has added a significant financial burden; and has affected her marriage adversely. It has disrupted educational and vocational goals and has introduced functional limitations in mobility. It has disrupted social contacts and has promoted an excessive fear reaction to riding in an automobile on the freeways. Susan's initial adjustment to these issues has followed a normal course from depression and emotional lability to anxiety about the future. She is also more easily upset according to her husband.

Educational and/or Training Experiences

After dropping out of high school for personal/family reasons, Susan later obtained a G.E.D. She states that her grades in high school (B's, C's, and D's) did not reflect her lack of interest or ability, but rather the conflicts at home. She reports preferring courses requiring reading as opposed to math. At approximately age 26, Susan began an Associate Degree program in nursing at a community college. She completed the full 60-hour program. Susan then transferred to a local university and changed her major to psychology. It was at this time that Susan's depression (over infertility) became worse and she left school. No other formal education or training experiences are reported.

Vocational Experience

Susan reports working at various jobs both before and after leaving high school. She could not recall all of the jobs held or their specific sequence, but did relate that she had worked as a transcriptionist at a hospital for a year and at one time had worked as an aide with blind children. Her last job prior to the accident was selling cars for a dealership.

Following the accident, Susan received general rehabilitation services from a state vocational rehabilitation agency including a vocational evaluation from a local rehabilitation facility for the blind. She was not pleased with these services because they did not lead to remunerative employment. However, she did meet a person through contacts at the state agency that employed her as a telephone solicitor. She stated that she liked her employer, but left after almost two years because of very low pay and transportation problems. Money is a problem now, so employment is a more immediate goal for Susan than continuing her education.

Results of Neuropsychological and Vocational Evaluation

Standard psychological and neuropsychological tests, as well as special instrumentation for the blind were administered. In general, Susan performed about as well on visual versions of the tests as she did on special tactile versions. Exceptions to this observation are noted. Susan was cooperative and attempted all of the tests presented to her. Given the comprehensiveness of the evaluation and Susan's stamina, three separate testing sessions were required. The present results are considered a valid representation of Susan's actual abilities and limitations.

Intelligence/Cognitive

Susan's full scale IQ of 93 on the WAIS-R is in the low normal range of intellectual functioning. There is a significant difference between the verbal and performance IQ's; verbal (100), and performance (84). Considering the possible effects of her visual impairment on the performance subtests, the CTB was also administered. This test correlates highly with the WAIS-R, but requires no vision. The total CTB standard score of 88 is in the low normal range and is generally consistent with the WAIS-R full scale IQ. In contrast, the CTB verbal standard score of 90 is lower than the WAIS-R verbal IQ. This may be explained by differences in the subtest content of the two instruments. The CTB Verbal (and performance) section includes subtests of active memory, problem solving, and learning in addition to long-term stored information or highly practiced skills. Therefore, it tends to be more sensitive to brain damage than the WAIS-R VIQ. Figure 1 presents the WAIS-R results.

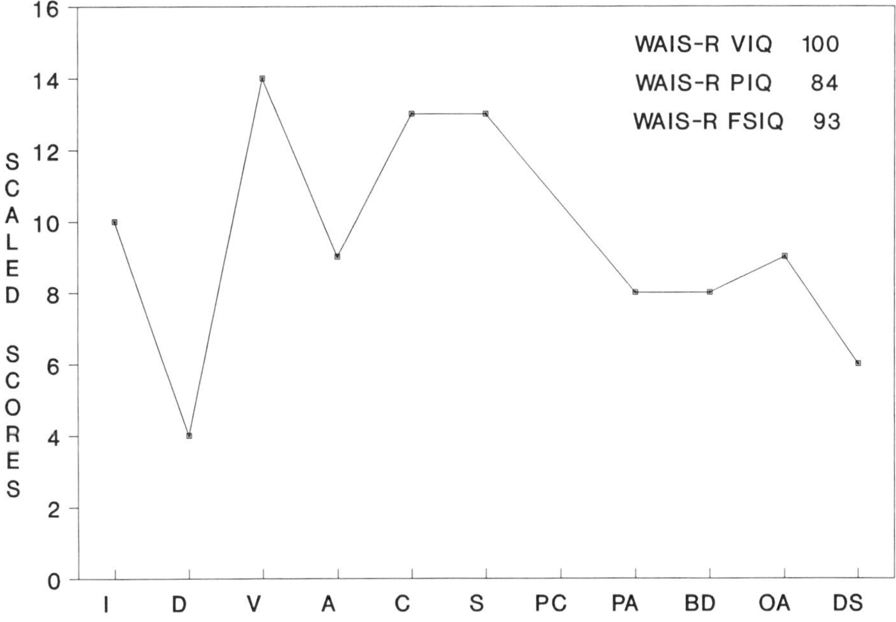

Fig. 1. WAIS-R Profile

Several of the WAIS-R verbal subtests are considered to be somewhat more sensitive to premorbid functioning in contrast to the CTB subtests that require active processing and memory of new verbal information. For example, the WAIS-R vocabulary, comprehension, and similarities subtests may be relatively unaffected in late chronic recovery from brain damage, unless such damage includes an extensive lesion of the left temporal lobe. Indeed, Susan's WAIS-R subtest profile reveals relative elevations on these particular subtests (vocabulary = 14, comprehension = 13, and similarities = 13). These verbal subtest scaled scores are above the mean for the general population and suggest that Susan's premorbid abilities (at least in terms of verbal intelligence) are bright-normal to superior. This observation is also consistent with her premorbid educational attainment (e.g., straight A's in college work).

Commentary

> To fully understand the affects of brain trauma on cognitive functioning for a given patient, it is necessary to derive an estimate of premorbid intellectual functioning. This is accomplished by considering educational/vocational history and performance levels on tests/subtests that are less sensitive (more "resistant") to the affects of brain damage. Sociotraditional measures of intelligence, such as the WAIS-R, may alone no longer provide an accurate estimate of what a person "can learn" (e.g., the correlation to potential academic achievement often "breaks down").

In contrast, her other verbal subtest scores requiring attention, concentration, and memory (digit span = 4, arithmetic = 9) were either below normal or at the average level. The information subtest scaled score of 10 was also average.

Susan's CTB performance standard score of 79 is somewhat lower than the WAIS-R performance IQ, but only slightly. This may suggest that, in general, there was little, if any, effect of Susan's visual impairment to performance on the WAIS-R or CTB. Therefore, the WAIS-R performance subtests may be more reliably interpreted as reflecting her actual visuospatial abilities. However, it should be noted that one WAIS-R subtest requiring the most detailed visual analysis (picture completion) was not administered. The remaining WAIS-R performance subtests were all low average or below (picture arrangement = 8, block design = 8, object assembly = 8, and digit symbol = 6). Figure 2 presents the CTB results.

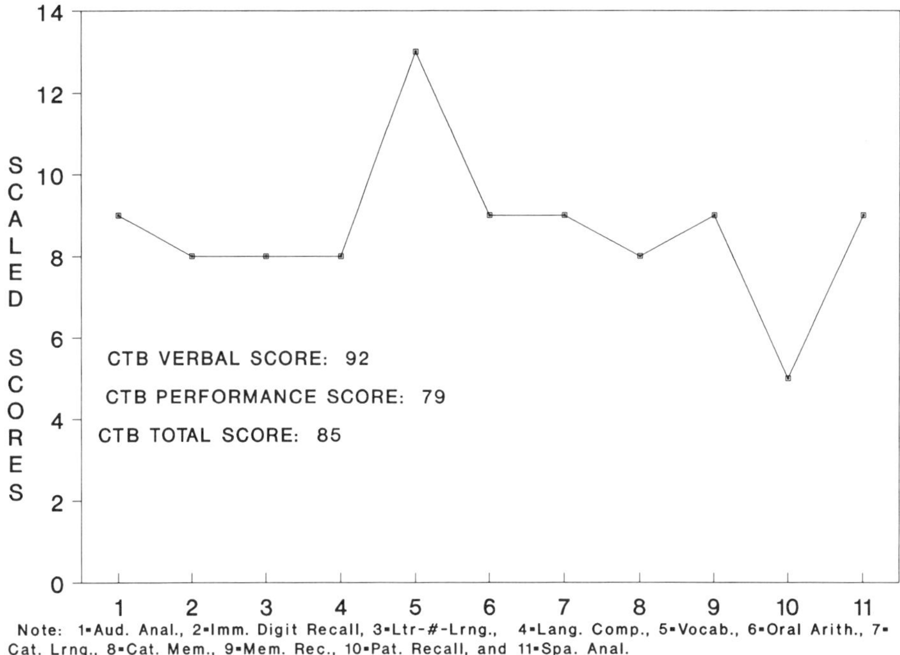

Fig. 2. CTB Profile

The WAIS-R findings are further supported by the CTB factor standard scores as follows:

1. Conceptual (94). A nonvisual measure of abstract thinking using touch senses to learn and solve problems. Only one of two subtests contributing to this factor was used, since feedback was previously given on a visual version of the other subtest (i.e., the Booklet Category Test [BCT]). Susan made 73 total errors on the BCT which is well over the cut-off for brain-damaged samples (51).
2. Learning (94). Verbal and nonverbal learning tasks. Susan performed in the average range on this factor.
3. Verbal memory (88). Susan performed in the low average range on this factor.
4. Nonverbal memory (88). Susan also performed in the low average range on this factor.
5. Language (94). Susan's performance on this factor is in the average range and is consistent with her WAIS-R verbal IQ.
6. Spatial (79). Susan's performance on this factor is below average and is also consistent with her WAIS-R performance IQ.

In summary, Susan is performing intellectually at a low average level. Her present intellectual abilities are probably significantly less than premorbid estimates. She processes some verbal information better than spatial information and tasks which require new learning in contrast to those depending primarily on existing funds of information will be more difficult for her. Tasks which require attention, concentration, and immediate or short-term memory will be performed less well or will require repeated trials for learning.

Commentary

Susan's verbal-spatial cognitive/intellectual profile is consistent with the medical reports and history of cranio-cerebral trauma; and administration of the visual version of the Intellectual/Cognitive Tests did not enhance or impede her performance.

Academic Achievement

Susan's WRAT-R standard score of 106 in reading is in the normal range and indicates a reading recognition grade level of greater than 12. This finding is generally consistent with estimated premorbid intelligence, but is slightly lower than would be expected based on her academic history. The use of the regular print version and mild relative effects of left hemisphere dysfunction may have affected her performance. Spelling and arithmetic standard scores of 98 and 97, respectively, are also in the normal range and consistent with the above findings. Figure 3 presents the academic achievement results from the WRAT-R.

	Raw Score	SS	% ile	Grade
Reading	75	106	66	12+
Spelling	34	98	45	12B
Arithmetic	35	97	42	12E

Fig. 3. WRAT-R Profile

Considering that Susan has been out of the academic environment for some time and that her visual impairment is an obstacle to reading, the present levels might be improved slightly with practiced use of visual aides. However, it should be noted that "reading comprehension," which requires verbal memory, was not assessed in the present evaluation and would likely yield a lower standard score.

Sensory

The regular presentation of the BVMGT revealed no scoreable errors. Susan reproduced the designs in the upper portion of the paper. The quality of her reproductions was slightly less than would be expected for a "normal" adult (i.e., no visual, perceptual, or motor impairment). In Susan's case, the quality of her performance can probably be attributed primarily to her visual impairment. No obvious visual-motor impairment was evidenced on this test. Figure 4 presents Susan's BVMGT drawings.

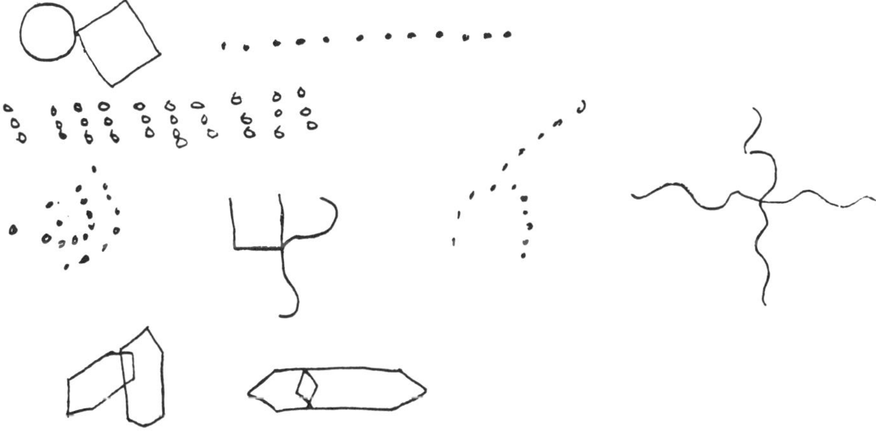

Fig. 4. BVMGT Drawings

The HVDT was administered to measure Susan's ability to integrate touch senses with vision. The test is primarily sensitive to parietal lobe functioning, but may be affected by impairment to the visual system as well. Susan's right and left hand presentations of the HVDT revealed standard scores of 82, which is below average for the sighted population. Mild deficits in parietal lobe functioning may be indicated bilaterally by these results. Her most impaired subtest performance was observed in the discrimination of sizes (52 on both the right and left sides of the body). Relatively higher and symmetrical performance was observed on the other HVDT subtests (shapes = 115; textures = 88; and configurations = 73). This pattern of subtest performance is often seen clinically when impairment is lateralized to some extent to the left cerebral hemisphere. Figure 5 presents Susan's HVDT profile.

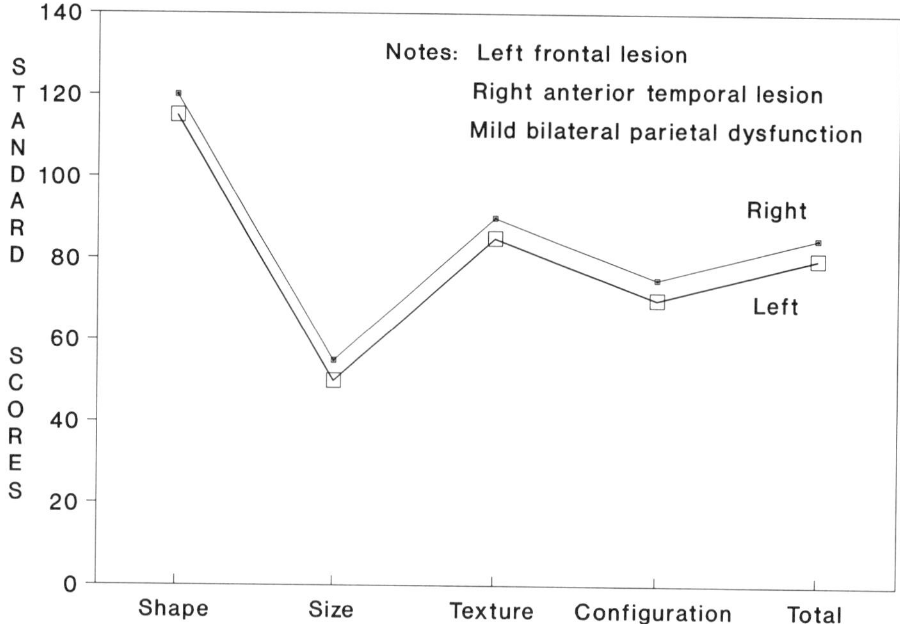

Fig. 5. HVDT Profile

To control for the possible effects of visual impairment on the HVDT performance, the HSDT was administered. This test correlates well with the HVDT, but does not involve the use of vision. It measures, instead, tactile memory matching skills and is also sensitive to parietal lobe functioning. Susan's right hand presentation of the HSDT revealed a standard score of 69 which is significantly below the norms for both sighted and blind individuals. Her left hand presentation revealed a standard score of 77, also below average. The combined HSDT total standard score of 73 is significantly lower than that obtained from the HVDT; however, the latter (HSDT) requires immediate to short-term memory, whereas, the former (HVDT) requires simultaneous visual recognition on a photographic plate of the particular shape, size, etc., that is being tactually explored under a screen. Therefore, the observed differences in scores may reflect mild tactile memory deficits.

Commentary

> The observed asymmetry between the right (69) and left (77) HSDT standard scores, in concert with relative deficit performance levels on both the HVDT and HSDT, would suggest mild parietal lobe dysfunction bilaterally with a slightly greater lateralization of dysfunction to the left cerebral hemisphere.

The Seashore Rhythm Test was administered to assess auditory analysis of nonlanguage patterns of sound, in this case, patterns of tones. The patient identifies whether two patterns presented one after the other are the "same" or "different." Susan was able to identify 24 patterns correctly, which is on the cusp of the brain-impaired cutoff. This level of performance is consistent with, though not conclusively, bright-normal individuals who have mild right anterior temporal lesions.

In conclusion, the present sensory findings would suggest a mild diffuse impairment to posterior cerebral structures in addition to the primary lesions identified by the CAT scans and described in the medical reports. Functionally, this impairment, though mild, may affect new learning; may require additional time in a training or educational process to achieve at the same level as others; and may limit the degree of complexity of what is learned, at least under ordinary circumstances. This would appear to be particularly relevant if further academic pursuits are considered in the future.

Motor

The MAND was administered to assess Susan's fine and gross motor functions. Her performance on this test was compared to both the sighted and visually-impaired/blind norms (VIB). When compared to the VIB norms, Susan's total motor standard score (NDI) of 74 suggests mild impairment in neuromuscular skills; in contrast to the sighted norms, her NDI reveals moderate impairment (62). Figure 6 presents Susan's MAND profile.

Susan performs in the normal average range on the persistent control (PC) factor using VIB (90) or sighted (85) norms. The PC factor is a measure of slow, carefully controlled movements, particularly of the upper body. Susan's muscle power (MP) standard scores of 60 (VIB) and 45 (sighted) would suggest moderate impairment in muscle power. This impairment is most evident in upper body strength on the right side. Moderate deficits were observed on the kinesthetic integration (KI) for both the VIB (65) and the sighted (50) norms. The KI factor measures balance and gross coordination. In contrast, Susan performed in the normal range (105) on the bimanual dexterity factor.

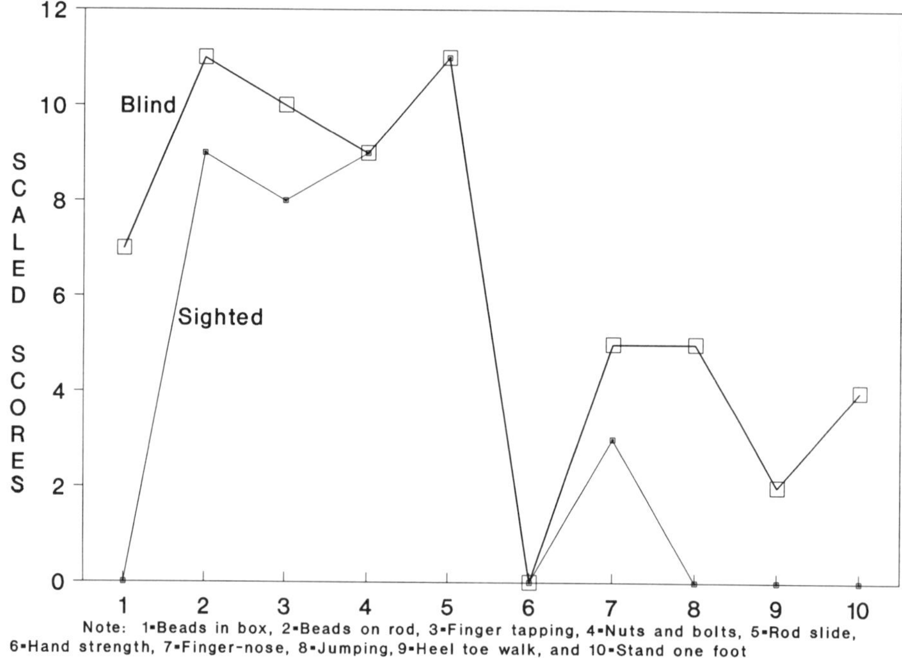

Fig. 6. MAND Profile

Commentary

> Susan's right side performance on both the finger tapping and hand strength subtests was less than that observed for the left. This pattern, for a right preferred individual, is suggestive of a possible left frontal lesion. In Susan's case, such is evident from both the CAT scans and the medical records.

The Trail Making Test (Forms A and B) was administered to measure visual-motor performance on what is, essentially, a simple cognitive test. Form A requires the individual to draw a line as rapidly as possible in numeric sequence from one to 25. The numbers are randomly scattered on a standard sheet of letter-sized paper. Form B is similar, but requires alternate shifting from numbers in order to letters in order — "an additional shifting of cognitive sets." Figures 7 and 8 present Susan's Trail Making test results.

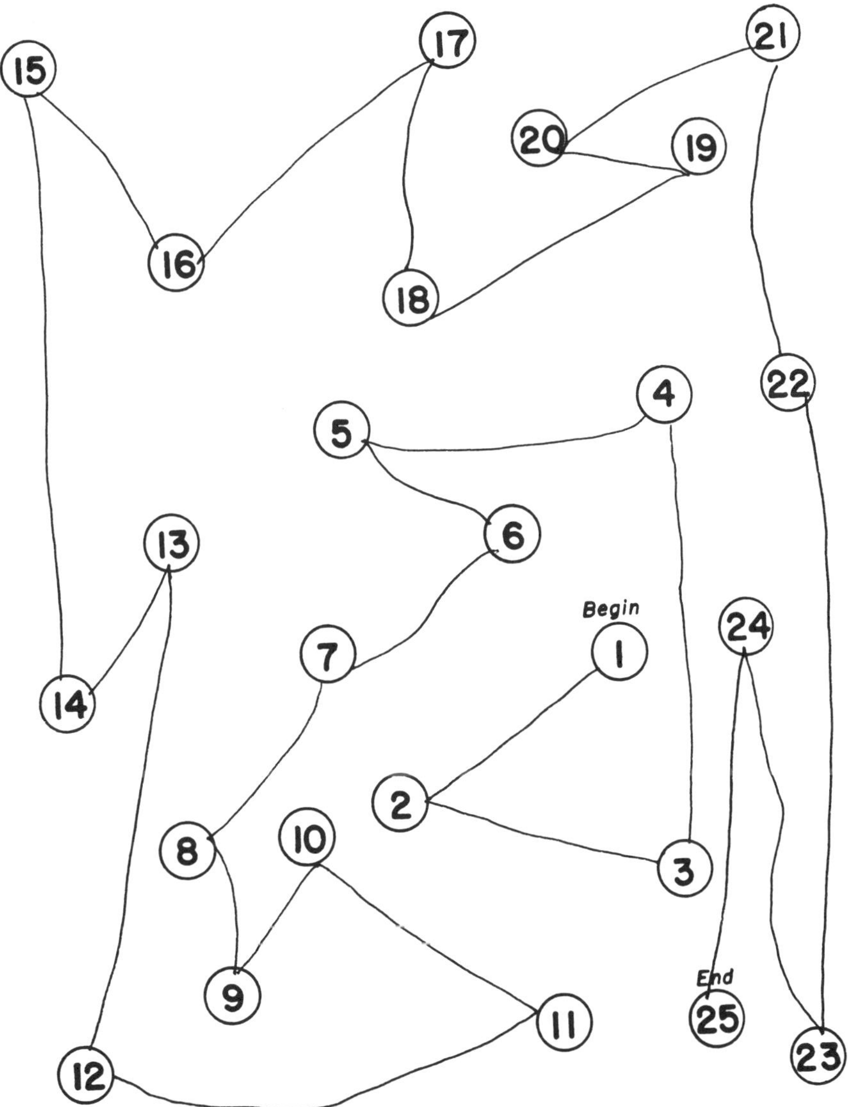

Fig. 7. Trail Making-A. Susan's score of 87 seconds significantly exceeds brain damage cut-off of 39 seconds. No errors observed.

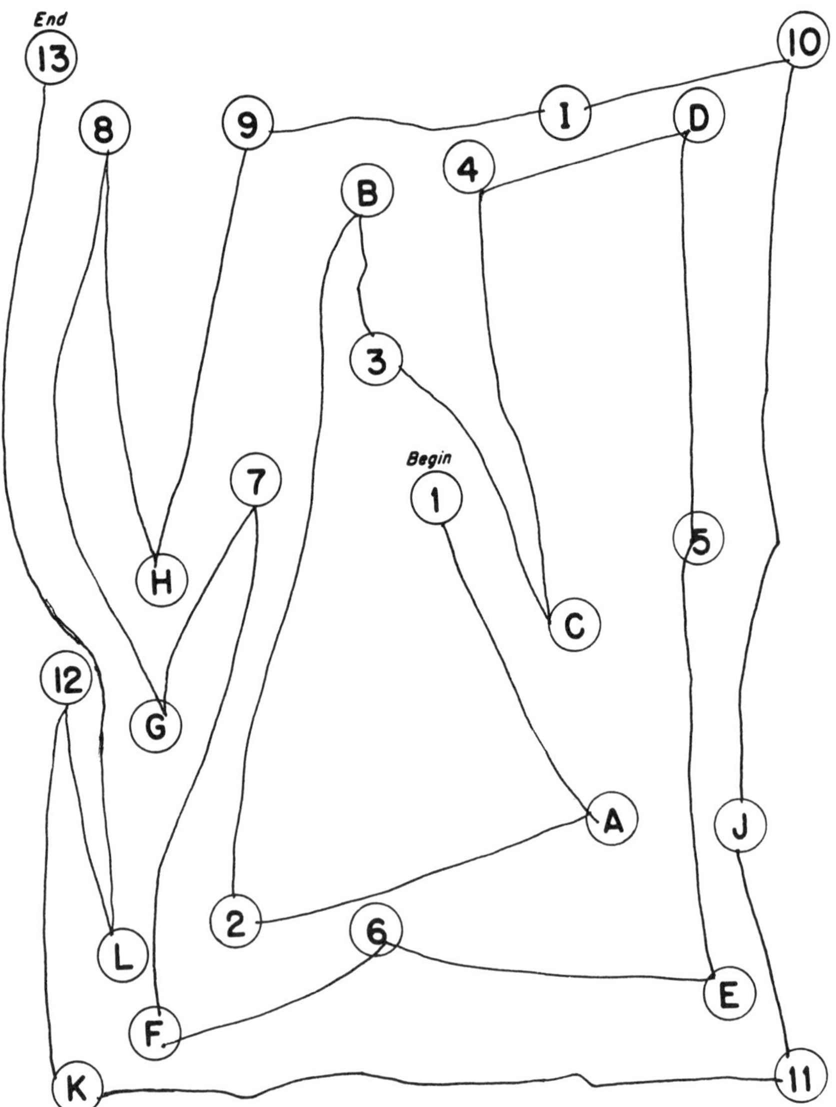

Fig. 8. Trail Making-B. Susan's score of 174 seconds significantly exceeds brain damage cut-off of 86. No errors observed.

Susan exceeded the time cutoffs on both tasks (form A = 87, norm = 39; form B = 174, norm = 86) by a considerable margin. Her deficit performance would appear to reflect cognitive-motor slowing, as well as visual searching problems.

In summary, Susan's motor profile is consistent with a chronic anterior frontal lesion of the left hemisphere. However, the motor cortex would appear to be minimally involved. Motor strength in the hands and arms has been adversely affected in contrast to the norms, but there was no observed spasticity or other hard signs and no medical reports of such observations. Nevertheless, Susan's loss in muscle power may impair moderate to heavy lifting, carrying, pushing, or pulling of weight. It is also possible that she might improve these functions with adequate, medically approved exercise. Of more concern in the present evaluation is the observation of moderate impairment in balance and gross coordination even when comparing her performance to the visually-impaired/blind norms. Excess weight can, in part, contribute to a lower score on this factor, but not usually to the extent observed in Susan's performance. This aspect of the profile may reflect a mild diffuse dysfunction that includes the vestibular system as well. Regardless, the functional concommitants of her balance/coordination deficits would suggest limitations in climbing, balancing, stooping, or other movements around potential hazards in an occupational or other environment. Preference should be given to occupations or settings which would accommodate this problem.

Emotional Behavioral Status

Susan's responses to the MMPI would suggest that she is experiencing much unexpressed anger and depression. Her profile indicates that she is likely to have had these feelings for a long time. The source of Susan's anger may be family members and may involve feelings of rejection. She is likely to have strong needs for approval, particularly from those closest to her. It may be difficult for Susan to form close personal friendships and she may be hypersensitive to rejection.

Her relationship with her husband, though enduring, may involve a significant degree of interdependency. Susan may be able to verbalize sources of conflict or anger, but tends to repress these feelings. In the interview Susan stated that she had been very depressed over her husband's change in feelings toward her, but that "things were much better now." However, her responses in the interview and to the MMPI would suggest that she still feels very upset and angry about this change. She is likely experiencing this change as a significant rejection, but has much difficulty expressing her feelings.

There would also appear to be a loss in functional abilities associated with the MVA. Susan still has not adjusted completely to her disabilities. This lack of adjustment may impede further progress in her rehabilitation. Psychotherapy or counseling is indicated, but the prognosis is one of a slow and possibly lengthy course of recovery. Susan's MMPI profile is depicted in Figure 9.

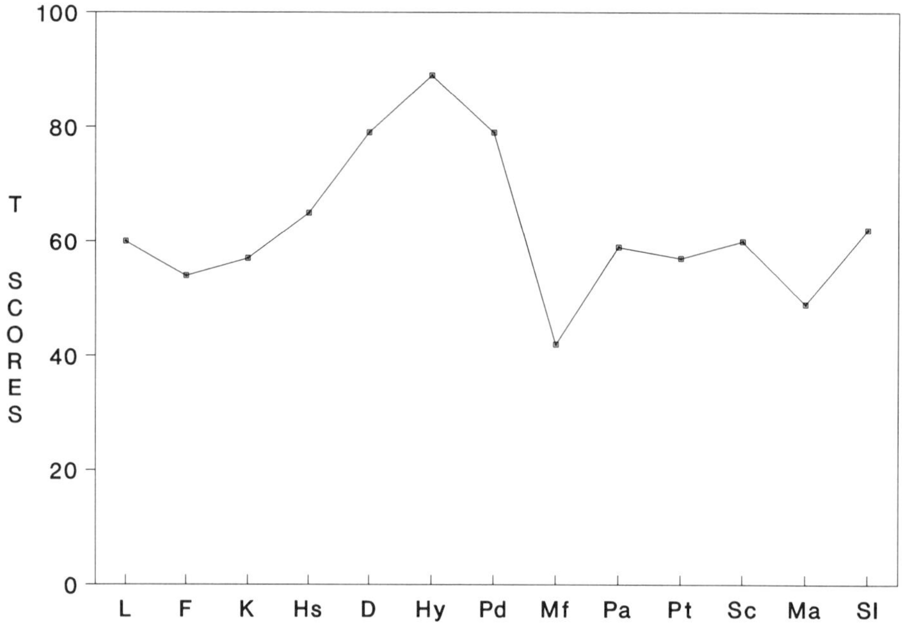

Fig. 9. MMPI Profile

Results from the EBC and OEI-R would suggest essentially normal emotional behavioral functioning, despite the underlying issues mentioned above. Susan has developed mechanisms for coping with her problems that help her function reasonably effectively on a day-to-day basis without overt dysfunctional behaviors, but which, nevertheless, perpetuate poor adjustment – namely, repression and denial.

Adaptive Behavior

The SFAB was rated from interview and behavior observations made during the testing sessions. This scale measures practical behaviors related to everyday living. Susan's total SFAB standard score of 90 is in the average range for the adult sighted and visually impaired populations. For the most part, Susan would appear to be able to manage most day-to-day activities assuming sufficient accommodations were provided for orientation, mobility, and other tasks that require visual processing. A mild relative deficit was observed in the "Daily Living" section of the scale suggesting the need for particular accommodations in such areas as transportation. In contrast, Susan was rated higher on the "Functional Academics" section of the scale which measures such tasks as measuring skills, practical arithmetic, simple reading, etc. Vocational skills and behaviors were rated in the low average range with specific needs for visual accommodations. Susan may also have some restrictions as to lifting, climbing, balancing, etc.

Data Obtained from Other Sources

The Luria-Nebraska Neuropsychological Battery (LNNB) was administered as an adjunct assessment in the present evaluation. Only two scales of the LNNB (visual and right hemisphere) were elevated above the critical level (adjusted for years of education). Several other scales approached this level including "impairment," "pathognomonic," "intermediate memory," and "intellectual." It is not unusual for the LNNB to reveal a false negative finding in late chronic lesions involving unilateral

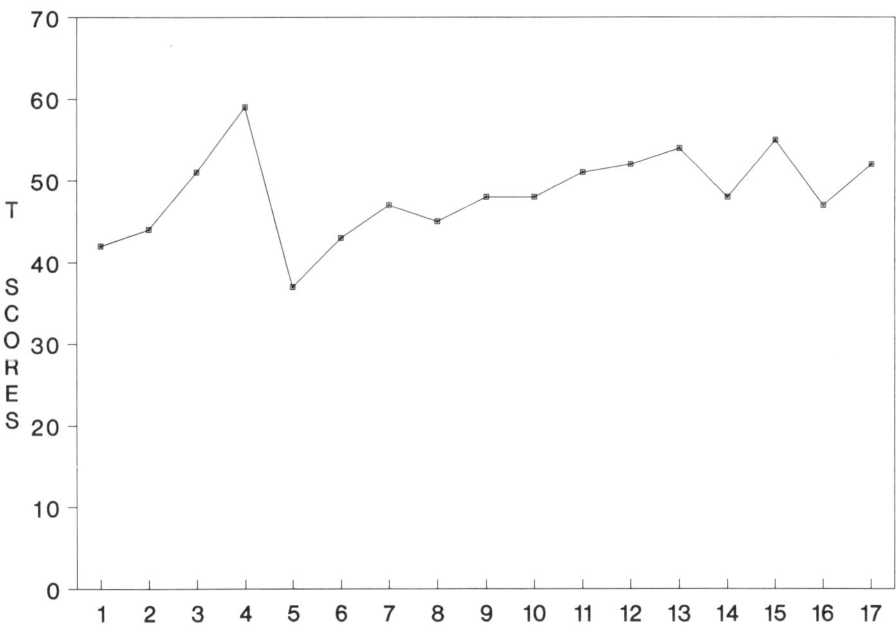

Fig. 10. LNNB Profile. Note: 1=Motor, 2=Rhythm, 3=Tactile, 4=Visual, 5=Receptive, 6=Expressive, 7=Writing, 8=Reading, 9=Arithmetic, 10=Memory, 11=Intellectual, 12=Intrmed. Mem., 13=Pathognomonic, 14=Left Hem., 15=Right Hem., 16=Elevation, and 17=Impairment

lesions of the frontal lobes, particularly when the motor cortex is minimally involved and when the individual has a relatively higher premorbid educational level. Therefore, the present findings on the LNNB tend to underestimate Susan's actual level of impairment as demonstrated both in the medical and other neuropsychological findings. Figure 10 presents Susan's LNNB profile.

Vocational Interests

Susan's vocational interests include becoming a psychologist and working with children or adolescents, sales, and office work using computers. She would like to return to college eventually and complete a degree in psychology, but financial concerns dictate employment as a more immediate goal. She has also expressed some fear of not being able to perform in college as before. Susan's interest profile using Holland's model would suggest occupational exploration in the social, enterprising, or conventional areas.

Commentary

It is important to note, however, that responses to "interest tests" typically include projections of psychodynamic or personality features of the individual which may present a false elevation on one or another of the Holland codes. For example, Susan's elevated "social" scale may depict personal needs for attention, affection, friendship, and intimacy. These needs may conflict with adequate adjustment to many occupations included in the social category. It is important for the evaluator to integrate other information, such as social-emotional history, MMPI results, etc., with the interest profile prior to making special recommendations for training or job placement. Furthermore, the evaluator should consider expressed interests in light of measured aptitudes, functional strengths and limitations, and prior work history or training. Susan's cognitive profile may argue against considering occupations requiring a four- to six-year college program, while her emotional-personality profile would depict a more "conventional" person. Initially, occupations in the conventional area might be considered (e.g., clerical, secretarial, receptionist, data entry positions). Jobs in this interest area, in general, would not require a degree, would utilize Susan's existing skills, are available in the local area and would provide more structure, initially, in the work environment. A secondary consideration might be given to enterprising jobs, such as sales. Susan has demonstrated the ability to perform telephone solicitation and may, with accommodations, be able to perform in other sales positions. A third consideration might be given to social interest areas. Jobs such as teacher's aide, therapist technician, caseworker aide and other entry level human service positions may be appropriate.

Susan's interest in "psychology" (which involves investigative interests as well) may be better actualized by considering a shift to the human service or rehabilitation field. Professional level entry positions in this field can be obtained at the bachelor degree level, whereas, practical entry into the field of psychology requires at least a master's degree. Considering Susan's present abilities and limitations, a vocational goal that requires graduate study is probably unrealistic. In fact, the completion of a bachelor's degree will likely be a considerably difficult and stressful task for Susan at this time. However, such a possibility (given sufficient accommodations) cannot be ruled out.

Summary and Impressions

Susan's overall neuropsychological profile is consistent with the primary left frontal and right temporal lesions reported in the medical records and/or evidenced in the CAT scans. However, in addition to these lesions, the present results would suggest a mild diffuse dysfunction involving posterior cortical structures as well; particularly, the parietal lobes with some greater lateralization to the left cerebral hemisphere. Plate C presents a recent CAT scan of Susan's brain.

This condition appears to be chronic and static. Such a condition may impair learning of complex material and affect educational/vocational goals. This would appear to be particularly relevant in reference to Susan's stated goals and estimated premorbid functioning. In addition, Susan appears to have a history that includes bouts of depression. It is questionable whether the issues underlying this condition were completely resolved prior to the accident, but the disabling effects of the MVA and the change in her husband's feelings toward her since the accident has intensified this psychological state. There appears to be much

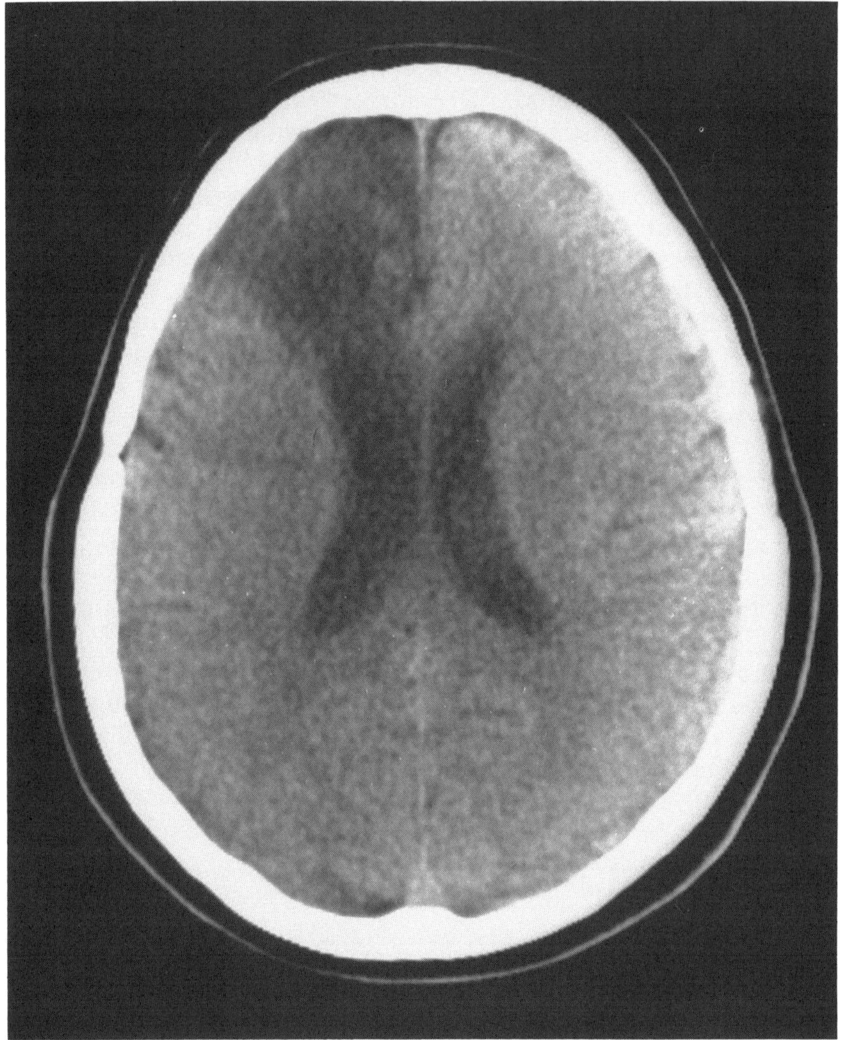

Plate C. Recent CAT scan.

repressed anger and denied depression at this point and Susan has not yet made an adequate adjustment to changes in her life.

Commentary

Diagnostic impressions may not be necessary or appropriate when conducting a traditional vocational evaluation, but are included when a combination neuropsychological and vocational evaluation is conducted. The more important feature is the inclusion of a summary listing of functional limitations and strengths that may be useful when conceptualizing rehabilitation programming.

Diagnostic Impressions

AXIS I:	294.80	Organic Mental Disorder-NOS
	311.00	Depressive Disorder-NOS (Recurrent depressive disturbance that does not meet the criteria for Dysthymia. During acute presentations, Susan's condition has probably met the criteria.)
	V62.20	Occupational problem – due to visual impairment and OMD.
AXIS II:	NO DIAGNOSIS	
AXIS III:	Visual impairment - see medical records	
AXIS IV:	Psychological stressors: visual impairment, mobility problems, relationship problems Severity: 3-4 moderate to severe	
AXIS V:	Global assessment of functioning Current: 55 Highest in past year: 55	

Commentary

A summary of functional strengths and limitations is constructed by considering all sources of data for each of the MDS (or CVES) factors. The evaluator should review case history, behavioral observation, and standardized test results when formulating a list of strengths and limitations. Contradictory information from different sources (e.g., history versus test results) must be reconciled. For example, Susan's history would suggest a much higher cognitive ability than was observed in the testing. However, this disparity is easily reconciled by considering the nature of her lesion (e.g., mass, chronicity, location). The evaluator may wish to begin with the person's general profile of strengths and limitations as defined by the overall test results. This is easily accomplished with the aid of computer software that supports the MDS, CVES, and/or LNN Batteries. The following example of Susan's profile is extracted from the EPARS program which supports the CVES Battery. EPARS converts raw data to standard scores, constructs the individual profile and predicts the person's levels of vocational and residential functioning using the MDS model. Figure 11 presents Susan's EPARS Profile.

DEFICITS, PROBLEMS AND/OR FUNCTIONAL LIMITATIONS

1. Visual impairment-see medical records
2. Immediate/recent memory loss-mild
3. Loss in upper body strength, particularly on the right side of the body-mild to moderate
4. Loss in balance and gross coordination-moderate
5. Deficit in sensory integration skills-mild
6. Weight gain-significant
7. Relationship problem-see text
8. Transportation problem-see text
9. Vocational problem-see text
10. Social/interpersonal problem-see text
11. Adjustment difficulties-see text

STRENGTHS AND/OR ABILITIES

1. Recent increase in "optimistic outlook"
2. Improvement in general functioning over last two years
3. Friendly presentation
4. Increased motivation to work
5. Increased motivation to consider vocational education/training
6. Can perform routine household tasks
7. Functional vision remains in left eye/nasal field
8. Fine motor skills (particularly, bimanual dexterity)
9. Verbal-language skills (CTB, WAIS-R, VIQ)

INDIVIDUAL EVALUATION PROFILE FOR THE
VISUALLY-IMPAIRED/BLIND

Name: SUSAN TUCKER   Age: 37Y/5M   Sex: F
Program: TRANSITIONAL   Residence: SEMI-INDEPENDENCE

```
-------------------------------------------------------------------------
|                  |Score  MDS-T  30   40   50   60   70   80   90  100 |
| MEASUREMENT      |       STD    25   40   55   70   85  100  115  130 |
|                  | Raw          :...:...|...:...:....|..:.....:       |
|------------------|-----|--------------------------------------------- |
| WAIS Verbal IQ   | 100 | 100    :...:...|...:...:....#..:.....:      |
| CTB - Total      |  90 |  90    :...:...|...:...:#...|..:.....:      |
| CTB - Verbal     |  90 |  90    :...:...|...:...:.#..|..:.....:      |
| CTB-Performance  |  91 |  91    :...:...|...:.#.:....|..:.....:      |
| HSDT - Right     |  18 |  69    :...:...|...#...:....|..:.....:      |
| HSDT - Left      |  20 |  77    :...:...|...:.#.:....|..:.....:      |
| HSDT - Total     |  38 |  73    :...:...|...:#..:....|..:.....:      |
| Fine Motor       | 402 | 101    :...:...|...:...:....#..:.....:      |
| Gross Motor      | 161 |  60    :...:...|.#.:...:....|..:.....:      |
| Total Motor      | 563 |  81    :...:...|...:..#:....|..:.....:      |
| EBC              |   2 |  94    :...:...|...:...:..#.|..:.....:      |
| OEI - R          |   5 |  95    :...:...|...:...:..#.|..:.....:      |
| SFAB             | 232 |  90    :...:...|...:...:.#..|..:.....:      |
|------------------|---------------------------------------------------|
| AVG STD SCORE,   |     |   SP mean ->   |            |<-GP mean      |
| All FACTORS      |     |  78 :....:......|...:..#.:....|..:.....:     |
| PREDICTED        |     |     :....:......|...:.######.|..:.....:     |
| VOCATIONAL       |                                                    |
| LEVEL            |                                                    |
-------------------------------------------------------------------------
|             Daycare <---                        -  Semi-Skill         |
|                Work Activity ---                  - Skilled           |
|                  Extended --  --                   ---------->        |
|SP is Special Population          Transitional ---  Technical/         |
|GP is General Population                            Professional       |
-------------------------------------------------------------------------
```

Susan's predicted level of vocational functioning is within the Transitional range (79.3). The standard score range for this vocational level is > = 75 < 90. The Transitional Training program is designed to provide employment and or training of a temporary duration for individuals. After suitable work adjustment training and exposure to a work environment, these persons may be expected to move into competitive employment.

Susan's predicted level of residential functioning is within the Semi-Independent range (83.3). The standard score range for this level is > = 72 < 85. Monitoring by counselors may be necessary; residents are generally employed in community settings or in work training centers.

Fig. 11. EPARS Profile

Recommendations

1. Counseling/therapy is recommended to help Susan adjust to disability and to help her gain insight into and learn to appropriately express negative/angry feelings.

2. Consideration should be given to marital counseling.

3. Vocational rehabilitation services may be more appropriately rendered at this time with greater probability of success than before. Career development counseling and placement assistance would be helpful.

4. Low vision evaluation for visual aides is recommended. Protective eye glasses should be worn at all times.

5. Initial vocational placement should consider Susan's conventional or enterprising interest areas first, perhaps followed by social interests. Considering her previous experience, good bimanual dexterity skills and ability to read a computer display, placement in secretarial work (word processing, running computer applications, etc.) would be appropriate.

6. Return to college, if considered, should be on a gradual basis with maximum accommodations and minimum course loads. A consideration should be given to a change in majors from psychology to a related field that would have better employment opportunities for entry level at the bachelor's level.

7. Susan should be encouraged to take part in social activities or social organizations outside of the home to help increase her contacts with other people.

8. Susan should be encouraged to join a health club and develop a routine exercise program under medical advisement.

9. Accommodations for memory deficits should be considered (e.g., calendars, written lists, pocket computers, datebooks).

10. New employment situations should allow for extra time/trials for learning new tasks, work schedules, etc.

11. Alternative means of transportation should be explored through the Commission for the Blind.

Chapter Summary

This chapter presented the case study of Susan Tucker, who was involved in a moving vehicle accident that resulted in significant brain damage. This case study was selected to illustrate the integration of vocational and neuropsychological assessment information into a single report useful for conceptualizing an effective rehabilitation program. The report includes demographic information, history, behavioral observations, and test results. Diagnostic conclusions are formulated on the basis of the person's history and present findings. The report focuses on issues regarding return-to-work in addition to the traditional clinical findings. Four major evaluation batteries were administered to Susan and data from each were discussed. A summary profile of strengths and limitations was constructed from the CVES battery and sample recommendations were enumerated. Obviously, the opportunity may not exist nor would it be appropriate in every case to conduct such an extensive evaluation. Nevertheless, the present case study provides an excellent opportunity to compare and contrast several major neuropsychological batteries and to illustrate their application in a vocationally oriented report.

5

An Ecological Approach to Vocational Evaluation

Fong Chan
Jack G. Dial
Robert Schleser
Brian T. McMahon
Linda R. Shaw
Michelle Marmé
Chow S. Lam

5

An Ecological Approach to Vocational Evaluation

Fong Chan
Jack G. Dial
Robert Schleser
Brian T. McMahon
Linda R. Shaw
Michelle Marmé
Chow S. Lam

Head Injury Rehabilitation: A Vocational Emphasis

Traditionally, work is considered therapeutic and essential for both the physiological survival and psychological well-being of people in contemporary societies (Dawis, 1987; Osipow, 1968). Recognizing the importance of work, vocational rehabilitation (VR) professionals have

---

Funds for the preparation of this chapter were provided in part by a Rehabilitation Services Administration Experimental and Innovative Training Grant (#H129T00022) and a contract (#RIRC255551IIT) from the Midwest Regional Head Injury Center for Rehabilitation and Prevention.

consistently advocated for work as a fundamental human right of people with disabilities (Rubin & Roessler, 1987; Wright, 1980). Ultimately, effective job placement at the highest possible level is the goal for each client with traumatic brain injury (TBI) served by a VR program. A second but equally important benefit of aggressive VR programming within the overall operation of the TBI treatment program is its capacity to provide traction, focus, and meaning to other therapies or services. In this sense, VR is best regarded as a "pull factor" and, as such, is distinguished from other "push factor" therapies (i.e., those from which the client will hopefully become independent) (McMahon & Fraser, 1988).

The probability of successful placement is enhanced when all therapies can be related to work, and vice-versa. McMahon and Fraser (1988) provided specific suggestions regarding how all interdisciplinary team members might approach their respective duties to maximize the level and stability of ultimate job placement. Fawber and Wachter (1987) argue that traditional VR, which typically occurs at the end of the treatment continuum, is insufficient for effecting successful placement for persons with TBI. Rather, they argue for a "treatment-oriented placement process (with) concomitant treatment of cognitive and psychosocial sequelae of severe head injury" (p. 28). Such a pervasive VR approach seeks to distribute responsibility for VR outcomes among all interdisciplinary team members. Typically, such an approach can be successfully accomplished only when accompanied by a strong management commitment and consistent staff training. When this approach is successfully employed, however, the TBI program is able to achieve an effective VR effort without the expenditure of significant funds for what is regarded, regrettably and sometimes erroneously, as a nonreimbursable service component.

The process of assessing and placing persons with TBI into the world of work is very complicated and tends to be compounded by many factors including, most notably, the disability itself. The impact of severe disability on work personality and performance varies significantly from one individual to another, and across different work settings (Dunn, 1974). Therefore, effective assessment of persons with TBI tends to require a comprehensive approach and may occur at all three levels including screening, clinical case study, and vocational evaluation (Vocational Evaluation and Work Adjustment Association [VEWAA], 1975).

LEVELS OF REHABILITATION ASSESSMENT

In general, most rehabilitation clients go through a basic assessment process which can be termed *screening* (VEWAA, 1975). This is essentially similar to vocational guidance procedures used by high school or college counselors involving one or two interviews. The vocational needs of clients are derived on the basis of a subjective description of work values, interests, and skills. These data are then supplemented with job history and medical information including residual physical capacities.

The second level of assessment is the *clinical case study*, or in-depth vocational counseling approach (VEWAA, 1975). In addition to the methods used in screening, this method involves securing a detailed personal history, synthesizing the findings of other agencies and professionals, delivering a full range of psychological tests (interest, personality, achievement, and aptitude), and conducting several hours of personal interviews. This level of assessment is required to identify transferable job skills and retraining potential.

The third level of assessment is the *vocational evaluation* (VEWAA, 1975). It is most appropriate for people with severe disabilities (such as TBI) and limited work history. In addition to screening and clinical case study, this level involves assessing the vocational potential of disabled clients in real or simulated work settings utilizing a combination of psychological testing, job analysis, work samples, and situational assessment approaches (Neff, 1966; VEWAA, 1975). This level of assessment typically requires two or more weeks of comprehensive evaluation as well as the observation of work behavior in a community-based setting.

Prerequisite Knowledge

GENERAL INFORMATION

To perform an evaluation appropriately, the work evaluator must be knowledgeable about:

1. current vocational assessment theories and associated technologies;
2. medical and psychosocial aspects of disabilities;
3. vocational implications of different disabilities;
4. work demands and requirements of different occupations;
5. job trends and training opportunities in the local and national economy;
6. development and availability of job accommodation methods and assistive devices; and
7. community resources (Roessler & Rubin, 1982).

Because of the degree of complexity and difficulty, vocational evaluation for people who are severely disabled is time-consuming, expensive, and comprehensive in scope. The vocational evaluator must have a thorough understanding of both the dynamics of the world of work and the impact of disability on work and human behavior (Neff, 1966). It is imperative for the vocational evaluator to have an integrated theoretical framework for vocational evaluation to systematically evaluate the vocational development and rehabilitation programming needs of people with disabilities. The Minnesota Theory of Work Adjustment (Dawis, 1987) is one example of a useful framework.

INFORMATION SPECIFIC TO HEAD INJURY

It is also critical that the work evaluator possess additional knowledge regarding salient vocational issues in TBI rehabilitation. For example, it is generally acknowledged that VR is more effective when all interdisciplinary team members understand that *the primary impediments to vocational recovery are the clients' cognitive and psychosocial deficits*. Accordingly, those team members whose primary responsibilities are for cognitive and psychosocial remediation will generally experience more interaction with VR personnel than other team members, and appropriately so (Fraser & McMahon, 1988).

It is generally agreed that *VR interventions (especially work evaluation) should be directed at the entire work repertoire* including work behaviors (e.g., skill proficiency, work rate, work quality, work endurance); work adaptive behaviors; work values; work interests; learning style; and motivation.

Perhaps the single largest explanation for the failure of most VR programs with TBI clients is their excessive emphasis on the development of skill proficiency, typically manifest by elaborate training services. On balance, greater benefits will be realized when services are focused on work adaptive behaviors, especially the abilities to relate to coworkers and supervisors (Fraser, Clemmons, & McMahon, 1990).

In each step of the VR process there exist *unique considerations which, if implemented, can significantly enhance the effectiveness of VR interventions* (Fraser, McMahon, & Vogenthaler, 1988). In work evaluation, for example, these include:

1. the avoidance of group interventions;
2. the minimal use of commercially available work samples;
3. the expectation of frustration and anger;
4. the testing of limits;
5. the flexibility of test administration;
6. the avoidance of attribution of all errors to neurogenic causes;
7. the focus on known correlates of vocational success;
8. the pre-eminence of situational assessment, on-the-job evaluation, and occupational trials.

With reference to Chapter 2, it should be obvious how outpatient *day programming is naturally consistent with these recommendations* because the "face validity" of the evaluation experience is naturally improved and the range of occupational opportunities considered is typically expanded beyond what is available in remote residential settings. Conversely, one potential danger of day programming is the tendency to subcontract vocational evaluation services to extant VR facilities in which reliance on prepackaged, commercially available work samples is commonplace. This practice often leads to the underestimation of vocational potential for individuals with TBI.

Whenever possible, the work site should be utilized as the primary site of all rehabilitation activity. All assessment, work skills training, and work adjustment training may be provided either at the work site, or in as normalized an environment as possible such as neighboring vocational-technical schools, employer on-the-job training programs, occupational trials, projects with industry, apprenticeship programs, and the like. Rehabilitation facilities and hospital-based work hardening programs should be utilized only as a last resort, as none can compare to the workplace for face validity and the broadest possible range of occupational and training experiences.

One might consider that when a child becomes disabled, there follows automatically every effort to reintegrate that child into the school environment at the earliest possible moment and to expect that school to accommodate that child and become the logical site and vehicle of redevelopment (not just educational redevelopment). Similarly, the preinjury work site should serve a similar function for the adult with TBI whenever possible.

JOB PLACEMENT INFORMATION

It is also helpful if the work evaluator has some understanding of the unique considerations in job placement for clients with TBI. A job placement decision-tree has been described which delineates how work evaluation results may be used to prescribe the appropriate job placement approach (Fraser, Clemmons, & McMahon, 1990). More traditional job placement approaches (e.g., selective placement and job seeking skills training) have many inherent limitations when applied to persons with TBI. Specifically, the inefficiency of the former and the didactic nature of the latter are problematic. The "systems selling" approach (McMahon & Spencer, 1979) is likely to experience a resurgence of interest in the post-ADA *(Americans with Disabilities Act)* era. This approach involves a straightforward exchange of VR consultation and technical assistance to employers in exchange for preferential hiring considerations for a segment of rehabilitation clientele.

For the near future, it appears likely that traditional job placement approaches will be used in tandem with supported employment interventions. Supported employment is defined as paid work, typically in a variety of settings, in which disabled workers are integrated with nondisabled workers, and in which supports are provided to ensure that the disabled client/worker will succeed. Eligible workers are those who would not otherwise succeed without such supports, defined as any activity designed to improve client competitiveness. While a full evaluation of the efficacy of supported employment for TBI clients is far from complete, the advantages of this approach are numerous and are remarkably similar to the advantages of outpatient over residential treatment. Much of the preliminary success of the supported employment approach can be traced to its roots in applied behavior analysis.

The following section is a discussion of the specific factors and appropriate tools required to systematically assess vocational potential and programming needs of people with disabilities and of people with TBI in particular.

Basic Approaches to Vocational Evaluation

Vocational evaluation is defined as a systematic process that utilizes real or simulated work as a major focus for assessing the vocational potential of people with disabilities (Pruitt, 1986). There are four major approaches to vocational evaluation including standardized testing, job analysis, work samples, and situational assessment. Each plays an unique role in measuring the vocational behaviors of people with TBI.

THE STANDARDIZED TESTING APPROACH

Psychological testing has evoked more criticism than any vocational evaluation procedure. Berven (1979) summarized these criticisms as follows:

> *Criticism of the value of psychometric assessment is often related to essential differences between the assessment situation and work and training situations. Psychometric tasks are often highly abstract, the samples of behavior are very brief, and attempts are made to maximize motivation and concentration, all of which differ from work and training situations—the criterion situations of interest. (p. 48)*

However, psychometric assessment does have several distinct advantages over other approaches (Neff, 1966). It can provide the vocational evaluator with objective indices of work-related cognitive, affective, and psychomotor traits quickly and inexpensively (Berven, 1979; VEWAA, 1975). Therefore, psychometric assessment is frequently used early in the evaluation process to obtain baseline information about an individual client and to provide direction for subsequent assessment efforts.

Aptitude and interest matching is frequently used in the standardized testing approach (Menchetti & Flynn, 1990). Interest matching requires the use of needs/values and personality/interest instruments to identify vocational interests (e.g., the Minnesota Importance Questionnaire). Aptitude matching is characterized by the use of aptitude instruments (e.g., the Apticon) to measure various vocational aptitudes. The results are compared to Occupational Aptitude Patterns which the U.S. Department of Labor suggests are related to various jobs. A list of jobs balancing the client's needs and abilities can be generated by cross-referencing jobs identified through aptitude matching and interest matching. The resulting job list can then be thoroughly investigated in subsequent evaluation using other vocational evaluation approaches.

THE JOB ANALYSIS APPROACH

Job analysis focuses primarily on the description of work to be performed and only secondarily on characteristics of the worker. In vocational evaluation, job analysis enables the vocational evaluator to better understand the realistic demands of a job in the workplace. By focusing on the nature of the task to be performed, the vocational evaluator can determine the job modification and accommodation needs of the client in the real world. In addition, by conducting job analyses of high-demand occupations in the community, the vocational evaluator will be able to develop work samples that are realistic and responsive to local employment opportunities.

THE WORK SAMPLE APPROACH

The work sample is probably the most popular approach used in vocational evaluation. Work samples can be grouped into trait-oriented and work-oriented instruments (Menchetti & Flynn, 1990). Trait-oriented work samples are similar to multiple aptitude batteries in that they are designed to measure a number of traits inherent in a job or a variety of jobs. The major differences between trait-oriented work samples and aptitude tests are that: (a) work samples tend to focus on measuring motor responses through the use of complex and more expensive apparatuses; (b) there is less focus on general intellectual and academic abilities in the work samples; and (c) many work samples are designed to be used independently and need not be administered as part of a larger battery (Menchetti & Flynn, 1990).

Work-oriented work samples utilize simulated work such as drill press operation and electronic assembly to measure performance on specific tasks. These work samples have higher face validity since they approximate real work activity. In general, work samples focus on assessing work potential for skilled, semi-skilled, and unskilled jobs.

THE SITUATIONAL ASSESSMENT APPROACH

While psychometric assessment, job analysis, and work samples tend to emphasize specific employability skills, situational assessment focuses on general employability skills and work adaptive behaviors (Neff, 1966). Situational assessment is based on an effort to simulate actual working conditions with an orientation toward work behavior in general. The vocational evaluator uses different means to structure the work environment so that general work behavior can be observed. As noted earlier, situational assessment is the generally-preferred mode of work evaluation for persons with severe TBI.

Information obtained from situational assessment is designed to help the vocational evaluator answer such questions as, "Can the worker work at all? Can he or she conform to customary work rules? Can he or she respond appropriately to supervision? Can he or she produce at an acceptable rate both in terms of quality and quantity?" Situational assessment is the most appropriate method for answering these questions while assessing potential behavioral problems in the work site.

Toward an Ecological Approach to Vocational Evaluation

In many aspects, the vocational evaluation of clients with TBI is similar to other disability groups. The vocational behavior of a client with TBI can be systematically evaluated using the same theoretical and operational framework mentioned above. However, as pointed out by McMahon and Fraser (1988), issues related to the treatment of persons with TBI are very complex, variable, and in constant flux. Clients with TBI tend to manifest sets of behavioral problems that are quite different from people with mental retardation, learning disabilities developmental disabilities, or strict physical disabilities.

Ben-Yishay, Silver, Piasetsky, and Rattok (1987) found in their review of the employment outcome literature that between 40% and 60% of people with TBI cannot achieve re-employment without ongoing support. They further noted that sheltered employment is far from a satisfactory solution for this population. As a result, supported employment as a job placement and training option has gained significant popularity and is fast becoming the preferred vocational programming arrangement for persons with TBI.

Given the significantly varied impact of TBI on work and independent living, and the rapid emergence of community-based employment approaches in the VR of clients with TBI, traditional vocational evaluation may not be totally appropriate for this population. Conceptually, the three levels of traditional assessment described above may still be applicable for the TBI population, and the degree of comprehensiveness of the evaluation may still depend on the severity of the brain injury. However, the emphasis of assessment approaches (e.g., situational assessment as preferred to work samples) used in vocational evaluation must be shifted to meet the different vocational programming needs of the TBI population. As Cook (1990) notes:

> *Vocational evaluation of the individual with traumatic brain injury is a different process than that used with other disabled populations. Effective vocational evaluation requires individualized planning, flexible and varied procedures in actual/realistic job situations, and repeated evaluations over time and under varying conditions. (p. 497)*

Additionally, the inclusion of neuropsychological evaluation and family support data and a stronger focus on the ecological model of vocational evaluation may be required (Menchetti & Flynn, 1990; Szymula & Schleser, 1986).

It is clear that when evaluating clients with TBI, the concern shifts dramatically to the ways in which functional limitations (especially the cognitive and psychosocial) are manifest in work settings. These behaviors cannot be effectively evaluated within the controlled and often protective environment of a rehabilitation facility, and must be evaluated within a larger environmental context (i.e., individual, family, school, occupation, and society). The emphasis of assessment approaches used in traditional vocational evaluation may need to be changed to meet the different vocational programming needs of the TBI population. Specifically, an ecological-based evaluation model may be more appropriate for this population.

Supported employment has emerged as one of the most successful vocational programming options for persons with TBI. Wehman et al.

(1988) and Fraser et al. (1990) described in great detail how the supported employment concept — including job placement, job-site training and coaching, and long-term follow-up — can be modified to fit the needs of persons with TBI. This emphasis on community-based evaluation and training underscores the importance of adapting an ecological model of vocational evaluation for TBI clients.

An ecological systems approach explains behavior as a multisystemic interaction involving the individual, family, school, occupation, and society (Davidson & Rappaport, 1983). The defining attribute consists of concern with effective coping strategies through the identification and development of strengths, instead of focusing on maladjustment or pathological conditions (Jeger & Slotnick, 1982). The ecological systems perspective encompasses three important facets. These include cultural relativity, individual diversity, and person-environment "fit." Cultural relativity demands that individual differences be viewed from their cultural context. Diversity requires respect for others' opinions, preferences, and physical statuses despite personal discomfort. Finally, person-environment fit concentrates on the identification of those key variables which contribute to the best possible adjustment between the person and the social/physical environment (Rappaport, 1977).

Several implications emerge out of the ecological systems perspective. First, behavior can be understood by watching how individuals interrelate with their environment. Second, identification of the systems most important and most troublesome to the individual must precede any effective intervention. As Henggeler (1982) noted, abnormal or deviant behavior may serve an adaptive function as the only means of dealing with stress. Third, faulty interaction between a person and the environment leading to adjustment problems can be modified by altering aspects of either the individual or the environment.

An ecological system approach differs from a traditional rehabilitation perspective in that the former emphasizes showing people how to acquire the necessary social, political, or psychological resources to improve their condition while the latter emphasizes the provision of treatment and services. As a result, traditional rehabilitation may foster an attitude of personal dependence instead of providing an opportunity for individual responsibility. However, rehabilitation does advocate, while not always providing the means, for resource allocation. From an ecological systems perspective for vocational evaluation, the key point is the incorporation of the three areas of relativity, diversity, and person-environment fit as an operational philosophy toward persons with TBI. This means that the measurement of vocational potential and the definition of successful adjustment requires an assessment of both the individual and the environment, not merely a preset, standardized assessment of the individual alone.

There are several implications of the ecological systems perspective for vocational evaluation. First, the assessment must try to identify the strengths of the individual and base recommendations on the best utilization of assets. It is too easy to compile a list of weaknesses which vastly outnumber assets for persons with severe TBI. Second, vocational evaluation must consider systems beyond an individual level (such as the family, community, and society) as influencing factors both during and after the process. Third, failure to utilize environmental measures such as job analysis, labor market surveys, or on-site assessment increase the chance of poor adjustment between a TBI client and the work setting. Fourth, limitations of traditional vocational assessment procedures with the TBI population must be recognized to avoid inaccurate conclusions regarding individual ability.

A fifth and final concern is the relative nature of vocational outcomes. Seemingly successful solutions may later turn into unexpected problems. Individuals may lose jobs as a result of changing economic condition. A compliant person in a training program may, in reality, be too passive for a particular employment setting. Thus, strategies must continuously be adapted to environmental changes and as a result will require frequent reappraisal.

Measures of the Environment in Vocational Evaluation

Vocational evaluation viewed from the ecological systems perspective takes on a new emphasis and depth that are important in the evaluation of the TBI client. The ecological viewpoint, stressing proper fit between person and setting can serve as a validity criterion by identifying the content appropriate for assessment. One advantage of this perspective is the increasing reliance on environmental measurement. Specifically, measurement in this context requires the measurement of the social climate or ecology of the workplace (Menchetti & Flynn, 1990). Menchetti and Flynn pointed out that work environments have unique "personalities" just like people; some are more supportive than others. Chadsey-Rusch and Rusch (1988) suggested that by accurately measuring the ecology of the workplace, a vocational evaluator can facilitate a good match between a client and the job.

According to Menchetti and Flynn (1990), there are several dimensions which should be considered when measuring the ecology of supported employment settings: (a) the physical ecology, (b) the social ecology, and (c) the organization ecology. Other dimensions, such as transportation requirements, family support, work disincentives (e.g., SSI or SSDI benefits), and the availability of external incentives (e.g., targeted jobs tax credits) must also be considered (Menchetti & Flynn, 1990; Szymula & Schleser, 1986).

These dimensions of the ecology of a workplace are interactive and constantly change as a result of this interaction. The assessment of these dimensions allows VR specialists to determine the adaptability of the environment to meet the needs of an individual. The adaptability of the environment can be compared with the TBI client's abilities to determine the degree of person-environment fit. Decisions about the client's work potential in that environment can be made in terms of accepting the person, accepting the person with support, or recommending a specific alternative (Menchetti & Flynn, 1990). Chapter 8 by Robert Fraser exemplifies an ecological perspective as applied to supported employment.

Summary

Because the ability to work is strongly valued in contemporary society, vocational rehabilitation is seen as critically important. Whether viewed as a means toward the goal of successful vocational placement or as a "pull factor" which motivates clients to become invested in their overall rehabilitation programs, appropriate vocational services may be viewed as a critical and integral treatment component.

Persons with TBI generally require a comprehensive assessment which includes three levels of assessment: screening, clinical case study, and vocational evaluation. Because of the complexity of TBI, vocational evaluation tends to be a time-consuming, complex process requiring the evaluator to possess considerable prerequisite knowledge about evaluation principles and techniques, placement issues, and specific considerations for the TBI population.

While many different assessment approaches may be utilized, it appears that the situational assessment is the best-suited to the needs of clients with TBI. Even this approach has limited utility, however, given the complex and ever-shifting needs of the TBI client. Consequently, the authors propose an ecological approach to vocational evaluation.

The ecological approach explains behavior as a multisystemic interaction involving the individual, family, school, occupation, and society. The ecological approach to vocational evaluation requires that the evaluator consider systems beyond the individual client, resulting in a more thorough understanding of the client-environment interaction.

To provide specifics and substance to the foregoing discussion, a comprehensive TBI evaluation protocol which includes vocational evaluation is presented in the appendix which follows.

Appendix A

Extended Evaluation Program Components

The final product of the evaluation process is a prescriptive plan for community re-entry. This will include:

1. a summary and integration of all the assessment information provided by individual specialists as described below;
2. an identification of individual assets, deficits, and functional goals;
3. an identification of treatment and support services necessary to achieve identified goals; and
4. projected reasonable treatment timelines and outcomes which could be realistically expected given the assessment findings and the approval and provision of necessary treatments.

I. Health and Physical Therapy Assessment

Standard medical history and physical examination by appropriate medical or physical restoration specialists to include complete assessments of:

Overall physical health
Ability to regulate and manage own health status
Musculoskeletal and body movement
Range of motion
Muscle strength
Posture
Functional balance
Functional mobility
Gait

II. Psychological Evaluation

Standard mental status examination by appropriate psychiatrist, psychologist, or mental health counselor to include emotional and social behavior, with observations preferably conducted in the home and community environment. May also include the following if consideration is given to subject's cognitive status:

Minnesota Multiphasic Personality Inventory
Michigan Alcoholism Screening Test

III. Neuropsychological Evaluation

Standard neurological evaluation plus standardized neuropsychological battery to address specific referral questions. May also include the following:

Wechsler Adult Intelligence Scale
Galveston Orientation and Amnesia Test
Wide Range Achievement Test
Wechsler Memory Scale
Wisconsin Card Sorting Test

IV. Assessment of Cognitive Status

Woodcock-Johnson Psychoeducational Battery
(Subtests of Cognitive Functioning)
Ross Information Processing Assessment
Stroop Test
Modified Trail Making Test
Key Math
Audiological and eye examinations (if indicated)

V. Assessment of Communication Skills

Boston Naming Test
Peabody Picture Vocabulary Test
Boston Diagnostic Aphasia Examination
Woodcock-Johnson Psychoeducational Battery
(Language Subtests)
Oral and Voice Examinations
Modified Barium Swallow Test (prn swallowing problems)
ENT Examination (prn voice/airway dysfunction)

VI. Therapeutic Recreation

Leisure Diagnostic Battery
State Technical Institute Leisure Assessment Process
Treatment Screening B (Functional Skills and Leisure)

VII. Occupational Therapy Assessment

Situational assessment within residence and community to assess activities of daily living and community living skills such as shopping, banking, transportation, etc. May also include the following if consideration is given to the subject's cognitive status:

- Visual-Perceptual
  - Hooper Test of Visual Organization
  - Motor Free Visual Perception Test
  - Benton 3-D Block Design
- Physical Restoration
  - Hand Strength: dynamometer, pinch meter
  - Dexterity/Coordination
  - Jebson-Taylor Hand Function Test
  - Box and Black Test
  - 9-Hole Peg Test
  - Minnesota Rate of Manipulation Test
  - Spasticity and Muscle Tone Evaluation
- Activities of Daily Living
  - Klein-Bell ADL Test
  - Independent Living Checklist

VIII. Vocational Evaluation

Must include job analyses, labor market analyses, and job market analyses of targeted jobs if appropriate. Situational assessment for minimum of 10 working days involving community-based employer to evaluate work adaptive behaviors. May also include the following if consideration is given to the subject's cognitive status:

- Vocational Interests and Values
  - Strong Campbell Interest Inventory
  - Vocational Research Institute Interest Inventory
  - Minnesota Importance Questionnaire
- Vocational Aptitudes and Abilities
  - Micro-Computer Evaluation and Screening Assessment
  - McCarron-Dial Evaluation System
  - APTICON
  - Vocational Transit Evaluation System
- Physical Capacities
  - Valpar 19: Physical Capacities Workstation
  - Medical identification/substantiation of work restrictions

References

Ben-Yishay, Y., Silver, S. M., Piasetsky, E., & Rattok, J. (1987). Relationship between employability and vocational outcome after intensive holistic cognitive rehabilitation. *Journal of Head Trauma Rehabilitation*, Vol. 2, 25-48.

Berven, N. L. (1979). Psychometric assessment in rehabilitation. In B. Bolton (Ed.), *Rehabilitation client assessment* (pp. 46-64). Baltimore, MD: University Park Press.

Chadsey-Rusch, J., & Rusch, F. R. (1988). Ecology of the work place. In R. Gaylord-Ross (Ed.), Vocational education for persons with special needs (pp. 234-256). Mountain View, CA: Mayfield.

Cook, J. V. (1990). Returning to work after traumatic head injury. In M. Rosenthal, E. R. Griffith, M. R. Bond, & J. D. Miller (Eds.), *Rehabilitation of the adult and child with traumatic brain injury* (2nd Ed.) (pp. 493-505). Philadelphia: F.A. Davis Company.

Davidson, W., & Rapport, J. (1983). Advocacy and community psychology. In G. Weber & G. McCall (Eds.), *Social scientists as advocates* (pp. 67-97). Beverly Hills, CA: Sage.

Dawis, R. (1987). A theory of work adjustment. In B. Bolton (Ed.), *Handbook on the measurement and evaluation in rehabilitation* (2nd ed.) (pp. 207-217). Baltimore, MD: Paul H. Brooks.

Dunn, D. (1974). *Placement services in the vocational rehabilitation program.* Menomonie, WI: Research and Training Center, Stout Vocational Rehabilitation Institute, University of Wisconsin-Stout.

Fawber, H. L., & Wachter, J. F. (1987). Job placement as a treatment component of the vocational rehabilitation process. *Journal of Head Trauma Rehabilitation*, *2*, 27-33.

Fraser, R. T., McMahon, B. T., & Vogenthaler, D. R. (1988). Vocational rehabilitation counseling with head injured persons. In S. E. Rubin & R. T. Roessler (Eds.), *Foundations of the vocational rehabilitation process* (3rd ed.) (pp. 217-242). Austin, TX: PRO-ED.

Fraser, R. T., Clemmons, D. C., & McMahon, B. T. (1990). Vocational rehabilitation. In J. S. Kreutzer and P. H. Wehman (Eds.) *Community integration following traumatic brain injury* (pp. 169-184). Baltimore: Paul H. Brookes.

Henggeler, S. (1972). The family ecological systems theory. In S. Henggeler (Ed.), *Delinquency and adolescent psychopathology* (pp. 1-10). Boston: John Wright.

Jeger, A., & Slotnick, R. (1982). Community mental health. In A. Jeger & R. Slotnick (Eds.), *Community mental health and behavioral ecology* (pp. 7-24). New York: Plenum.

McMahon, B. T., & Fraser, R. T. (1988). Basic issues and trends in head injury rehabilitation. In S. E. Rubin & R. T. Roessler (Eds.), *Foundations of the vocational rehabilitation process* (3rd ed.) (pp. 197-216). Austin, TX: PRO-ED.

McMahon, B. T., & Spencer, S. A. (1979). A systems selling approach to job development. *Journal of Rehabilitation, 45*(2), 68-70.

Menchetti, B. M., & Flynn, C. C. (1990). Supported employment: New directions for vocational evaluation. In F. R. Rusch (Ed.), *Supported employment: Models, methods, and issues* (pp. 111-130). Sycamore: Sycamore Publishing.

Neff, W. S. (1966). *Work and human behavior.* Chicago: Aldine.

Osipow, S. H. (1968). *Theories of career development.* New York: Appleton-Century-Crofts.

Pruitt, W. A. (1986). Vocational evaluation. Menomonie, WI: Walt Pruitt Associates.

Rappaport, J. (1977). *Community psychology.* New York: Holt, Rinehart, and Winston.

Roessler, R. T., & Rubin, S. E. (1982). *Case management and rehabilitation counseling.* Austin, TX: PRO-ED.

Rubin, S. E., & Roessler, R. T. (1987). *Foundations of the vocational rehabilitation process* (3rd ed.). Austin, TX: PRO-ED.

Szymula, G., & Schleser, R. (1986). A reappraisal of vocational evaluation from an ecological systems perspective. *Rehabilitation Literature, 47*, 224-229.

Vocational Evaluation and Work Adjustment Association. (1975). *Vocational evaluation project final report.* Menomonie, WI: Materials Development Center, Stout Vocational Rehabilitation Institute, University of Wisconsin-Stout.

Wehman, P. Kreutzer, J., Wood, W., Morton, M. V., & Sherron, P. (1988). Supported work models for persons with traumatic brain injury: Toward job placement and retention. *Rehabilitation Counseling Bulletin, 31*, 298-312.

Wright, G. N. (1980). *Total rehabilitation.* Boston: Little Brown.

6

Applied Behavior Analysis and Work Adjustment Training

Frank D. Lewis
Craig F. Bitter

6

Applied Behavior Analysis and Work Adjustment Training

Frank D. Lewis
Craig F. Bitter

Work is one of the most highly valued roles in our society (Schneider & Ferritor, 1982). Work is a means for achieving independence and life goals. One's occupation can be a significant source for positive social interactions and may serve as the context within which lasting friendships are made. The consequences of prolonged unemployment, therefore, impact not only economic status, but also one's social and interpersonal well-being.

The absence of work is a major complaint of TBI survivors (Roessler, Schriner, & Price, 1990). The majority of head injuries occur to young males between the ages of 18 and 35 when they are beginning or establishing their work role. Most of these persons can expect to live a normal life span, but for many, residual deficits in cognitive, physical, and interpersonal functioning will preclude return to competitive employment. As a result, they lose a primary means of validating personal value and self-worth and may face the prospect of a lifetime of dependency.

Severe brain injury has a devastating impact on an individual's ability to meet the intellectual and social demands of the work place. Unemployment rates for TBI survivors are high (Brooks, McKinlay, Symington, Beattie, & Campsie, 1987; Jacobs, 1988; Prigatano et al., 1984; Prigatano, Klonoff, & Bailey, 1987). Following a review of the literature, Haffey and Lewis (1989) concluded that return-to-work rates for severely brain-injured persons who have not received specialized post-acute rehabilitation ranges on average from 23 to 30%. Unfortunately, studies of outcomes following specialized vocational TBI rehabilitation have reported only modestly better return-to-work rates (Ben-Yishay, Silver, Piasetsky, & Rattok, 1987; Pepping et al., 1989; Prigatano et al., 1984). Even with comprehensive post-acute rehabilitation the majority of severely head-injured individuals are unable to obtain and maintain employment. Those who do return to work typically do so at fewer hours, in less demanding positions, and at lower pay. The current status of vocational outcomes following TBI underscores the need this population has for lifelong support and follow-up.

Due to this need for ongoing support and intervention, supported employment has gained increased popularity in TBI rehabilitation (Wehman, Kreutzer, Wood, Morton, & Sherron, 1988). Briefly, supported employment is a "place and train" model of rehabilitation in which clients are placed in a job consistent with their interests and are paid wages comparable to those of nondisabled employees in similar positions. Rehabilitation therapies are conducted at the job site by a trained job coach. Assistance and support are faded as the performance standards are met, although help is available throughout clients' job tenure. A major advantage of the supported work model is that training is provided in the natural environment. Clients, therefore, learn to apply newly acquired responses to a wide range of real world situations which can promote more enduring behavior change (Sailor, Goetz, Anderson, Hunt, & Gee, 1988).

Wehman et al. (1988) reported placement rates and preliminary job retention data for 32 severely head-injured individuals referred for job coaching assistance. Persons in the sample were between the ages of 18 and 64, were not active drug users, and had a post-injury history of employment instability. Initial job placement rates were 47% (15 of 32). At the time of their report 73% (11 of 15) of the placed clients were still working. The mean length of employment was 9 months.

In a subsequent study, Wehman et al. (1989) reported the outcomes of five TBI adults with poor work records and histories of drug use and aberrant social behavior. Although all the clients were successfully placed, three lost their jobs after several weeks. Consecutive weeks of employment ranged from 12 to 59 weeks for those who lost their jobs. In both supported work studies, inadequate interpersonal skills (e.g., inability to control anger or emotions, bizarre or irritating behaviors, failing to follow supervisor instructions) were major factors contributing to job loss.

The supported work model appears to be a promising rehabilitation approach for returning TBI survivors to work. However, a major contributor to failed supported work outcomes is the presence of persistent behavior problems and poor social skills. Surveys of businesses that frequently hire disabled workers reveal that employers want employees who are dependable, get along with co-workers, carry out supervisor instructions in a timely fashion, and work steadily on assigned tasks (Wilms, 1984). Unfortunately, TBI survivors are often deficient in these important job retention skills. To improve return-to-work rates among TBI survivors, job coaches and vocational counselors must address these work adjustment problems.

There is a large body of literature supporting the efficacy of applied behavioral analysis (behavior management) in the treatment of work adjustment problems. The *Journal of Applied Behavior Analysis* is replete with articles addressing problems of distractibility, grooming, tardiness, social skills, and verbal and physical aggression in the work place. The behavior analytic approach is especially relevant in TBI rehabilitation because unlike other psychological therapies, its effectiveness is not dependent upon clients' ability to retain and process abstract verbal information. It has been used successfully with severely cognitively impaired TBI clients to modify maladaptive social behaviors (Foxx, Martelle, & Marchand-Martella, 1989; Lewis, Nelson, Nelson, & Reusink, 1988).

The purpose of this chapter is to illustrate specific behavior management procedures that can be applied in supported work and other training settings. The behavior management approach described includes functional analysis of work behavior and practical strategies to both reduce maladaptive behavior and increase prosocial skills in the work place. Procedures for enhancing the generalizability of adaptive behaviors are also presented. Although applied behavioral analysis has application for clients in the early (acute) stages of recovery, the focus of this chapter is clients for whom the period of post-traumatic confusion has been resolved and post-acute rehabilitation is appropriate.

Functional Analysis of Work Behavior

A functional analysis seeks to identify the causes of a problem by considering both the conditions under which the problem occurs and the consequences that follow it. Behavior can be changed by altering the antecedents (stimulus or setting events which may either precede or exist simultaneously with the behavior) and/or consequential events (events that follow a behavior). The first step in this process is defining the work adjustment problem.

PROBLEM DEFINITION

To perform a functional analysis the vocational counselor must define the work adjustment problem in behaviorally specific terms. This is important for two reasons: 1) accuracy in measurement, and 2) selection of the appropriate intervention. Rehabilitation professionals frequently use words such as impulsive, emotionally immature, irresponsible, inattentive, and others to describe the behavior problems exhibited by TBI clients. While such labels are useful in that they alert the work adjustment counselor that a problem exists, they lack the objectivity and clarity needed to accurately assess change and progress over time. It is much more difficult to gauge how often a person is "irresponsible" than it is to determine the frequency of reporting to work late or failure to complete assigned tasks. Ambiguous labelling requires observers to draw inferences about the occurrence of the behavior. These inferences can be affected by a variety of personal variables (e.g., mood of the observer, feelings toward the client, therapist desire to achieve a goal) and/or situational factors (e.g., behavior of others overshadowing that of the client). Without accurate data the vocational counselor is at risk of concluding that the intervention was effective when it was not (type I error) or that the intervention was not effective when it actually did improve behavior (type II error).

The other reason it is important to define work adjustment problems in behaviorally specific terms concerns selection of the intervention. To select an appropriate intervention the vocational counselor must know the following information about the target behavior: the frequency, duration, and/or intensity with which it occurs; whether it is a surplus behavior or a performance or skill deficit; the conditions in which it is most and least likely to occur; and the consequences following its occurrence and nonoccurrence. This information can be obtained only if the work adjustment problem is objectively defined.

An objective definition is formulated from a global label or description by asking what behaviors the client engaged in to merit the label. For example, a client may be characterized as disruptive in the work setting. A close examination of the client's actual behavior reveals that he or she yells obscenities when given corrective feedback. With this level of objectivity, the problem can be accurately measured and a treatment plan developed to address it through management of the environment (antecedents and consequences). In the example above, changing an antecedent condition, such as teaching the supervisor to speak slowly and in a neutral tone of voice when giving corrective feedback, may be sufficient to eliminate the client's obscene language.

One method to test whether the target behavior has been defined objectively is to assign two independent raters to observe the client simultaneously. The target response is objectively defined if the two observers consistently agree about the presence or absence of the behavior at any point in time.

The behavioral definition should also be complete. This means that the range of responses included in the definition should be specified along with any conditions in which the behavior would not be counted. For example, the target behavior "talking to co-workers during work periods" could be defined broadly to include any verbalization. Alternatively, it could be restricted to include only those comments that were not relevant to successful task completion. Some talking, such as offering suggestions to improve work performance or asking for clarification of instructions, may be considered appropriate even though it temporarily disrupts work. The more complex the target behavior, the more important it becomes to specify these boundary conditions to minimize ambiguity of the data.

TYPES OF BEHAVIORAL PROBLEMS

Behavior problems displayed by TBI clients can be classified as either behavioral deficits or surpluses. Behavioral deficits are behaviors that occur too infrequently to meet minimal performance standards required in a given situation. In contrast, behavioral surpluses are behaviors that occur more frequently than is appropriate for the situation. The causes of these problems are varied and may include environmental, premorbid (learning histories), and organic factors. Diffuse damage to specific brain structures almost always contributes directly or indirectly to behavior problems observed in the TBI population. For instance, damage to the medial cortex of the frontal lobes has been associated with flattened affect, lack of goal-directed behavior, loss of drive (adynamia), and loss of the sense of pleasure (anhedonia). In the work place these conditions can result in deficit behaviors such as poor grooming and hygiene, withdrawal from co-workers, and failure to follow instructions or complete assigned tasks.

Behavioral deficits may be further categorized into skill and performance deficits. Skill deficits imply that the target behavior is not in the individual's behavioral repertoire. Skill deficits require interventions to teach the client the desired behavior or strategies to compensate for its loss. Performance deficits refer to those behaviors for which the client has the requisite skills yet fails to adequately perform them. For example, the client has the strength to lift 50-pound bags of fertilizer on a truck but refuses to do it. Remediation of performance deficits involves modification of environmental contingencies to increase the probability that the desired behavior will occur at the appropriate time.

Perseverative verbal and motor behavior, social disinhibition, impulsiveness, and episodic aggression are classes of behavioral surpluses associated with damage to medial surfaces of the temporal lobes and the limbic system. In the workplace, these syndromes are manifested as excessive talking, frequent break-taking, aggressive outbursts in response to correction or change in routine, and obsessiveness in the performance of job tasks. Reduction of surplus behavior typically involves programming not only to reduce excess behavior but also to increase appropriate alternative responses.

MEASUREMENT

Once problem behaviors have been defined and identified as surpluses or deficits they must be measured along a dimension that yields quantifiable information sensitive to detecting meaningful clinical changes. Dimensions of behavior that may be measured include frequency (how often the behavior occurs during a specified period), duration (how long it last when it occurs), and intensity (the magnitude of the behavior). Bellack and Hersen (1988) provide a compendium of behavioral assessment techniques appropriate for measurement on each of these dimensions.

Assessment begins with a baseline period in which the target behavior is measured as it occurs naturally in the work setting without specialized intervention. This data is analyzed to determine whether a discrepancy exists between the client's performance and expectations established for the job. If a discrepancy exists, its significance is assessed by asking, "What would happen if the behavior remained unchanged?" If no significant negative consequences would result from leaving the behavior unchanged, then intervention is not necessary. It is unproductive to spend the time, effort, and cost required of intervention if the behavior does not impact negatively on job performance. However, intervention is necessary if the discrepancy threatens job stability. After the decision is made to intervene, measurement continues throughout the behavioral treatment and for some time beyond to assess the stability of the behavior change. Precise measurement of the problem allows for the detection of small changes in performance and for timely alterations in the treatment if appropriate. It also enables treatment staff to determine when the client's performance meets criterion of the work setting.

CONDITIONS ANALYSIS

Conditions or antecedent analysis is conducted to identify environmental events that precipitate or evoke the target behavior. This analysis should also include an assessment of neurochemical and neurophysiological damage on behavior. Neurochemical and neurophysiological processes determine how we perceive and respond to external and internal stimuli and therefore must be taken into account when developing behavior interventions for TBI survivors. As previously mentioned, many behavior disorders are a direct result of neurological damage. For example, it is widely believed that damage to the limbic system is associated with unpredictable aggressive outbursts. Seizure disorders are also common following TBI. Such conditions may necessitate pharmacological as well as behavioral intervention. Therefore, it is essential that data from neurological and neuropsychological assessments be included as part of the conditions analysis.

There are a large number of external antecedent events that can evoke problems in the workplace. A conditions analysis requires direct naturalistic observation to identify the events or situations that consistently predict the problem behavior. In other words, there may be certain situations in which the behavior always occurs and others where it never does. Events that trigger performance problems can include supervisor demands, interruptions, overstimulation caused by working in a noisy or crowded area, presence of specific co-workers or customers, unstructured break periods, and change in job tasks. Internal events such as fatigue from working continuously without a break, confusion and frustration from not understanding work assignments, and boredom caused by monotonous repetitive work can also evoke problem behavior. If the antecedent conditions that lead to maladaptive behaviors can be identified and then altered, the probability of the problem occurring in the future will be reduced. The topic of modifying behavior through antecedent control is addressed further in the stimulus change section of this chapter.

CONSEQUENCE ANALYSIS

The other component of functional analysis is the consequences, those events that follow the target behavior. There are two categories of consequences – reinforcers and punishers. Reinforcement involves receiving something of value (positive reinforcement) or escaping an unpleasant event (negative reinforcement) contingent upon the performance of a behavior. Punishers are unpleasant or aversive events that suppress or decrease the frequency of the behavior they follow. If a stimulus or event is a reinforcer it will increase the likelihood that the behavior it follows will reoccur. A consequential analysis is performed by observing the person in the work setting and noting the events that immediately follow the target behavior. The events that follow a surplus behavior may be reinforcers maintaining the behavior at high rates. For example, a client working as a proofreader in a newsroom repeatedly asked his job coach for assistance with tasks he was capable of performing independently. Each request for help was followed by a supportive or encouraging response from the job coach. Although the job coach did not actually assist with the task, the high rate of unnecessary requests were being maintained (reinforced) by the supportive statements.

A consequence analysis can also reveal when behaviors are maintained because they serve to remove a person from unpleasant circumstances. For example, each time a client who was working in a floral shop was asked to work with a group on an arrangement she yelled, cursed, and refused to cooperate. When this occurred she was reassigned to work independently. The swearing and uncooperative behavior was being maintained (negatively reinforced) by removing her from the undesirable group situation. Later in this chapter the ways in which consequent events can be altered to effect positive changes in behavior will be addressed.

In summary, the purpose of a functional analysis in the work setting is to identify factors that cause or contribute to behavior problems. The first step in the analysis is problem definition – specifying the behavior to be changed in observable and measurable terms. Antecedents (including biological factors) and consequences are then identified. Finally, the target behavior can be modified in the following ways: (1) altering the events that precipitate or evoke the behavior; (2) changing the consequence events that are maintaining the behavior; or (3) increasing alternative appropriate responses through reinforcement procedures.

Increasing Behavioral Deficits

Specific behavior management techniques can be used to promote adaptive work behavior in TBI clients participating in vocational retraining programs. Several of these techniques are described below. Principles and techniques of generalization programming are presented after each behavior management technique.

TASK ANALYSIS

A task analysis is an effective method to help TBI survivors develop or compensate for work-related skill deficits. Task analyses provide a precise description of the sequence of steps required to perform an activity. Activities selected for a task analysis are those that have functional significance for the learner. For example, one activity important for independent living is laundering clothes. Laundering clothes involves a sequence of behaviors that can be listed in a task analysis. Virtually any work-related activity is suitable for the task analysis method.

There are three steps to writing a complete task analysis (Popovich, 1981):

1. Write a behaviorally specific performance objective. This objective defines the task to be accomplished and includes the criterion for its successful completion.
2. Identify the client's initial level of performance. Record the number of steps the client performs correctly without assistance.
3. Sequence the steps between the client's initial performance and the completed tasks. In other words, list all the remaining steps the client must perform to complete the task.

Staff can determine the steps in a job task by physically performing the task and writing down each step in the sequence as it is completed. If the vocational specialist does not know how to do the task, he or she should recruit an expert to model the task and then write down each step as it is performed.

The following is an example of a task analysis for a janitorial job. The performance objective for the client is "Jim will wash the tile floor in the lobby until all black marks are removed." The sequence of steps to accomplish this objective include:

1. Pick up the bucket on the janitor's cart.
2. Take the bucket to the sink in the custodial room.
3. Fill the bucket half way with water.
4. Get the box of detergent and a measuring cup from the janitor's cart.
5. Pour detergent into the measuring cup.
6. Pour the cup of detergent into the bucket of water and stir.
7. Take the mop from the janitor's cart and dip it in the bucket and wring out.
8. Move the mop back and forth over the tiles.
9. When the mop dries, dip it in the bucket and wring out.
10. Apply the mop to each tile in the room.
11. Inspect the floor for black marks.
12. Rewash any tile with black marks.
13. After all the black marks are gone, rinse out the mop and return it to the janitor's cart.
14. Empty the bucket of dirty water in the sink.
15. Return the bucket to the janitor's cart.
16. Inform supervisor you have completed the task.

Task analyses may be structured in either a general or specific format. A general task analysis specifies the major steps required to do the task (e.g., the floor will not be washed if water is not poured in the bucket). The general task analysis allows latitude in how the steps will be performed. The specific task analysis includes many more smaller steps in the sequence (e.g., Place the bucket under the faucet and turn on the water.). A specific task analysis facilitates skill acquisition. The general task analysis is most appropriate for maintaining performance following acquisition. The number of steps in a task analysis is determined by the client's performance during baseline. As a general rule, the more errors the client makes the greater the number of steps required in the task analysis.

The steps of a task analysis may be presented in a variety of ways including index cards, notebooks, personal computers, or audiocassettes. The method of presentation of the task analysis depends on the client's cognitive and perceptual functioning. For most clients, written task analyses are easiest to follow when each step in the sequence is presented on a separate page or screen. In any case, the information should be presented in a fashion that is "user-friendly."

Generalization and Maintenance

The first consideration when programming for generalization and maintenance is selection of the job task to be analyzed. Job tasks most likely to be maintained are those that have high probability of evoking praise and feedback from the supervisor. The job coach should consult with the employer to identify the tasks that are most critical and the performance criteria for each of those tasks. Obviously, these tasks should be the primary focus of training.

Typically, clients learn task analyses more rapidly if the vocational counselor identifies and lists the stimuli associated with each response in the chain (i.e., the discriminative stimuli or S^Ds). In the task analysis above, the bucket and other cleaning materials on the janitor's cart are the S^Ds for the first response – picking up the bucket. The empty bucket in the client's hand is the S^D associated with Step 2, "Take the bucket to the sink in the custodial room." Each S^D cues or sets the occasion for the next response in the chain. When a behavior is emitted consistently in the presence of a certain stimulus and not at all or rarely in its absence, the behavior is said to be under stimulus control. Due to neurological damage sustained in a TBI, behavior may be too strongly associated with or controlled by specific stimuli in the environment. These persons often exhibit what is referred to as stimulus-bound behavior. Even small changes in the controlling stimulus can result in failure to emit the desired response. In the example above, when a bucket of a different color and size than the one used during skill acquisition is placed on the janitor's cart, the client asks the supervisor for help rather than filling the new bucket with water. When a different brand of detergent is placed on the cart the client stops working and reports not knowing what to do next.

In the workplace, features of the controlling stimuli change frequently. For example, a secretary may be asked to type on a computer that has a slightly different keyboard than the one he or she is accustomed to using. A bus boy in a restaurant must remove dirty dishes from tables on slow days when few customers are present and on busy days when many people are anxiously waiting to be seated. For the TBI client these changes can severely disrupt performance. Task analysis training, therefore, should be designed to promote stimulus generality – "...performance of the target response in the presence of stimulus conditions other than those in which it was directly trained...." (Cooper, Heron, & Heward, 1987). The following steps will help the vocational counselor promote stimulus generality:

1. Identify the relevant and irrelevant features of the S^Ds and teach these differences to the client. For example, relevant features of detergent on the janitor's cart are the box, the dry white powder, and the distinctive soap smell. Irrelevant features include the brand name and color, size, and shape of the box.
2. After the client has mastered the job using the task analysis, introduce variations of the critical S^Ds that may be encountered later on the job (e.g., different brands of tools used to do the job, various locations where the job may be done, changes in the number of persons present when the job is done, etc.).
3. Conduct as many training sessions as possible at the actual work site.

POSITIVE REINFORCEMENT

Positive reinforcement is a process that results in an increase in the probability of a behavior due to an increase in a contingent event. Steve, a new job coach for a paralegal in a law office, began praising his client for submitting his case reviews on time. Shortly thereafter, this reinforcement by praise greatly increased on-time case reviews. Positive reinforcement is the cornerstone of behavior management interventions. It has been used alone or in combination with other procedures to promote adaptive work behaviors across a wide range of client populations (Rusch, 1986).

Selection of the reinforcer is a critical process in developing an effective reinforcement program. TBI clients vary in their reinforcer preferences. A consequence that is reinforcing for one client may not be reinforcing for others. Some employees may enjoy being praised publicly by their supervisor, whereas, others may find such recognition embarrassing. The latter clients may prefer to receive recognition in a private meeting or in a memo. A work adjustment program will not be successful if the events or objects selected as reinforcers have little or no value to the client.

A number of stimuli or events can serve as reinforcers, including, food (e.g., a favorite snack at break), tokens, social attention, activities (e.g., assignment to a preferred work station, permission to leave work a few minutes early), positive feedback on performance, and money. There are several methods for identifying reinforcers. One of the most effective is to observe clients and note how they spend the majority of their time. Behaviors a client engages in frequently can be used to reinforce behaviors that occur less often (i.e., Premack Principle). A client may remain on task at his or her work station (low probability behavior) in order to earn time to socialize with staff (high probability behavior).

Another approach is to simply ask the client what he or she likes. The question may be asked in a variety of ways such as, "What do you like to do? What things make you happy? What is something you would be willing to work for? What would you hate to lose?" Typically, clients seek to provide input concerning their program and will readily provide a list of reinforcers. Other ways of discovering reinforcers include identifying workers with whom the client likes to work, activities engaged in during breaks, and activities or things enjoyed by people similar to the client.

Money is the primary motivation for going to work for many people. However, as the high job loss rate among TBI survivors indicates, receiving a paycheck periodically does not guarantee that a person will engage in the work behaviors needed to maintain employment. Although highly valued by almost everyone, money is typically not used as reinforcement for promoting adaptive work behaviors. As a reinforcer, its effectiveness is enhanced when given contingently and closely following behaviors to be increased. For example, Hermann, deMontes, Dominuez, Montes, and Hopkins (1973) reduced tardiness among 131 factory workers by providing small financial incentives each day for those employees who arrived to work on time.

Praise from supervisors is a common and potentially powerful reinforcer in the workplace. Most employees value recognition from their boss and it is a consequence that can be delivered contingently and immediately following the behavior to be increased or maintained. Also, praise and positive feedback occur naturally in the worksetting which facilitates the transfer from training contingencies to real-world contingencies.

For some TBI clients, however, verbal praise may not be reinforcing. Cognitive impairments, such as receptive aphasia, interfere with comprehension of spoken communication. Verbal praise to aphasics may be a source of confusion and frustration rather than a positive event. Other forms of praise and feedback, such as performance graphs or "thumbs up" gestures, may be effective in these cases.

There are several other factors which might limit the effectiveness of praise as a reinforcer. For example, clients that deny having any performance deficits may view the praise as trite or condescending. Older clients with years of pre-injury supervisory experience may resent praise from a younger person whom they perceive as less qualified and knowledgeable in the job than themselves. In these situations strategies such as self-monitoring and self-reinforcement, which place control with the client, may be used effectively. For example, Eric was a personnel manager for a major manufacturing company for 15 years prior to sustaining a TBI in a plane crash. Eighteen months following the injury, the major barrier preventing Eric from returning to his former position was that he frequently argued with his boss over his and his department's performance. The job coach first taught Eric to identify those situations in which his boss was likely to critique his performance. Prior to those meetings he rehearsed his response. The response to be increased was paraphrasing corrective feedback (e.g., "I understand, you want me to reduce overtime hours in my department by 20%.") and calmly offering his own opinion. Eric reinforced himself by recording each successful use of the strategy in his appointment book. Six months following intervention, Eric was still employed and had recorded 52 successful meetings to only nine unsuccessful ones.

Adhering to the following guidelines will maximize the effectiveness of reinforcement programs:

1. Deliver reinforcers immediately after the response to be increased. Immediate reinforcement is much more effective than delayed reinforcement. The immediacy with which the reinforcer follows the target response is especially critical for TBI clients with short-term memory disorders. The longer the reinforcement delay, the more difficult it is to learn association between behavior and the reinforcer.
2. Reinforcers and the behaviors upon which they are contingent should be specified for the client. In general behavior, change occurs more rapidly if the client is told which specific behaviors yield reinforcement and which do not. Telling a client, "You may take a break after you clean your work station," is not as informative as saying, "You may take a break after all the tools are returned to the storage room and the sawdust is swept from the floor." Similarly, it is better to say, "John, you worked on your proofreading job for an hour without stopping to talk. Great work!" than to say, "John, you did a good job today."
3. Speak slowly and pause frequently when specifying reinforcers and behaviors to clients with attentional deficits.
4. For clients with sequencing deficits, break instructions down into small steps. After you have finished, ask the client to repeat the instructions and reinforce correct responses.
5. Use a variety of reinforcers. This helps to maintain the positive value of the reinforcers and prevents satiation.
6. Initially, reinforcers should be given on a continuous schedule of reinforcement (immediately after the occurrence of each target response). Research has shown that conditioning occurs relatively slowly in persons with diffuse head injuries. Wood and Eames (1981) suggest that for these persons, continuous schedules of re-

inforcement should be implemented for numerous trials (until the response is consistently emitted) before fading to intermittent schedules.

Generalization and Maintenance

While initial learning is facilitated when reinforcement is given on a continuous schedule, in the natural environment reinforcement comes much less frequently. As stated above, once the client has acquired the response, the vocational counselor should shift from reinforcing it on each occurrence to reinforcing it after a variable number of occurrences. Behaviors that are reinforced intermittently will endure longer after reinforcement is completely withdrawn. Two types of intermittent reinforcement that produce steady rates of responding and which are resistant to extinction are variable ratio (VR) and variable interval (VI) schedules. On a VR schedule, reinforcement is delivered after a variable number of target responses. A client working in a mail room on a VR 10 schedule might receive reinforcement after first sorting one piece of mail correctly and then after each of 10, 20, 15, and 4 pieces were sorted. The average number of responses to earn reinforcement is 10.

On a VI schedule the reinforcer is delivered following the first response after a time interval has passed. The length of the time intervals between reinforcement varies randomly. A data entry clerk on a VI five-minute schedule is reinforced first after one minute, then again after seven, four, and eight minutes. At the end of each interval the client had to be working to receive reinforcement. The client did not know when the reinforcement would occur, but associated it with working at a steady rate.

With variable schedules of reinforcement, the time intervals or responses that are required before a single response is reinforced are gradually increased as the target behavior strengthens. Thinning the reinforcement schedule too rapidly can weaken performance. Return to reinforcing more frequently if the client's performance deteriorates on the leaner reinforcement schedule. The vocational counselor can never ensure that a target behavior will continue to be reinforced under natural work contingencies. It is critical, therefore, that the schedule of reinforcement be thinned out during training. This practice will promote more lasting behavior change increasing the likelihood of successful placement.

Another approach to enhance skill generalization is to utilize reinforcers that occur in the everyday work environment. Often the reinforcers used in training (tokens, points, special privileges, etc.) are not available in the natural environment. If behaviors have been developed with reinforcers specific to the training environment, there must be a transition in which those behaviors can be maintained with reinforcers common in the worksetting. As discussed earlier, money delivered contingent upon performance can be a very effective reinforcer. Also observe other workers at the job site to determine the nature and frequency of reinforcement in the natural environment. After skill acquisition is demonstrated, gradually shift from training reinforcers to more natural reinforcers. This transition is facilitated by pairing the naturally occurring consequences with the contrived reinforcers until those consequences are sufficient to maintain behavior.

Another way to promote skill generalization is to teach functional target behaviors that will have a high probability of being reinforced when they occur in the natural environment. In the workplace this would include classes of behavior such as punctuality, acceptance of new job responsibilities, acceptance of supervision, and prosocial behaviors. For example, workers who have learned to be congenial and cooperative are reinforcing to other people. Therefore, they are more likely to receive reinforcement from peers and supervisors than persons who are disagreeable or annoying. Similarly, workers who accept new job roles without argument are likely to elicit positive responses from their supervisors. This reinforcement serves to maintain these adaptive work behaviors.

Again, there are no guarantees that contingencies in the natural environment will reinforce appropriate behavior and extinguish maladaptive ones. In fact, oftentimes it is the maladaptive behavior that is reinforced by peers and staff. Therefore, a critical component of generalization programing is teaching supervisors, peers, and family members to identify and reinforce adaptive behaviors. In addition, clients can be taught to self-monitor and self-reinforce their behavior.

SHAPING

A supervisor might never have an opportunity to reinforce a behavior because it occurs so infrequently or not at all. This is especially true for complex behaviors requiring a sequence of responses. Shaping is a procedure for developing new behaviors that are not currently in the client's repertoire. It is a process in which "the terminal behavior is achieved by reinforcing small steps or approximations toward the final response rather than reinforcing the final response itself" (Kazdin, 1980, p. 139). Shaping begins by reinforcing responses already in the client's repertoire that either approximate or are the initial requisites of the desired behavior. As steps in the sequence are mastered, the criterion for reinforcement is gradually increased to a response that more closely approximates the terminal behavior.

The following case illustrates shaping to increase voice volume and intensity of a 34-year-old male construction worker who sustained a closed head injury in a motor vehicle accident. The client could meet the physical demands of his job as a roof trusser, but he exhibited severe "aphonia," a condition in which his voice volume and intensity were so low that his speech was barely audible. The condition interfered with his ability to communicate at work and threatened his employment. The terminal target behavior was to speak in a voice of normal intensity and volume. The shaping procedure began by having the client read aloud scripted vignettes of conversations among his co-workers while on breaks and at meetings. Initially he was reinforced for any audible words. On subsequent trials he was prompted to read louder. Each time the client read louder, he was given enthusiastic praise and approval by his job coach. If his voice dropped to a lower volume reinforcement was withheld. The procedure continued until he was reading the vignettes in a clear, audible voice. In the next phase, the job coach and the client role-played vignettes of social and instructional situations at work. The shaping process was repeated in this context until he was speaking at normal levels. In the final phase, the job coach arranged for conversations to occur between the client and his co-workers at the job site. Audible speech was maintained by positive responses from the client's co-workers and others.

An important question to consider in a shaping program is the size of each step in the shaping sequence and how much practice is required at each step. In general, if the client is consistently meeting the criterion for reinforcement at each successive step, then the length of the step and the amount of practice is appropriate. If performance begins to deteriorate to the point where the client's responses do not yield reinforcement, then the incremental steps are too large. Large numbers of nonreinforced trials can be frustrating and retard the learning process. The shaping schedule should be one that affords the client a great number of successes.

The effectiveness of shaping can be maximized by following these steps:

1. Behaviorally define the terminal behavior.
2. Behaviorally define the current performance level.
3. Reinforce a behavior in the client's repertoire that approximates the terminal behavior.
4. Withhold reinforcement for behaviors that are incompatible with or do not approximate the terminal behavior.
5. After a step in the sequence is mastered, increase the criterion for reinforcement to a response that represents a closer approximation to the terminal behavior. No longer reinforce behavior occurring earlier in the sequence.
6. Reinforce the terminal behavior on a continuous schedule.
7. Fade to an intermittent schedule of reinforcement when the terminal behavior is occurring consistently.

Generalization and Maintenance

Each of the generalization and maintenance strategies (i.e., selection of functional target behaviors, intermittent and natural reinforcement, self-monitoring) discussed in the positive reinforcement section apply to behaviors that have been established through shaping programs. In addition, as the delivery of reinforcement is being thinned to intermittent schedules, enlist relevant persons from the work or training site to give reinforcement. In the previous example, the job coach gained the support of the client's co-workers to reinforce normal speech and to ignore inaudible speech (i.e., they did not ask the client to repeat or speak louder if speech was not audible).

CONTINGENCY CONTRACTS

A contingency contract is a formal agreement between the vocational counselor and the client. It specifies which behaviors the therapist expects from the client and which reinforcers the client can earn by performing those behaviors. Contracts may be written or recorded on audio or videotape.

A contingency contract should include the following pieces of information:

1. Clearly defined target behaviors and reinforcers to be earned for those behaviors.
2. Consequences for failure to meet the terms of the contract stated in unambiguous language.
3. The conditions in which the target behaviors are to be performed so that it is clear when the terms of the contract have been met.
4. Schedules for the delivery of reinforcers.
5. Procedures for tracking the rate in which reinforcers are earned so progress can be monitored.

The contract should be written simply in a language that the client understands. Emphasis is placed on the positive consequences to be gained from performing the target behavior. The client and supervisor should work together to determine target behaviors, reinforcers, and consequences for not meeting the terms of the contract. After agreeing to the terms of the contract, both parties sign it.

The following illustrates the use of contracting to increase productivity and reduce complaining in a TBI client who had a job assembling aluminum vents for air conditioning and heating systems. The client complained frequently to co-workers and supervisors that he deserved a pay increase. The rate of complaining was so high it reduced his and others' productivity. The target behaviors selected by the job coach and agreed to by the client were: (1) increase the number of correctly assembled vents from an average of 30 per day to a minimum of 50 per day, and (2) reduce comments about pay increases to no more than two per day. Data on productivity and complaints were recorded and graphed each day by the job coach and supervisor. The contract stipulated that the client would receive a 10-cent per hour increase after two consecutive weeks of meeting the daily criterion for both behaviors. Each week thereafter for the next four weeks he could earn an additional 10-cent per hour increase provided target behaviors were maintained at criterion. Failure to meet the criterion resulted in no pay increase for that week. Six weeks after the contract was initiated the client had earned the maximum 50-cent per hour raise.

Generalization and Maintenance

One way a contract can promote generalization and maintenance is as a self-monitoring tool. The absence of self-monitoring skills contributes to the failure of performance gains to generalize across settings and persons (Koegel & Koegel, 1988). The contract promotes self-monitoring in several ways. First, the client assists in selection of target behavior(s). This shifts the client from a passive to an active role in the therapy process, increasing motivation to monitor progress. Second, the behavioral objectives are stated in concrete, observable terms which simply makes self-monitoring easier because the client knows what to monitor. Third, the client can use the contract as a cuing or prompting strategy by carrying it while working. Lastly the contract can stipulate that the client record and graph targeted behaviors. In the example above, the client could record his own productivity and complaint data. The reliability of this data could then be assessed by comparing it to the data kept by the supervisor and job coach. The degree of agreement between the two sets of data provides a measure of the client's awareness of his or her behavior and the impact it has on others.

SOCIAL SKILLS TRAINING

The head-injured survivor's attempts at social interactions with others often result in punishing consequences which serve to suppress overall social responding or lead to inappropriate behaviors that are reinforced. This learning history and underlying cognitive impairments can contribute to severe skill and performance deficits in which appropriate social behaviors rarely, if ever, occur in the worksetting. Therefore, the efficacy of shaping techniques at the actual work site are limited.

Social skill training programs (SST) are typically conducted in controlled settings where clients receive high density reinforcement and have a safe context to rehearse and develop target social responses. There are several advantages to teaching complex social responses in social skill training classes:

1. Clients can make mistakes without fear of punishment.
2. Shaping processes can be carried out more efficiently than in the work setting environment. Even the most basic social responses (e.g., eye contact with supervisor) can be heavily reinforced in the training session.
3. Audio and visual modeling can be used to demonstrate correct skill execution.
4. Critical social cues that signal when responding is appropriate and when it is not can be emphasized in training (e.g., supervisor smiling and greeting the employee vs. him or her frowning and not speaking).
5. Clients are given an opportunity to rehearse newly learned skills until they are mastered.
6. Training environments can be created that incorporate critical stimuli from work (e.g., a simulated restaurant with staff playing the role of customers could be created for a client learning to be a waitress).

The specific training methods employed in SST programs include: (1) instruction, (2) modeling, (3) role-play, (4) feedback and positive reinforcement, and (5) homework. Each training lesson begins with specific instructions to the clients about how to use the target skill. Clients are told when and where to use the skill and are given reasons why the skill is important. Kelly (1982) recommends that the clients recite the steps involved in using the skill and the benefits to be gained from using the skill. This actively involves the clients in the learning process and enables the instructor to identify students who are having difficulty comprehending the lesson. Instructions may also include a summary of previous lessons and an explanation of how the current skill adds to the skills already in the client's repertoire.

Modeling is the next step in SST programs. Modeling is used to demonstrate both correct and incorrect execution of the target behavior (Kelly, 1982). The skill may be modeled *in vivo* by trainers or presented on video or audiotape. Modeling is especially helpful when trying to explain complex aspects of social behavior, such as the correct timing of responses (e.g., when to ask for help, when to interject your opinion in a conversation). Whether the modeling is live or presented on tape, the actors should attempt to emulate as closely as possible the situation clients find troublesome. Research has identified several characteristics of models that enhance observational learning. Observers are more likely to imitate behavior of models that are similar in age, of the same sex, exhibit behavior that reflects warmth, receive positive outcomes from the interaction, and exhibit behavior closer to that of the observer than of highly competent persons (Bandura, 1969).

After observing models demonstrate the skill, clients rehearse it in role-play situations with trainers or other clients. Role-playing provides a means of practicing target behaviors in a variety of situations. Typically, role-plays include a description of a social situation followed by the delivery of a prompt line by the trainer. The role-play performance is repeated until the client's performance matches the criterion established by the trainer. Then, the client performs several additional errorless repetitions of the skill to promote mastery. The number of additional rehearsals should not exceed the client's tolerance level. Research with other populations has shown that too many repetitions may be frustrating and diminish the effectiveness of training (Hulicka & Weiss, 1965).

Immediately following role-plays, clients are given individual feedback on their performance. The feedback is directed toward specific behaviors (e.g., "Very good! When you corrected your co-worker's performance you were looking at him and spoke in a calm, clear voice."). First, positive feedback is given for behaviors role-played correctly. Then, behaviors performed incorrectly are pointed out and examples of appropriate alternatives are provided (e.g., "Jim, rather than looking at the floor, you will appear more attentive if you look your supervisor in the eyes when he is giving instructions."). To prevent information overload, feedback should be limited to the component behaviors taught in current or previous lessons. Most often, clients' role-play performance must be gradually shaped to meet the criterion set by the trainers. In some cases, trainers must begin by reinforcing participation in role-plays before providing feedback on specific target behaviors. Feedback on style and delivery aspects of social responses can be given after clients have mastered the specific behavioral components required of the interaction (i.e., teach what to say first, then teach how to say it).

Homework is the final step in SST programs. Clients are given assignments to use newly acquired skills in the worksetting. Specific instructions are given concerning where and when to use the skills. Homework assignments can be carried out individually and in pairs. Initially the job coach should accompany the client on a homework assignment to provide feedback and support and to conduct a functional analysis of the performance.

Generalization and Maintenance

The failure of social skills to generalize is often due to target behaviors being under the control of a limited range of stimuli. In other words, the client learns to perform the target responses, but only in the presence of specific training stimuli (e.g., the job coach, the training room, in role-plays). For example, the client responds appropriately to corrective feedback when it is given by his social skill teacher, but swears and yells when corrected by his supervisor at work.

As discussed in the section on task analyses, generalized responding is more likely when behavior is under the control of relevant features or stimulus classes rather than specific idiosyncratic stimulus elements. Relevant stimulus features are the characteristics that define membership in the stimulus class. For example, relevant stimulus features of corrective feedback situations include: assignment to a task; presence of an authority figure, such as a supervisor, job coach, and/or a teacher; and a request by the authority figure to change performance. Those elements define corrective feedback situations. These situations will differ on several irrelevant features, such as type and location of the task, and sex and appearance of the authority figure. Irrespective of these variations, the appropriate response includes looking at the supervisor, communicating in a clear way, acknowledging the feedback, and, if appropriate, changing performance.

General case programming (Horner, Sprague, & Wilcox, 1982), is a method of instruction designed to bring behavior under the control of stimulus classes. The method involves identification of the critical stimuli that define a stimulus class. Then, multiple teaching examples are presented that show the correct skill usage under a variety of stimulus conditions. Negative teaching examples may also be presented to teach the client when the performance of the target behavior is not appropriate. Here the use of minimum difference examples, where it is not readily apparent that performance of the behavior is inappropriate, yields more precise response generalization. A minimum difference example for corrective feedback situations might be a co-worker instructing the client to perform the task in a way that is contrary to the supervisor's original instructions. In this situation, the co-worker is not an authority figure and acknowledging the correction and changing performance is a generalization error that could result in a reprimand.

Overlearning or overpractice is another technique to enhance the generalizability of social skill training. Overlearning is a procedure in which the response to be learned is performed "over more trials than are necessary to produce initial desired changes in the subjects behavior...." (Lopez, 1980, p. 287). During skill training overlearning can be incorporated into role-play practice by requiring multiple errorless repetitions of the target skill. Practicing the skill with increased speed and fluency also enhances generalization (Koegel & Koegel, 1988). Following skill acquisition the job coach can time the speed with which clients responded during role-plays. Shaping procedures can then be applied to gradually increase the speed of responding. This will facilitate more natural and automatic performance in the workplace.

Reducing Behavioral Surpluses

As mentioned previously, behavioral surpluses are undesirable behaviors that must be reduced or eliminated if the client is to succeed in the workplace. The subsequent sections will describe the following behavior management techniques for reducing maladaptive social behavior in the workplace: stimulus change, differential reinforcement, extinction, time-out from reinforcement, overcorrection restitution, and overcorrection positive practice. Each of these procedures also involves reinforcing prosocial behaviors to take the place of maladaptive responses. The generalizability of competing prosocial behaviors can be enhanced using the techniques described previously.

STIMULUS CHANGE

All behavior occurs in the presence of a complex set of stimuli. The physical surroundings of the workplace, activity level, and tone of the supervisor's voice are all stimuli which can have an effect on behaviors that follow their presentation. Typically, maladaptive behaviors occur in the presence of some stimuli and not others. For example, a client may consistently behave aggressively when assigned to a noisy or crowded work area. The same client, when assigned to a quiet area, never engages in maladaptive behavior. In this case, the noisy, crowded environment evoked the aggressive behavior. The stimulation is aversive to the client and his aggressive behavior always results in his being removed from the area. The maladaptive behavior can be reduced simply by assigning the client only to a quiet work area. This procedure is referred to as stimulus change (Sulzer & Mayer, 1972).

As noted earlier, sometimes stimuli fail to occasion the behavior we desire. For example, the instruction "time to go to work" may be followed by inappropriate avoidance behavior (e.g., talking to co-workers, taking a cigarette break) rather than work. Through a process of stimulus change and reinforcement the instruction can come to exert the desired control over behavior. In the example above, the first step is to switch the client's job task from sanding plywood, which he found aversive, to operating the drill press which he found reinforcing. Now the instruction "time to go to work" is followed by a task that is reinforcing to the client, increasing the probability that desired target behavior, compliance with the instruction, will occur. Instructional control is established following numerous trials in which compliance with instructions results in a positive outcome. Once compliance is established with high probability behaviors, the instruction to engage in less desired activities can be given with a greater likelihood of success. The probability of compliance is further enhanced by task-analyzing the activity and reinforcing compliance to work on the component steps.

EXTINCTION AND DIFFERENTIAL REINFORCEMENT

Many maladaptive behaviors can be reduced or eliminated by withholding the reinforcers that follow them. Extinction is a simple but effective procedure "in which reinforcement for a previously reinforced behavior is discontinued" (Sulzer & Mayer, 1972, p. 290). For example, excessive arguing is often reinforced by the attention it brings from staff. Due to cognitive deficits associated with a TBI, staff often feel compelled to respond to a client's arguing with thorough and lengthy explanations. Rather than clarifying the client's understanding, these explanations may only serve to increase the likelihood that arguing will occur again the next time the client is given instructions. The staff member who responds to arguing by breaking eye contact and not talking to the arguing client, has put the behavior on extinction. Extinction, however, will only be effective if all staff respond in a similar fashion.

Although extinction produces long-stable changes in behavior, the effects are not immediate. This is especially true for long-standing behaviors that have a history of intermittent reinforcement. If negative behavior has had a long reinforcement history, it will continue to occur for a period of time after reinforcement has been discontinued. In fact, initially the frequency may increase somewhat. Consistent application of the extinction, however, will result in cessation of negative statements.

Effective extinction programs include the following elements:

1. Reinforcers maintaining the maladaptive behaviors are identified and withheld.
2. The extinction procedure is applied consistently and is maintained over time. (It should be noted that for certain behaviors, such as physical aggression or destructiveness, extinction should not be used. In most cases, aggressive or destructive behaviors cannot be ignored. Techniques discussed in subsequent sections are generally more appropriate to treat those behaviors.)
3. The extinction procedure is used along with positive reinforcement for other appropriate behaviors.

Differential reinforcement of other behaviors (DRO) combined with extinction results in a rapid reduction in maladaptive behavior. DRO is defined as reinforcement for any performance the client emits except for one particular response (the response to be decreased) (Ferster & Perrott, 1968, p. 524). The job coach who reinforces the argumentative client after each instruction in which he or she does not argue is using a DRO schedule of reinforcement.

Differential reinforcement of low rate of responding (DRL) is a variation of the DRO technique. DRL is a procedure in which low rates of responding are reinforced while high rates are not. This procedure is effective when the goal is to reduce, but not eliminate, a behavior. For example, a supervisor may want to reduce, but not necessarily eliminate, a client's social talking while working on an assembly line. In a DRL procedure, talking would only be permitted after a specified period of quiet working. In this case, the supervisor would have to ensure that other workers on the line ignored talking except at designated times.

Other variations on differential reinforcement are differential reinforcement of incompatible behaviors (DRI) and differential reinforcement of alternative behaviors (DRA). In the DRI procedure, reinforcement is withheld except for selected responses that are incompatible with the inappropriate behavior. For example, a DRI procedure would involve reinforcing the client for remaining at his or her work station, which is incompatible with or the opposite of leaving. Reinforcing a client for taking a deep breath and counting to 10 when feeling frustrated as an alternative to verbal abuse is an example of a DRA procedure.

TIME-OUT FROM REINFORCEMENT

Time-out refers to the removal of the opportunity to receive positive reinforcement (Kazdin, 1980, p. 167). It typically involves removing the client to a place where reinforcers are not available. For example, a client who enjoys his job as a telephone switchboard operator is removed to a less desirable work station for a brief period each time he makes an inappropriate flirtatious remark to female callers. Time-out may involve removing a client to either an area where he or she cannot see others engaged in reinforcing activities or one in which he or she can. Time-out may also involve the withdrawal of reinforcers or reinforcing events without removing the client (inclusionary time-out).

Hinman and Marr (1982) describe an application of time-out for a client in a sheltered workshop who had extremely poor grooming and personal hygiene skills. The intervention included instruction on the importance of grooming and cleanliness for success in work and training in basic personal hygiene. The time-out component involved requiring the client to work in an isolated area of the workshop if he arrived to work with unpleasant body odor.

The following steps will maximize the effectiveness of time-out (Marr, 1982, p. 140):

1. Time-out should be applied immediately after the inappropriate behavior.
2. Specify to the client the inappropriate behavior for which the time-out is being implemented.

3. Time-out should be limited to five to 10 minutes. Longer periods of time-out have not been shown to increase the effectiveness of the procedure.
4. The time measurement begins and continues only when the client ceases inappropriate behavior (screaming, arguing, complaining, etc.).
5. At the conclusion of time-out, tell the client what behaviors earned that consequence and that he or she will be timed-out again if the behavior occurs again.
6. Make sure all staff are trained to carry out the procedure and that they carry it out the same way each time.
7. Use time-out along with positive reinforcement for alternative appropriate behaviors.

OVERCORRECTION RESTITUTION AND POSITIVE PRACTICE

An overcorrection restitution procedure is one that requires the client to restore, clean, or repair the environment that was damaged by his or her behavior. Typically, the duration of the restitution activity should not exceed five to 10 minutes and should be a natural or logical consequence of the maladaptive behavior (Marr, 1982). For example, if the client becomes angry and overturns his worktable, he would be required to return the table to its upright position, return all work materials to their proper place, and straighten other tables and chairs in the immediate work area.

Overcorrection positive practice requires repeated rehearsals of an appropriate response that is incompatible with the behavior to be reduced. This procedure should be limited to three to five minutes. Positive practice can be a potent intervention with TBI survivors with cognitive deficits because it involves repetition of a desired behavior. Therefore, in addition to being a punishment procedure that suppresses maladaptive behavior, it also has an educational function that promotes new appropriate responses.

Positive practice is often used along with restitution. For example, the client who became frustrated and overturned his desk, after rectifying the physical damage, might also have to rehearse a more appropriate response to frustration, such as asking the supervisor for help. Positive practice is also an effective procedure for reducing surpluses that have no obvious negative effects on the environment, such as maladaptive verbal behaviors. A client who engages in high rates of complaining to the supervisor might be required to rehearse steps to appropriately schedule an appointment to discuss work problems.

Several points should be considered to maximize the effectiveness of overcorrection procedures. First, they should be applied consistently and immediately after each occurrence of the target behavior. Each of the steps outlined for the implementation of a time-out program also apply when carrying out an overcorrection consequence. Second, overcorrection procedures often require physical and/or verbal guidance to help the client through the task. Overcorrection procedures are designed to reduce the frequency of behaviors they follow. Therefore, care should be taken that the attention accompanying verbal and physical guidance is not reinforcing the behavior the procedure is intended to reduce. Staff verbalizations should be limited to feedback on performance and delivered in a neutral, direct manner. Third, if clients are physically resistive or combative during overcorrection, other treatments for reducing the behavior should be considered (e.g., DRO, time-out, contracting).

Conclusion

The most recent outcome studies reveal that post-acute rehabilitation programs providing short-term (three to nine months) intensive rehabilitation have had only limited success in returning TBI survivors to productive activity. TBI survivors must cope with lifelong impairments and disabilities. These problems require long-term intervention and follow-up. Research suggests supported employment is the most promising model to achieve better vocational outcomes for TBI survivors. However, to be effective, job coaches must have strategies to deal with the persistent cognitive and behavior problems that threaten job stability. Examining work adjustment problems from an applied behavioral perspective, this chapter has presented several principles and practical interventions to help rehabilitation professionals more effectively treat TBI survivors in worksettings.

References

Bandura, A. (1969). *Principles of behavior modification*. New York: Holt, Rinehart, & Winston.

Ben-Yishay, Y., Silver, S. M., Piasetsky, E., & Rattok, J. (1987). Relationship between employability and vocational outcome after intensive holistic cognitive rehabilitation. *Journal of Head Trauma Rehabilitation, 2*, 35-48.

Bellack, A. S., & Hersen, M. (1988). *Behavioral assessment: A practical handbook* (3rd ed.). Elmsford, New York: Pergamon Books, Inc.

Brooks, N., McKinlay, W., Symington, C., Beattie, A., & Campsie, B. A. (1987). Return to work within the first seven years of severe head injury. *Brain Injury, 1*, 5-19.

Cooper, J., Heron, T., & Heward, W. (1987). *Applied behavior analysis*. Columbus, OH.: Merrill Publishing Co.

Ferster, C. B., & Perrott, M. C. (1968). *Behavior principles*. New York: Appleton-Century-Crofts.

Foxx, R. M., Martelle, R. C., & Marchand-Martella, N. E. (1989). The acquisition, maintenance, and generalization of problem solving skills by closed head-injured adults. *Behavior Therapy, 20*, 61-76.

Haffey, W. J., & Lewis, F. D. (1989). Programming for occupational outcomes following traumatic brain injury. Special issue: Traumatic brain injury rehabilitation. *Rehabilitation Psychology, 34*(2), 147-158.

Hermann, J., deMontes, A., Dominuez, B., Montes, F., & Hopkins, B. (1973). Effects of bonuses for punctuality on the tardiness of industrial workers. *Journal of Applied Behavior Analysis, 6*, 563-570.

Hinman, S., & Marr, J. N. (1982). *Cases in behavioral consultation in rehabilitation*. (Research Report). Arkansas Rehabilitation Research and Training Center, Fayetteville, AR.

Horner, R., Sprague, J., & Wilcox, B. (1982). Constructing general case programs for community activities. In B. Wilcox & G. T. Bellamy (Eds.), *Design of high school programs for severely handicapped students* (pp. 61-98). Baltimore: Paul H. Brookes Publishing Co.

Hulicka, I. M., & Weiss, R. L. (1965). Age differences in retention as a function of learning. *Journal of Consulting Psychology, 29*, 125-129.

Jacobs, H. E. (1988). The Los Angeles head injury survey: Procedures and initial findings. *Archives of Physical Medicine and Rehabilitation, 69*, 425-431.

Kazdin, A. (1980). *Behavior modification in applied settings* (2nd ed.). Homewood, IL: The Dorsey Press.

Kazdin, A., & Straw, M. K. (1976). Assessment of behavior of the mentally retarded. In M. Hersen & A. Bellack (Eds.), *Behavioral assessment: A practical handbook* (pp. 337-368). New York: Pergamon Press.

Kelly, J. (1982). *Social skills training*. New York: Springer Publishing Co.

Koegel, R., & Koegel, L. K. (1988). Generalized responsivity and pivotal behaviors. In R. Horner, G. Dunlap, & R. Koegel (Eds.), *Generalization and maintenance* (pp. 41-66). Baltimore: Paul H. Brookes Publishing Co.

Lewis, F. D., Nelson, J., Nelson, C., & Reusink, P. (1988). Effects of three feedback contingencies on the socially inappropriate talk of a severely brain-injured adult. *Behavior Therapy, 19*, 203-211.

Lopez, M. A. (1980). Social skills training with institutionalized elderly: Effects of precounseling structuring and overlearning on skill acquisition and transfer. *Journal of Counseling Psychology, 27*, 286-293.

Marr, J. N. (1982). Behavioral analysis of work problems. In B. Bolton (Ed.), *Vocational adjustment of disabled persons* (pp. 127-147). Baltimore: University Park Press.

Pepping, M., Roueche, J. R., Epler, E., Heilbronner, R. L., Ayers, M., Smith, M., & Marshall, K. (1989). Long-term follow-up after neuropsychological rehabilitation for brain injury: Outcome study III. Unpublished manuscript.

Popovich, D. (1981). *Effective educational and behavioral programming for severely and profoundly handicapped students*. Baltimore: Paul H. Brookes Publishing Co.

Prigatano, G. P., Fordyce, D. J., Zeiner, H. K., Roueche, J. R., Pepping, M., & Wood, B. C. (1984). Neuropsychological rehabilitation after closed head injury in young adults. *Journal of Neurology, Neurosurgery and Psychiatry, 47*, 505-513.

Prigatano, G. P., Klonoff, P. S., & Bailey, I. (1987). Psychosocial adjustment associated with traumatic brain injury: Statistics BNI neurorehabilitation must beat. *BNI Quarterly, 3*, 10-17.

Roessler, R. T., Schriner, K. F., & Price, P. (May, 1990). *Employment concerns of people with head injuries*. Paper presented at the President's Committee on Employment of People with Disabilities, Washington, DC.

Rusch, F. R. (1986). *Competitive employment: Issues and strategies*. Baltimore: Paul H. Brookes Publishing Co.

Sailor, W., Goetz, L., Anderson, J., Hunt, P., & Gee, K. (1988). Research on community intensive instruction as a model for building functional, generalized skills. In R. Horner, G. Dunlap, & R. Koegel (Eds.), *Generalization and maintenance* (pp. 67-98). Baltimore: Paul H. Brookes Publishing Co.

Schneider, M. J., & Ferritor, D. E. (1982). The meaning of work. In B. Bolton (Ed.), *Vocational adjustment of disabled persons* (pp. 21-37). Baltimore: University Park Press.

Sulzer, B., & Mayer, R. (1972). *Behavior modification procedures for school personnel*. New York: Holt, Rinehart, & Winston.

Wehman, P., Kreutzer, J., Stonnington, H., Wood, W., Sherron, P., Diambra, J., Fry, R., & Groah, C. (1988). Supported employment for persons with TBI: A preliminary report. *Journal of Head Trauma Rehabilitation, 3*, 82-93.

Wehman, P., Kreutzer, J., Wood, W., Morton, M. V., & Sherron, P. (1988). Supported work model for persons with traumatic brain injury: Toward job placement and retention. *Rehabilitation Counseling Bulletin, 31*, 298-312.

Wehman, P., West, M., Fry, R., Sherron, P., Groah, C., Kreutzer, J., & Sale, P. (1989). Effect of supported employment on the vocational outcomes of persons with traumatic brain injury. *Journal of Applied Behavior Analysis, 22*, 395-406.

Wilms, W. (1984). Vocational education and job success: The employer's view. *Phi Delta Kappa, 65*, 347-350.

Wood, R. L., & Eames, P. (1981). Application of behaviour modification in rehabilitation of traumatically brain-injured patients. In G. Davey (Ed.), *Applications of conditioning theory* (pp. 81-101). London: Methuen.

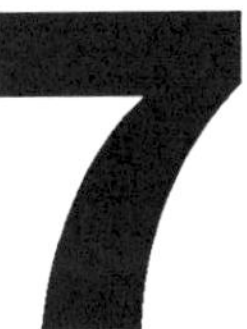

Supported Employment and the Vocational Restoration Process

David P. Mahaffey
Mary P. Ridgely

7

Supported Employment and the Vocational Restoration Process

David P. Mahaffey
Mary P. Ridgely

The vocational restoration process may be conceptualized as a "narrowing" process, both as it applies to persons with traumatic brain injury as well as to other disability groups (Lynch, 1983). Specifically, it is the task of the Vocational Rehabilitation Specialist, working with the client, the client's family member(s) or advocate, employer, physician, and various rehabilitation professionals and paraprofessionals, to identify that occupation or range of occupations for which the client is best-suited. Hypothetically, a given client is capable of performing any of a broad variety of occupations. The Vocational Rehabilitation (VR) Specialist begins to narrow this spectrum in a variety of ways, starting with the Diagnostic Interview.

Diagnostic Interview

The diagnostic interviewing process is critical to the success of vocational restoration efforts with persons who have sustained a traumatic brain injury. The client's self-report of psychosocial, cognitive, and related strengths and deficits, coping style, and vocational plans or lack thereof provides significant information to the VR Specialist. Given the nature of head injury and the potential for memory deficits, lack of insight, and organic denial of disability, it should be standard practice to solicit input from family members, friends/advocates, and other members of the rehabilitation treatment team as well (McMahon & Fraser, 1989).

The diagnostic interviewing process includes the following elements:

1) **Medical Background**: date of injury; surgical history; anticipated future surgical intervention; hospitalization history (including noninjury-related hospitalizations such as those for chemical dependency); rehabilitation history; current medical intervention, including medication; physical, cognitive, communicative, psychosocial, self-care, and behavioral assets and limitations; visual status, dominant hand; and mobility and ambulation limitations.

2) **Vocational Background**: current employer; contact person; dates of employment; job titles and duties, including physical, cognitive, and psychosocial requirements; union status; wage and salary history; military history; a review of the client's hobbies, interests and special skills, especially "pre-learned" skills which may translate to a potential job; and a review of the client's stated vocational plan or lack thereof.

3) **Educational Background**: academic and technical training; most and least preferred subject matter; attitude toward retraining; plans for future schooling or training.

4) **Demographic Data and Miscellaneous Areas**: marital status; number and ages of dependents; spouse's job status; current sources of family income; driving status; access and ability to use public transportation; litigation status; the presence of disincentives regarding return-to-work; the client's perception of what must occur pursuant to a return-to-work; and a review of potential positions available with the previous employer, if applicable.

Vocational Assessment

Following the Diagnostic Interview, the VR Specialist may begin the process of narrowing the range of occupational choices by more closely examining the client's interests, aptitudes, work values, temperaments, and academic skills. Assessment information gathered from the TBI transdisciplinary team, including Speech, Occupational, and Physical Therapies, Neuropsychology, Physiatry, and other medical specialties will provide needed data pertaining to various client assets and limitations. Specific cognitive functions, (e.g., attention and concentration, thinking and reasoning, information processing speed); psychosocial assets and limitations (e.g., decreased alcohol or drug tolerance, social isolation, impulsivity); communicative assets and limitations (e.g., functional communication status, functional academic skills status, interpersonal pragmatics); and independent living skills assets and limitations (e.g., community mobility status, self-care status) are typically included as a portion of such an assessment (Wachter, Fawler, & Mason, 1987).

A functional assessment, utilizing individualized situational assessment and on-the-job evaluation is generally the preferred method for obtaining the most useful information regarding work behaviors, quality, rate, endurance, skill acquisition, and interests. Placement readiness can be further augmented by utilizing volunteer work, job tryouts, or work trials (McMahon & Fraser, 1989).

The range of targeted occupations can be further narrowed by taking into account the job market within a given location, the client's earning requirements, and the employer's expressed versus actual job requirements and related factors (Lynch, 1983). It is worth noting that throughout the course of the vocational rehabilitation process, the client may be engaged in a variety of concurrent activities including, but not limited to, job seeking skills training, job analysis, work hardening services, vocational counseling, labor market survey data, and so forth. It is beyond the scope of this chapter to detail the ways in which these services are tailored given the special needs of individuals with traumatic brain injury.

Placement Hierarchy

It is the task of the Vocational Specialist, in conjunction with those parties noted earlier, to determine the most effective and efficient means of returning the TBI client to gainful employment utilizing the process outlined above. If it is determined that supported employment is the most likely method for meeting these criteria, it is at this point that such services are typically offered. Supported employment services are offered within the context of a hierarchy of return to competitive employment. This hierarchy is conceptualized as follows:

1. return to work in previous job with previous employer;
2. return to work in previous job with supports, with previous employer;

3. return to work in new job with previous employer;
4. return to work in new job with supports with previous employer;
5. return to work in new job with new employer;
6. return to work in new job with supports with new employer;
7. training;
8. affirmative industry placement; and
9. volunteer placement.

The Vocational Specialist, client, transdisciplinary team, previous employer, internal and/or external case manager, union business agent, and others may provide input regarding the hierarchical level to which initial vocational restoration efforts should be directed.

Characteristics of Supported Employment

As specified in the Federal Register, Supported Employment is defined as "(i) Competitive work in an integrated work setting with on-going support services for individuals with severe handicaps for whom competitive employment (A) has not traditionally occurred; or (B) has been interrupted or is intermittent as a result of severe handicaps;" (*Federal Register*/Vol. 52, No. 157/August 14, 1987, Part 363.7). This document further clarifies the characteristics of supported employment:

(1) "Competitive work means work that is performed on a full-time basis or on a part-time basis, averaging at least 20 hours per week for each pay period and for which an individual is compensated" [at minimum wage or above];

(2) "Integrated work setting means job sites where most co-workers are not handicapped; and individuals with handicaps are not part of a work group of other individuals with handicaps;... or have regular contact with non-handicapped individuals, other than personnel providing support services, in the immediate work setting";

(3) "On-going support services means continuous or periodic job skill training services...[and] other support services provided at or away from the work site, such as transportation, personal care services, and counseling to family members..."

Types of Support

Supported employment is often considered to be synonymous with the provision of job coaching services in the work site. In fact, job coaching is but one type of support available to the client. Broadly speaking, any type of intervention which enables the client to maintain his or her competitive employment status may be considered "support." Examples of both on- and off-site supports include, but are not limited to, the following (Tooman, Revell, & Melia 1987):

1. informed supervision (i.e., the on-site presence of a client's supervisor who is knowledgeable as to how the consequences of TBI affect the ability of the supervised worker to successfully carry out his or her job duties);

2. transportation (e.g., provision of specialized transportation services such as wheelchair adapted vehicle);

3. training (e.g., on-the-job skill training);

4. counseling (e.g., on-the-job behavioral counseling);

5. job engineering;

6. job restructuring;

7. alternative work schedules (e.g., gradual re-entry scheduling, "flex" time, permanent part-time, compressed workweek);

8. barrier removal;

9. employer education;

10. job coaching;

11. job modification; and

12. natural supports (e.g., co-workers who take an interest in assisting the client in carrying out his or her job duties).

It is important to note that each of the above supports are provided *throughout the course* of the employment experience. Additionally, the number, type, variety, frequency, and nature of the supports offered may well change during the course of the supported employment placement. This is particularly true for individuals with traumatic brain injury who are often subject to nonlinear courses of recovery in several functional areas for many months or years following the date of injury. Finally, most of the supports noted constitute "reasonable accommodations" as specified in the recently enacted *Americans with Disabilities Act.*

Advantages of the Supported Employment Approach

Among the potential advantages of using a supported employment approach with persons with traumatic brain injury are the following (Mank, Rhodes, & Bellamy, 1986):

1. The "place and train" approach (i.e., the client is placed in a supported employment position even if that client is not considered to be "job ready") as opposed to the more traditional "train and place" approach allows for immediate re-entry into a "real work" setting.

2. It affords the opportunity to assess and remediate those cognitive and psychosocial deficits – and in particular, behavioral limitations – which so often impede successful re-entry into the competitive work force.

3. It allows for on-site advocacy and timely intervention with the client's work supervisor in the event of work-related problems.

4. Ongoing assessment can be accomplished and the effectiveness of compensatory strategies devised by such professionals as speech, occupational, and physical therapists can be evaluated in a vocational context.

5. It restores the client's identity as a worker.

6. It provides financial compensation for real work.

7. It affords the opportunity for training on the actual job site versus in a less realistic clinical environment. The increased face-validity of the training environment minimizes the risks of poor generalization of treatment effects.

8. It provides a real-world context for the provision of other therapies thereby potentially enhancing the functional orientation of those therapies.

Potential Barriers to Supported Employment for Persons with Traumatic Brain Injury

These issues must be addressed for successful supported employment:

1. Supported employment can be costly. The provision of such ongoing supports as job coaching, barrier removal in certain instances where substantial work site renovation is required, transportation, and so forth may be costly both financially as well as in time required by both the employer and support personnel. The establishment and implementation of guidelines enforcing the provisions of the *Americans with Disabilities Act* recently passed by congress will provide data regarding the cost of providing supported employment services during the next five to 10 years.

2. Employment retention is historically moderate.

3. On-site intervention may be obtrusive or may be perceived as such by the client, the employer, and/or the co-workers.

4. The client may feel the on-site intervention will call attention to his or her disability.

5. Difficulties may arise in the areas of union guidelines and collective bargaining agreement precedent-setting. Resistance may be encountered in certain instances where supports provided to an individual with brain injury may be sought by other workers who are attempting to reintegrate into the competitive work force. Such issues may arise regardless of whether or not the client has experienced a work-related injury.

6. Resumption of paid employment may result in the discontinuation of workers' compensation and other disability benefits, as well as the assumption of liability for previous medical conditions by a new employer. Careful planning can alleviate these concerns and eliminate problems.

7. The availability of structured training for job coaches is currently limited.

8. Funding for job coaching and employer education is inadequate.

The Wisconsin Supported Employment Project

The following is a summary of the *Supported Employment and Traumatic Brain Injury First Year Report*, conducted by the Wisconsin Department of Health and Social Services (WDHSS), Division of Vocational Rehabilitation (WDVR) (Ridgely, 1990). This project was supported by a grant from the National Institute on Disability and Rehabilitation Research.

BACKGROUND

The WDHSS Brain Injury Task Force conducted a two-year survey of Wisconsin residents who had experienced a traumatic brain injury. Approximately 900 responses were received from head injury survivors, their families, and/or advocates. According to the final report published on April 6, 1988, of those surveyed "nearly sixty percent (60%) were supported by their own earnings before the injury, but less than twenty-five percent (25%) were [self supporting] after the injury. Before the injury less than two percent (2%) were receiving Social Security Disability Income. Following the injury, almost fifty percent (50%) were receiving disability payments. Vocational training and job placement were identified by respondents as the most needed services, followed by supported employment, work adjustment, vocational rehabilitation, education, financial assistance, behavior management programs and social skills training." (p. iii).

In response to the clearly documented need, the primary objective of the supported employment program developed by WDVR was to generate successful employment outcomes for clients who had previously been referred to the state vocational rehabilitation system, but whose files had been closed as "unsuccessful rehabilitant." The clients' cases had been closed for a variety of reasons, including: (1) the client did not meet eligibility criteria (e.g., determined not feasible for competitive employment); (2) the vocational rehabilitation plan was not implemented; and (3) the plan was implemented but services did not result in employment. The pilot project was located in Dane County, Wisconsin. This area was chosen primarily for its long-standing commitment to the supported employment concept and the availability of vendors. A review of clients with head injury residing in Dane County whose files were closed between 1984 and 1988 for the reasons listed above and a review of active cases notable for their extended length of involvement with the state vocational rehabilitation system generated a list of 43 potential project participants. An in-depth file review was conducted to confirm the diagnosis of traumatic brain injury, determine the current employment status of the individual, and to evaluate the need for long-term support services. The following criteria were applied when considering participants for the project:

1. demonstration of a willingness to participate in the project;
2. the need for long-term support, to be provided by the County Human Service Agency;
3. medical stability; and
4. availability of a "natural" support system (e.g., family, advocate).

A Project Coordinator was identified during the initial grant year, project vendors were solicited via proposal requests, and a training program was developed for direct service providers. Two vendors were selected to receive grant awards effective August 1988. These providers are referred to as Agency A and Agency B. Both selected agencies have ongoing contracts with the county human service agency responsible for providing the long-term support to persons with head injury in Wisconsin. This was critical to the success of the individual participants, since each would be transitioned to the county for long-term support following a period of 12 months in the project.

Each agency agreed to place five project participants per year into supported employment settings. Using the above-mentioned selection criteria, 10 individuals were referred to the project agencies in October 1988. These individuals presented with a mean age of 22 years at the time of injury, and a mean age of 30 at the time of referral. Mean length of time in coma was 58 days, with a range of less than 24 hours to 210 days. Seventy percent of the injuries were secondary to alcohol-related incidents. Thirty percent of the participants had some college-level experience, 60% were high school graduates, and 10% did not complete high school prior to their injury. Ninety percent of the participants received some form of public assistance during the first project year, and 30% had received some form of financial settlement secondary to a past legal action. Table 1 provides an overview of demographic data for project participants.

A two and one-half-day comprehensive training program was provided for direct service staff, county case managers, and VR Counselors prior to initiating client service delivery. Appendix A contains the **Model Training Outline**. Literature and technical assistance were provided to project staff on an ongoing basis by the Project Coordinator.

Project activities were documented on a daily basis and were tabulated by the Project Coordinator. Additionally, project staff were required to complete the **Wisconsin Supported Employment Information System** (WSEIS) forms. Appendix B contains examples of these forms. A "TBI

Table 1

Demographic Data of SE/TBI Project Participants

Persons Served Year 1	Years Since Injury	Age at Injury	Age at Enrollment	Cause of Injury	Alcohol Related	Length of Coma (Days)	Level of Education	Previous Setting	DVR Services Provided	Public Assistance		Living Arrangement
1	5	25	30	MVA	YES	21	G.E.D.	NONE	Driving Assmnt Funct. Capacities	SSI SSDI	99.72 377.00	W/PARENTS
2	8	31	39	Diabetic	YES	90	H.S.+	NONE	NONE	SSI SSDI	340.16 237.00	ALONE
3	9	20	28	MVA	YES	63	H.S.+	Employed (LTE)	Placement Evaluation Psychological	NONE		ALONE
4	4	18	21	Motorcycle	NO	210	H.S.	NONE	NONE	SSI	470.72	W/ATTEND.& ROOMMATE
5	6	21	27	Pedestrian	NO	29	H.S.+	NONE	Evaluation, Placement, Job Coach	SSDI	292.50	ALONE
6	3	35	37	MVA	YES	1	>H.S.	NONE	NONE	SSDI INS	557.00 977.00	ALONE
7	9	18	27	MVA	YES	42	H.S. (After Inj.)	NONE	Evaluation, Trans. Employment, Homecrafter	SSI SSDI	186.00 260.00	ALONE
8	14	17	30	MVA	YES	14	H.S.	NONE	Evaluation, Trans. Employment, Placement	SSDI	632.00	W/PARENTS
9	4	20	23	Motorcyle	YES	20	H.S.	NONE	Evaluation, AOOA Assessment	SSI SSDI	168.00 323.00	W/PARENTS
10	18	18	37	MVA	YES	90	H.S.	NONE	Evaluation, Mobility Trng., Clerical Trng., Situational Assessment, Placement	SSI SSDI	423.00 67.52	ALONE
Averages	8	22	30			58						

MALES=8 FEMALES=2

x age at injury = 22
x yrs since injury = 8
x age at enrollment = 30
x days in coma = 58

% alcohol-related injuries = 70%
% receiving public assistance = 90%

Level of Education:
Less than H.S. = 10%
H.S. Grad or equiv. = 60%
Some college = 30%

Supplement" was added to this system and was utilized by all supported employment providers around the state to provide information concerning clients with head injury in their programs.

METHODS

The research component of the grant involved a comparison of employment outcomes for participants pre-injury, post-injury, and following the provision of supported employment services. The length of time since the date of injury ranged from three to 18 years. Six clients had competitive work histories prior to their injuries; the remaining four were students or recent graduates at the time of their injuries. One individual was employed in a limited-term position at the time of referral. Four participants had previously been competitively placed through traditional vocational rehabilitation intervention, however, none of the jobs lasted more than six months.

Following intake, project staff conducted a review of all background information on each participant. A Functional Assessment provided information on functional abilities in a variety of settings, including activities of daily living. If appropriate, a work trial was developed to assess the client's interests, skills, assets, and limitations. Work trials were limited to nonprofit businesses/organizations, and were generally one to six weeks in duration.

PROJECT OUTCOMES: FIRST YEAR

Work Status of Participants

Table 2 describes the pre- and post-employment status of each client since the onset of their involvement with the project.

One participant was terminated before job development due to excessive drug usage and medical instability. Of the remaining nine clients, eight became employed from October 1, 1988 to September 30, 1989. One client relocated out of the project area, returned, and reapplied for services. Consequently, active job development on this individual's behalf did not begin until August 1989.

Two participants discontinued their jobs, and their involvement in the project, two to three months after job placement. Both of these individuals had substance abuse issues; one, in fact, was charged with Driving While Intoxicated and was ordered into treatment. (He subsequently reapplied for project services, which were reinitiated in January

Table 2
Employment Status of SE/TBI Project Participants

Persons Served	Preinjury Job Title	Preinjury Wage	Post-injury Job Title	Post-Project Job Title	Date Hired	Weekly Hours	Hourly Wage	Total Hrs. Intervention	Total Months Worked as of 10/1/89	Reason for Separation	Work Trials/ Dates
Agency A											
1	Groundskeeper County Suprv	unknown unknown	not employed	n/a	n/a	0.00	0.00	167.75	0.00	Term. from Project	
2	Furniture Mover	5.25	not employed	Counter sales	3/27/89	40.00	5.25	273.00	8.00		Art Rm Asst, Teacher Aide, Counter sales
3	Lab Animal Caretaker	4.00	Maintenance Janitorial	Maintenance Housekeeping Laundry	7/88 4/5/89 9/25/89	20.00 40.00 24.00	6.25 6.25 5.00	178.50	9.00 3.00 .25	LTE Behavior	Lab Animal Caretaker
4	Student	0.00	not employed	Clerical	6/7/89	12.00	0.00	474.75	4.00		Art Rm. Asst.
5	Student	0.00	Stock clerk Food service	Counter sales Asst Technician	3/14/89 6/12/89	20.00 18.00	4.25 4.25	350.00	2.00 3.50	New job	Elect. Assem. Parts Clerk
6	Nursing Asst.	2.10	Clerical	Clerical	1/1/90	15.00	5.28	53.00	0.00		Clerical
Agency B											
7	Student	0.00	not employed	Clerical	6/26/89	20.00	3.75	214.00	3.00		
8	Laborer	8.00	not employed	Lunchrm Asst Janitor	5/1/89 7/13/89	3.00 20.00	5.25 4.00	265.00	1.00 2.00	LTE Behavior	Lunchrm Asst.
9	Student	0.00	Clerical	Dough roller Clerical	5/1/89 7/6/89	20.00 20.00	4.00 4.00	340.00	1.50 3.00	Slow rate	
10	Construction	8.00	not employed	Clerical	6/26/89	20.00	4.25	132.00	3.00	Disliked job	

1990.) Two additional clients separated from their initial jobs, and were subsequently placed into other positions. The reasons for separation included behavioral problems on the job, unsatisfactory work rate, and expressed job dissatisfaction.

Allocation of Client Project Hours

Table 3 shows a comparison of each participants' total time in the project with the number of hours spent in work trials, volunteer placements, and paid employment.

Table 3

Total Time in Project Compared with Time in Work Trials, Volunteer and Paid Work; Time Spent in Work Activity as a Percentage of the Total Hours in Project

Client	Hrs. in Project	Work Trial Hours	Volunteer Hours	Hours in Paid Work	%
1	824	0	0	0	0
2	1880	216	0	1082	69
3	1544	40	0	528	37
4	1704	153	144	0	17
5	1224	40	0	325	30
6	528	24	0	0	5
7	2048	0	0	276	13
8	2048	39	0	219	13
9	2048	0	0	392	19
10	1704	0	0	256	15

The amount of time participants were involved in work activity as a percentage of the total number of possible hours of service varied from five percent (services for this participant began late in the project year) to 69% (this client worked 40 hours per week). One client was terminated before job development began, as indicated earlier, indicated by a zero at the top of the table.

Allocation of Staff Project Hours

Table 4 shows the relationship between staff intervention hours and the number of hours worked (in paid employment) by participants from October 1, 1988 to September 30, 1989.

Table 4

Hours in Paid Employment Compared with Hours of Staff Intervention Per Client

Client	Paid Work	Direct Service	Indirect Service	Support Service	Total Services
1	0	29.5	119.75	18.5	167.75
2	1042	160.25	79.25	33.5	273.0
3	528	84.0	47.75	46.75	178.5
4	0	311.5	107.0	56.25	474.75
5	325	311.25	33.75	5.0	350.0
6	0	39.5	11.0	2.75	53.25
7	276	278.6	171.25	67.0	516.85
8	219	85.04	174.75	85.0	344.79
9	392	344.09	175.25	41.5	560.84

Participants served by Agency A spent a total of 1,895 hours in paid employment, while those served by Agency B worked 1,168 hours. Overall, clients doing paid work received DIRECT services 61% of the time; INDIRECT services were provided 34% of the time; and SUPPORT services were provided 13% of the time. A DAILY MONITORING FORM lists the services in each category, and was completed each day by the job coach or employment training specialist. Under DIRECT services, the employment training specialist documents time spent *at the work site in direct contact with the participant*. Evaluation/assessment, skills training, behavior management, monitoring productivity, planning or counseling worker, job accommodation/modification, transportation/mobility, and employer/co-worker training and intervention are included in this category. INDIRECT services are those which do not require face-to-face contact, such as job analysis, job development, interagency consultation, coordination of services, staff training, and administrative duties (paperwork). SUPPORT services are those provided directly to the participant, but *away from* the work site (i.e., housing and residential assistance, transportation/mobility [non-job], health and medical needs, financial management, employment and career guidance, supportive counseling, planning with family or others, recreation and social assistance, support groups).

Factors which influenced job performance and retention most frequently were alcohol and other drug use, decreased anger control, job dissatisfaction, anxiety, and depression. Project staff spent significant amounts of time on service coordination – researching resources and making referrals to services agencies including chemical dependency programs, psychotherapy services, residential support services, adaptive recreation services support groups, and adult education and career counseling services. Time devoted to these activities is reflected in the incidence of indirect services provided to clients noted in Table 4.

The first year data from both agencies was compared relative to the *Total* and *Average* number of hours provided to project participants from October 1, 1988 to September 30, 1989. Agency A served a total of six clients, while Agency B served five clients. Job Coach intervention for Agency A included 925 hours of *direct*, 400 hours of *indirect*, and 150 hours of *support* intervention. Job Coach intervention for Agency B included 925 hours of *direct*, 650 hours of *indirect*, and 233 hours of *support* intervention.

Service Provision Guidelines

A review by the Project Coordinator and Project Advisory Committee in May 1989 of the hours of service reported by the two agencies in the three categories (direct, indirect, and support services) prompted the development of *Service Provision Guidelines* which were included in the second-year contract for services. These guidelines were modified for the county and state planners to use in developing new services for persons with traumatic brain injury. It is anticipated that this service model will be further modified as the project draws to a close in September 1990. Appendix C contains a copy of the Service Provision Model developed as a guide for VR Field Offices and County Managers.

Client Satisfaction, Substance Abuse, and Adjustment Counseling

A consumer satisfaction survey was conducted to determine the level of satisfaction among project participants served during the first project year. Participants were interviewed in their homes. Interview questions covered the following areas:

1) satisfaction with the job, its location, work environment, supervisor and co-worker relationships, and wage level;

2) satisfaction with the method of transportation to/from work;

3) satisfaction with the vendor agency, job coach, and level of assistance; and

4) general feelings about life/self since onset of participation in the project.

Seventy-one percent of the participants stated that they were satisfied with their current job, and 86% were satisfied with the number of hours that they were working. Forty-three percent were satisfied with the speed with which the vendor placed them in a job, and 71% were pleased with the level of assistance they received from a job coach.

Project staff were disturbed by the termination of one participant due to drug use. The individual had received five months of intensive services from project staff – contacting substance abuse professionals, coordinating medical appointments, meeting with home-care health professionals, counseling the individual – before the decision to stop services was made. When it became evident that other participants were actively using drugs and/or alcohol (eight out of the 10 admitted to using chemicals), the Project Coordinator invited substance abuse professionals to a joint meeting with head injury professionals to begin sharing information and discuss treatment alternatives. The monthly dialogue between the two professional groups resulted in a heightened awareness of the needs of this unique population, and made it possible for two project participants to obtain individualized services for alcohol and drug abuse, therefore increasing their chances for success on the job.

Another service need identified by project staff was adjustment counseling. Several of the participants voiced feelings of loneliness, depression, thoughts of suicide, and anxiety. Project staff located mental health clinicians in the Dane County area who were willing to develop expertise in serving persons with head injury to provide psychotherapy and related services. Often what appeared to be resistance on the part of project participants to job development efforts was actually fear of failure. In therapy, they could address their fears and, consequently, experienced positive changes at the job site. Even if the job was going well, often there were other issues (e.g., family dynamics, social/sexual needs, independent living, future planning) which needed to be addressed.

One example of this need to ensure access to adjustment counseling was an individual who was in the middle of divorce proceedings at the time of his referral to the project. Project staff recognized that little would be accomplished until he had dealt with his feelings about the divorce. Consequently, he was referred to a divorce support group. Project staff accompanied him to the meetings, and afterwards spent time reviewing the information shared. This experience proved to be extremely helpful to the participant, and the divorce group became a natural support network for him.

Discussion

Based upon this project review it would appear that a supported employment approach making use of informed selection criteria, offering a variety of required supports, and providing services using trained personnel is effective in restoring the client with head injury to the competitive work force. It also appears that this approach is effective with individuals who present with limited or nonexistent employment histories and those who have been unsuccessfully placed in the past through "traditional" vocational rehabilitation services offered by a state VR agency. The direct services provided in the form of a job coach were costly in terms of time and financial resources required to place and maintain individual clients on the job, and the level of indirect and support services was also considerable. Additionally, it is worth noting that services were offered in a geographic area that is noted both for its high quality and numbers of social services as well as experience with the supported employment approach.

The Wisconsin study underscores the need for a variety of support services offered in conjunction with those directly related to job placement and job maintenance. Specifically, the issues of substance abuse and social isolation were raised repeatedly by members of the project staff. These issues are not unique to this particular sample. Rather, they are representative of those psychosocial issues which present barriers to the successful reintegration of individuals with head injuries into the work force. These barriers have been discussed in detail elsewhere (Fraser, Clemmons, & McMahon, 1990) and commonly include the following:

1. major depression;
2. decreased initiative;
3. social isolation;
4. decreased alcohol/drug tolerance;
5. decreased sense of personal "responsibility";
6. irritability;
7. impulsivity.

The need for designated substance abuse programs for persons with head injury is apparent, as is the need for ongoing supportive counseling, identification, and/or development of a support network. Behavioral programming to eliminate negative behaviors and introduce those behaviors required to "get along" with one's co-workers is also essential.

Development of formalized training programs for Job Coaches and other personnel concerned with the implementation of supported employment opportunities for persons with traumatic brain injury is also of paramount importance to the successful reintegration of such individuals into the work force on a long-term basis. Vocational specialists and others will have the opportunity to impact on the development of specific implementation guidelines of the *Americans with Disabilities Act* as it pertains to the restoration of individuals with brain injury to competitive employment via supported employment.

Supported employment, combined with the impetus provided by the *Americans with Disabilities Act*, may well be used as a primary means of vocational re-entry for adults surviving brain injury in the 1990s and beyond.

Appendix A

Wisconsin Division of Vocational Rehabilitation Supported Employment and Traumatic Brain Injury Training Outline for Job Coaches and Direct Service Providers

I. BRAIN INJURY OVERVIEW

A. Definition of Brain Injury

1. The Wisconsin Act 307 (substitute own state legislation)
2. Causes
3. Incidence

B. Diagnosing the Damage

1. Types of impairments
2. The "invisible disability"
3. Impairments in executive functioning

C. Course of Treatment and Factors in Long-term Improvement

1. Acute medical treatment
2. Post-acute rehabilitation
3. Factors affecting long-term improvement
4. Myths of recovery

II. WORKING WITH FAMILIES/SIGNIFICANT OTHERS

A. Understanding the Affect of Brain Injury on the Family

1. Scenario (story of local family)

2. Other concerns (have group generate list)

B. Involving the Parent/Guardian/Spouse or Significant Other

1. Why is this important?

2. Strategies for increasing participation

III. GATHERING INFORMATION/INTAKE PROCEDURES

A. Sources of Information

B. What to Collect

1. Social/vocational history

2. Medical information

C. Using/Interpreting Information from Rehab Professionals

IV. INDIVIDUALIZED ASSESSMENT

A. Conducting the Assessment (using "FRIP" analysis developed by Stacy Graff under contract with Wisconsin Div. of Vocational Rehab)

B. Using Assessment Information

V. DEVELOPING A TEAM

A. Rehabilitation Services and Professionals

B. Definition of Service Categories

C. Local Resources

D. Service Coordination

VI. JOB DEVELOPMENT/TRAINING/FOLLOW-ALONG

A. Job Development

1. How it is similar to working with other disability groups

2. How it differs from other disability groups

B. Helping Employer/Co-workers Understand Brain Injury

1. Do's and Don'ts

2. *Hiring the Head Injured* - a manual for employers (DeBosky & Morin, 1986)

C. Place/Train/Follow-along

1. The place and train method

2. Follow-along

Appendix B

DEPT OF HEALTH & SOC SERVICES STATE OF WISCONSIN
DIV OF VOCATIONAL REHABILITATION
DVR-62 (Rev. 3/89)

ONE-TIME CLIENT DATA REPORT
SUPPORTED EMPLOYMENT
(WSEIS Manual, Form DVR - for Instructions for Completion)

1. Agency/Provider Name____________________________

2. County ____________________________

3. Client____________________________
Last name First name

4. Date of Report ____/____/____

5. Client Social Security No. ____________________________

6. Start date in program ____/____/____

7. DVR Client Account No.____________________________

8. DVR Counselor ____________________________

9. Client pre-employment benefits (circle those that apply) SSDI, SSI, PUBLIC ASSISTANCE, NONE, UNKNOWN, OTHER.

10. Total Amount of Cash Grant (Monthly) $__________ (From #9 above)

11. Disability (circle the P = primary and S = secondary next to the client's disability(ies)

Seizure disorder	P	S	*Traumatic Head Injury	P	S
Autism	P	S	Blind/Legally Blind	P	S
Cerebral Palsy	P	S	Physical/orthopedic	P	S
Schizophrenia	P	S	Sensory Impairment or Hearing-Impaired	P	S
Bipolar disorder	P	S	Learning disability	P	S
Personality disorder	P	S	Mental retardation	P	S
Other (identify)	P	S	Unknown	P	S
____________			Alcholism/Drug Abuse	P	S

*Complete DVR - if Traumatic Head Injury is the Primary or Secondary disability.

12. Living arrangement (check individual's current living arrangement)

_____ Independent
_____ Group Home
_____ DD Center or Mental Health Institute
_____ Unknown
_____ With parents/relatives
_____ Semi-independent setting (e.g., supported appartment)
_____ Nursing Home
_____ Other (explain) _______________________

13. Previous program setting (check the one which describes the individual's setting immediately prior to enrolling in the supported employment program)

_____ Adult education/Vocational school
_____ Other Supported Employment Program
_____ Institution
_____ Work activity program
_____ Employed
Special Education
    _____ segregated school
    _____ integrated school
    _____ formal transitional program
_____ Volunteer employment
_____ Sheltered work
_____ Day activity program
_____ No program
_____ Other (explain)
____
_____ Unknown

14. Use of public transporation (check those that apply)

_____ Driver's license
_____ Uses public transport with assistance & prompts
_____ Uses public transport independently
_____ Does not use public transport
_____ Not applicable/public transport unavailable
_____ Other (explain) ____

15. Form completed by (last name) ____

16. Phone no. (____)____________________

DEPT OF HEALTH & SOC SERVICES STATE OF WISCONSIN
DIV OF VOCATIONAL REHABILITATION
DVR-63 (Rev. 3/89)

EMPLOYMENT INFORMATION
SUPPORTED EMPLOYMENT
(WSEIS Manual, Form DVR - for Instructions for Completion)

1. Agency/Provider Name ________________________________

2. Dates covered in report ____/____/____ to ____/____/____.

3. Participant/Client ________________________________
Last name First name

EMPLOYER DATA (report only when the individual is first placed with the employer. If the individual has more than one employer, please complete a DVR-63 for each employment setting).

4. Employer/Business name ________________________________

5. Employer location (city only) ________________________________

6. No. of employees at this site ____________

7. Employment start date ____/____/____

8. Job located by (check the one that applies)

____ Job developer/coach
____ Lead from friends, family of participant
____ Employer initiated contact
____ Other (explain)
____
____ Combined efforts of SE staff
____ Corporate Initiative/Job Development Network
____ Newly created/expanded business under Dept. of Development/Supp Empl prog
____ Unknown/none

9. Type of employer (check the one which applies)

____ private not-for-profit ____ private for profit ____ public/government

10. Job title (given to the job by the employer) ________________________________

Please report the following each month:

11. Work site description (check description which best applies; see manual for descriptions)

____ Individual setting
____ Group setting
____ Cluster setting
____ Dispersed cluster
____ Mobile crew
____ Job sharing
____ Other (explain) ____

12. Hours work/week ____________________ 13. Pay/hour $ __________

14. Job restructured Y N 15. Job adaptations/technology Y N

16. Integration (check the description which best applies; see manual for descriptions)

____ No contact at job site
____ Opportunity, without social interaction
____ Incidental interactions
____ Parallel interactions
____ Systematic, significant
____ Extend beyond the work site

17. Employment benefits (check those that apply)

____ Vacation
____ Retirement plan
____ Sick Leave
____ Other
____ Health insurance
____ None

DEPT OF HEALTH & SOC SERVICES STATE OF WISCONSIN
DIV OF VOCATIONAL REHABILITATION
DVR-64 (Rev. 3/89)

SERVICE REPORT
SUPPORTED EMPLOYMENT
(WSEIS Manual, Form DVR - for Instructions for Completion)

1. Agency/Provider Name ______________________________

2. Dates covered in report ____/____/____ to ____/____/____.

3. Participant/Client ______________________________
Last name First name

4. Hours of direct service ____________________

Service provided this month (check all that apply; see manual for description)

____ Functional assessment
____ On-site job skill training
____ Community skill training
____ Work-related skill training
____ Planning with client
____ Supportive counseling
____ Behavior management @ work site
____ Employer/co-worker training/advocacy
____ Other (explain) ______________________________

5. Hours of indirect service ____________________

Service provided this month (check all that apply; see manual for description)

____ Interagency consultation
____ On-site observation
____ Job development
____ Coordination of services
____ Travel time
____ Planning with parent or significant other
____ Job analysis
____ Administrative duties
____ Staff training
____ Other (describe) ______________________________

Use the following *only* when recommended that DVR transition the client to long-term support system:

6. Check all that apply:

_____ Employed in the community
_____ Works 20 or more hours/week
_____ Works less than 20 hours/week
_____ Regular opportunities for interaction with nondisabled co-workers in an employment setting (of less than 8 persons with disabilities if it is a group site)
_____ Client/participant is satisfied with job
_____ Employer is satisfied with employee
_____ Client's training/stabilization plan is completed
_____ Long-term support is arranged with the following planned/anticipated services:
    _____ On-site job skill training @ _____ times per week/month (circle one)
    _____ Work-related skill training
    _____ Employer/co-worker training/advocacy
    _____ Subminimum wage certificate monitoring
    _____ Supportive counseling
    _____ Behavior management
    _____ Job development

7. Social Security Benefits (check those that apply)

_____ 1619 A
_____ 1619 B
_____ Work-related Expenses
_____ Self-Employment Plan
_____ Other (explain) ____________________
____

DEPT OF HEALTH & SOC SERVICES STATE OF WISCONSIN
DIV OF VOCATIONAL REHABILITATION
DVR-114 (Rev. 3/89)

ONE-TIME CLIENT DATA REPORT
TBI SUPPLEMENT

IF TRAUMATIC BRAIN INJURY WAS CIRCLED AS THE PRIMARY DISABILITY ON THE DVR-62, PLEASE COMPLETE THIS FORM TO THE BEST OF YOUR ABILITY.

1. Participant/Client ______________________________
Last name First name

2. Date of injury ____/____/____ 3. Age at time of injury: ______________

4. Cause of injury: (Check the appropriate cause)

____ Motorcycle accident
____ Automobile accident
____ Other vehicle (bicylce, ATV)
____ Pedestrian
____ Fall
____ Sports accident
____ Anoxia (near-drowning, etc.)

____ Gunshot
____ Assault
____ Tumor
____ Infection
____ Cerebral vascular accident
____ Other (please describe)
____

5. Alcohol/Drug-related

Individual with head injury ____ Y ____ N
Individual who caused head injury ____ Y ____ N
____ NA ____ Unknown

6. Other problems resulting from the injury:

____Seizure disorder
____ Visual impairments
____ Communication disorder
____ Behavior disorder

____ Physical/orthopedic impairments
____ Auditory impairments
____ Other sensory impairment (smell, taste)
____ Substance abuse (not premorbid condition)

7. Level of education:

_____ Less than high school	_____ High school graduate
_____ Some post-high school (college or technical school)	_____ College or technical school graduate
	_____ G.E.D.

8. If employed immediately prior to sustaining the head injury, indicate the job title and hourly wage: Put NA if not employed.

9. Job title ______________________________

10. Hourly wage $________________

Appendix C

Wisconsin Division of Vocational Rehabilitation Supported Employment and Traumatic Brain Injury Project

May 12, 1989

1. SERVICE PROVISION MODEL

Since the key to the research is tracking the individual *after* they begin working, the Committee recommends an emphasis on getting the person to work as soon as possible. The following guidelines were developed to accomplish this goal and to avoid delayed placement:

a. Placement into permanent employment, at least 20 hours a week at competitive wage, must occur within six months of the individual's start date in the project.

b. The initial assessment should last no longer than two months, and should include *at least one occupational trial*. Other job interests, service needs, and concerns can be assessed while the person is working. The occupational trials can be unpaid, or be incorporated into an existing transitional employment site, but should be no longer than two to three weeks if the person is working 20 to 40 hours per week.

c. The individual's job goal must be balanced with available job market information. Matching job interest is encouraged, but not to the extent that delays in placement are the result.

2. STAFFING

The Committee recommends that 75% of project staff time be spent in work-related activities (assessment, job development, training) versus case management, supportive counseling, etc. Due to the intensive nature of job coaching required by individuals and the difference in skills required for job development versus training, the Committee recommends a model of service allowing for job development to be done by someone other than the job coach/trainer. The proposed staffing pattern would involve a job developer working four to five hours per week, with the job coach working 35 to 36 hours per week.

3. ROLE CLARIFICATION

There has been some confusion on the part of project staff regarding the role of the VR Counselor versus the Project Coordinator. Seven VR Counselors are connected to clients in the project, and their level of involvment varies. Vendors have expressed concern regarding the number of meetings they are asked to attend in addition to the progress reports and other paperwork, which subtracts from the time they spend in job development activities. Ideally, the Committee feels that having only one or two Counselors involved in the project would be less confusing. The role of the Project Coordinator will be discussed/clarified with the Field Office Supervisor.

4. CRITERIA FOR TRANSITIONING TO THE COUNTY FOR LONG-TERM SUPPORT

a. Permanent employment, 20 hours/week average over a two-week pay period, at minimum wage or above;

b. Job Coach support at 25% or less;

c. Job should be stable, even if it is not the individual's optimal level of employment – a mechanism should be developed before transition for referring the individual *back* to DVR for additional services to upgrade employment.

References

DeBosky, D. S., & Morin, K. (1986). *A "how to handle" manual for families of the brain injured.* Tampa, FL: Hillsborough County Hospital Authority Printing and Graphic Services.

Federal Register (1987, August 14). Final Regulations, Vol. 52(157), pp. 30546-30552. Washington, DC: U. S. Government Printing Office.

Fraser, R., Clemmons, D., & McMahon, B. (1990). Vocational rehabilitation counseling. In J. Kreutzer & P. Wehamn (Eds.), *Community integration following traumatic brain injury.* Baltimore: Paul H. Brookes.

Lynch, R. (1983). The vocational expert. *Rehabilitation Counseling Bulletin, 27*(1), Special Issue: Private Rehabilitation.

Mank, D., Rhodes, L., & Bellamy, G. T. (1986). Four supported employment alternatives. In W. Kiernan & J. Stark (Eds.), *Pathways to employment.* Baltimore: University Park Press.

Ridgely, M. (1990). *Supported employment and traumatic brain injury, First Year Report.* Wisconsin Division of Health and Social Services, Division of Vocational Rehabilitation. Grant of the National Institute on Disability and Rehabilitation Research.

Tooman, M., Revell, W., & Melia, R. (1987). The role of the rehabilitation counselor in the provision of transition and supported employment programs. In S. Rubin and N. Rubin (Eds.), *Contemporary challenges to the rehabilitation counseling profession* (pp. 77-92). Baltimore: Paul H. Brookes.

Wachter, J., Fawler, H., & Mason, S. (1987). Treatment aspects of vocational evaluation and placement for traumatically brain injured adults. In M. Ylivsaker & E. Gobble (Eds.), *Community re-entry for head injured adults* (pp. 259-274). Boston: College-Hill.

8

New Avenues to Job Placement: The Advantages of Natural Supports

Robert T. Fraser

8

New Avenues to Job Placement: The Advantages of Natural Supports

Robert T. Fraser

Introduction

A BASIC PERSPECTIVE ON SUPPORTED EMPLOYMENT

In a recent review of supported employment models, Wehman (1990) summarized the major characteristics as real pay in community-based work activity for people with severe disabilities. Additionally, work activity should be integrated with and around nonhandicapped co-workers with permanent ongoing or intermittent support being provided for the duration of employment. This approach can be very appropriate for many individuals with traumatic brain injury (TBI) who have moderate to severe cognitive sequelae and sometimes even individuals with mild impairment (e.g., individuals with overall average to above average cognitive functioning, but with idiosyncratic memory deficits). In other instances, supported employment can assist in stabilizing clients with specific behavioral issues (e.g., verbosity, temper tantrums, or other social inappropriateness). To date, there have been a number of different models of supported employment developed. These include the following:

Enclave. This employment option involves a small group of workers (usually four to eight) with disabilities who are receiving long-term on-site supervision at a host company. In some instances, members of the enclave are working together (e.g., around a specific assembly task), but in other cases they may be conducting diverse tasks within a restaurant, mail-order company, or hotel, and receiving intermittent supervision.

Mobile work crew. Mobile work crews involve a team of four to six individuals working with a supervisor. They provide specific services such as landscaping, housekeeping, auto washing, janitorial services, and other hospitality industry services. Workers generally tend to be paid by a specific nonprofit organization set up for the purpose of providing this work or by a larger nonprofit organization for whom this activity is simply one of the services that it provides to the community. Wehman (1990, p. 189) indicates that this model is highly viable in rural areas in which the specific needs of the community can be identified and expeditiously met.

Small business option. This is another supported employment model in which a small group of disabled workers are paired with a nondisabled supervisor and/or other workers in one specific small business, such as lawn mower or snowmobile servicing, printing, or a mail-order operation.

Individual supported employment model. This model, as highly popularized by Paul Wehman and colleagues at the Medical College of Virginia, uses a "one-to-one" job coach to client support ratio. The model can be individualized to the job placement, training, and stabilization needs of a client with TBI.

There is no question that these diverse models of supported employment can be applied to clients with severe TBI. In a study sponsored by the National Institute on Disability and Rehabilitation Research (NIDRR) and completed at the Medical College of Virginia (Wehman et al., 1990), 77 percent of 59 clients were placed in competitive jobs using the individual job coach model. This is definitely a successful effort since the natural course of work return for those with similar disabilities is between 23 and 30 percent (Haffey & Lewis, 1989).

CONCERNS ABOUT ESTABLISHED SUPPORTED EMPLOYMENT MODELS

There have been, however, a number of concerns expressed about supported employment in our country today. These are generic concerns and not specific to clients with TBI, but worthy of review. Nisbet and Hagner (1988) highlight a number of these as follows:

a. Moderate supported employment retention rates at one year from placement with a range of 44 to 70 percent (Lagomarcino, 1986; Moss, Dineen, & Ford, 1986; Vogelsberg, 1986; Wehman, 1986).

b. The obtrusiveness of the job coach within the work site.

c. Interdependencies that develop between job coaches and clients.

d. The attention drawn to the client with the disability through the use of the job coach.

e. The undetermined cost-effectiveness of one-to-one job coaching and other models of supported employment.

f. Supported employment procedures were developed by disability specialists within traditional rehabilitation environments and facilities. These procedures are "externally imposed on natural work environments, often based on a very meager and superficial understanding of how these environments function" (Nisbet & Hagner, 1988, p. 261).

These authors also emphasize that informal interactions flourish at work, patterns of social interactions vary widely across and within work environments, and some support is available naturally within the work environment. Their work draws attention to some of the reasons for more carefully considering "natural support" approaches.

From work at the University of Washington (Fraser, Dikmen, McLean, & Temkin, 1988), it was found that in addition to some of the above concerns, the following difficulties were encountered when attempting to use the individual supported employment model with clients with TBI:

a. A number of the jobs were simply too complex for the level of sophistication of the available job coaches (e.g., electronics technician, attorney, journeyman carpenter, etc.). A number of clients sought return-to-work activities that were very difficult to coach. This concern is also underscored in findings from an earlier study (Fraser et al., 1988, p. 280) in which a review of the job backgrounds of 48 consecutive TBI hospital admissions revealed few patients with unskilled work backgrounds—only eight percent. Those employed were primarily in skilled (50 percent) or semiskilled work activity (42 percent). This situation represents different challenges than supported employment or job coaching with developmentally disabled persons for whom job goals are primarily at entry level.

b. Some individuals, although work motivated, were not receptive to having a job coach on the work site and were not interested in accepting this model. This, of course, was often related to denial of cognitive and interpersonal deficits, but in other cases it would really have been unwieldy to have a coach at the work site.

c. Some companies, although receptive to our program, felt that they were best equipped to do their own training. Consequently, despite the appropriateness of individual job coaching as a model, it was difficult to utilize coaching personnel in these situations.

The work of Nisbet and Hagner (1988) and the experiences of the author and other colleagues suggest that a consideration of "natural supports" in the work place is timely and may specifically benefit the segment of the rehabilitation population with TBI.

A Perspective on Alternative Placement Models: The Use of Natural Supports

The purpose of this section is to present some of the alternative placement models that have been used within the University of Washington project (Fraser et al., 1990) and also introduce some of the "natural support" strategies recently presented by Sowers (1989), from the Oregon Research Institute in working with individuals having severe cognitive and physical disabilities. The first two strategy categories relate to efforts piloted at the Oregon Research Institute under the direction of Dr. Sowers, while the last two involve models which were utilized in the recent "Vocational Re-entry of the Traumatic Brain Injured" demonstration project funded by NIDRR (Fraser et al., 1990):

1. **Forms of job modification.** In the recent Sowers (1989) review, the author describes job creation and task design strategies as approaches to actually modifying the job or job activities. Job creation involves task reorganization and restructuring so that the one or two tasks a person can competently perform will, in fact, comprise at least part-time job activity. Examples of these tasks include paper shredding, filing, or specified mailing or billing functions. Some of these jobs can actually be conducted at home with the work being brought to the client. Certain clients may be able to perform more than one part-time job, based upon segmented task groupings, which could be a more stable

employment situation for them. They may be less at risk for lay-off in the event of an economic downturn.

As described by Sowers and Powers (1989) there are five major types of job design strategies that can be used to accommodate individuals with severe disabilities. These include:

a. Redesigning the job so that difficult tasks are eliminated.

b. Identifying an alternate approach to accomplish a difficult movement or discrimination task.

c. Modifying or reengineering the work environment to increase the client's access to the job task.

d. Positioning the client so that movements may be made more easily.

e. Using assistive devices, such as jigs, vices, and other special equipment, so that the client can be accommodated on the job. In most cases, a rehabilitation engineer or occupational therapist should be consulted on making device-type recommendations. When outside consultation is required, requests may be sent to the Job Accommodation Network so that special equipment or modification approaches can be recommended.* This is a no-cost consultation service that is provided nationally to employers attempting to outreach and hire rehabilitation clients.

The concept of job modification has existed for many years in rehabilitation, but Sowers and Powers (1989) present a typology that can bring renewed interest to the area. Of particular interest is type 1(a), which involves the segmenting of less complex job tasks that can become part- or full-time positions.

2. **Co-worker assistance**. Shafer (1986) categorizes potential co-worker roles as those of advocate, observer, and trainer for workers with disabilities. As an advocate, the co-worker is described as handling both protective and communicative functions. Protection involves ensuring that the worker with a disability does not have his or her rights compromised by unsupporting co-workers (e.g., preventing a worker with TBI from being saddled with the least prestigious or most routine tasks [if this is inappropriate]; minimizing the frequency of practical jokes played on a client; or facilitating the handling of difficult confron-

* Job Accommodation Network, West Virginia University, 809 Allen Hall, P.O. Box 6122, Morgantown, WV 26507-9984, Phone: 1-800-JAN-7324.

tations that may occur) (Shafer, 1986, pp. 216-217). A large part of the advocacy function for clients with TBI involves the education of co-workers about the specific deficits experienced by the client. Their new co-worker needs to be understood as not simply a "brain-injured" person, but a person with specific types of memory or problem solving deficits (as examples) who can perform the necessary work tasks given specific prompts or compensatory strategies (e.g., lists, picture sequences). Co-workers who understand "nonvisible" deficits are more likely to be cooperative and better support the training mission.

The co-worker observer function, as described by Shafer (1986, p. 220) can involve both providing subjective ratings as well as gathering more discrete data to objectively evaluate worker performance. Shafer (1986) recommends that to avoid some of the more typical observational difficulties, such as observer "drift" and "bias," co-worker training becomes critical to the gathering of accurate information. Co-workers need to be focused on the appropriate behaviors, generally limited to one or two, and use observational systems that do not take them too far outside their regular duties.

Although the concept of one worker assisting another to learn job tasks is not a new one, it has only recently received expanded attention as a support mechanism for workers with disabilities (Curl et al., 1987; Sowers, 1989). In Sowers' review, she indicates that co-workers can provide the trainee with on-task or task initiation prompts, quality check the individual's work, provide physical assistance, routinely praise a co-worker, or otherwise coach the disabled worker in the completion of work activities. Based upon the amount of time involved, the company could be reimbursed or the co-worker paid directly for the hour or two per day that may be necessary to ensure that the work is completed. Until the worker reaches adequate production and quality criteria, the co-worker could be paid through state rehabilitation agency training funds or under the category of post-employment services.

In some cases, a support co-worker model could be used with a job actually being shared by a disabled and nondisabled individual. Sowers (1989) describes the Oregon Alternative Work Concepts Program contracting with a company for a fixed amount of work hours per week to which it assigns a disabled and nondisabled worker. The worker with the disability is paid based upon productivity. Through contract monies from the company and state rehabilitation agency training funds or supported employment monies, this arrangement becomes very feasible. In using this approach, it becomes necessary to identify jobs or tasks that an individual will be able to do independently or with minimal ongoing support. The Oregon program has teams involved in contracted photocopying work, sandwich delivery, drapery dry-cleaning, legal office tasks, and item unpacking and pricing.

Some individuals will need a long-term personal care attendant to assist on the job. This type of support can be funded through the Medicaid system in some cases. Under the Social Security Administration, the PASS (Plan for Achieving Self-Support) Program could be used through which a person can pay for support services on the job which are then claimed as a job-related expense and deducted when calculating earnings for SSI purposes. Although the PASS Program is time-limited, the Impairment Related Work Expenses (IRWE) is another Social Security work incentive option that may be used following expiration of the PASS time period. In her work, Sowers recommends the Association for Persons in Supported Employment (APSE) newsletter to learn more about developments in paying for job-related supported services.**

An avenue for funding personal attendants on the job site, as endorsed by Sowers, is the cost-sharing of the attendant's expenses among several individuals with disabilities. This sharing method can enable several individuals to work within one host company or within companies that are relatively proximate to share the capabilities of the attendant.

3. **The employer or supervisor as training mentor**. For a number of individuals with severe cognitive difficulties, the direct employer or supervisor can very adequately perform the training function, although education is often required relative to the cognitive assets and deficits of a brain-injured client. In addition, a job coach may be used to behaviorally frame the training or, in some cases, the behavioral management plan. On-the-job training funds can be used as a means of defraying the employer's or supervisor's training time, thus facilitating the establishment of this relationship.

4. **Use of a community training consultant**. For a number of jobs within the recently funded NIDRR demonstration project (Fraser et al., 1990), a subgroup of clients with severe TBI required intensive training which could not be fully accommodated within a classroom situation or by a relatively inexperienced job coach. In these cases, a trainer from the community (e.g., a welder) or a retired professional (e.g., a pharmacist) was retained to work with a client on a one-to-one basis until appropriate work productivity and accuracy criteria were achieved. In some cases an individual was able to attend a technical training program within a community college, but stayed after class each day for specific individualized instruction and took considerably longer to achieve skill competency than other technical school trainees (e.g., remaining in school for

---

** Association for Persons in Supported Employment (APSE), 5001 West Broad Street, Suite 34, Richmond, VA 23230.

a nine-month period versus six months for the nondisabled trainees). In most cases, due to "generalization" or transfer of learning deficits, clients with moderate to severe brain injuries will learn and adjust better at the actual job site.

Natural Supports: Training Considerations

In using co-worker, employer, or training consultants as in the previously discussed models, the importance of structured training sessions becomes apparent. Fortunately, some new materials have become available for these purposes (Curl et al., 1987), but they have chiefly been developed for programming with mentally retarded clients.

The co-worker training manual, *Put That Person to Work*, as developed by Curl et al. (1987) at Utah State University emphasizes the use of training scripts, verbal instructions and modeling, training tips for the co-worker (taping sessions, one-minute reminders, bonuses, warnings) and trainee aids (picture checklists, timers, work checking procedures). The manual also offers tips for advocating in the work place and evaluating job performance. Although the appendices provide specific task lists and scripts, most of these materials relate to a limited range of service industry jobs. The Utah State group underscores that the manual and accompanying tapes are meant to be used as supplementary materials to a formal co-worker training program and should not stand alone as an avenue to co-worker training.

Based upon his review of available programs, Shafer (1986, p. 222) indicates that co-worker training sessions should consist of three segments:

a. Discussion of the behaviors to be modified and the specific behavioral procedures to be used in training.

b. Modeling of the training procedure to be used with verbal description.

c. Behavioral rehearsal by the co-worker of the specific training procedure, either with the job coach/trainer or with an actual client as the actual trainee.

Periodic follow-up should be conducted in an unobtrusive manner to ensure that the co-worker's abilities as a trainer are adequate and are modified as necessary.

Implementing a Co-Worker Training Program

To effectively implement a co-worker training model, there are a number of issues that relate to the selection of co-workers as trainers, the commitment made by management and supervisors, and other areas of concern which, if addressed, can facilitate successful efforts by co-workers as trainers. Since co-worker training is a new area of rehabilitation services investment, it is important to review these identified areas of concern.

IDENTIFICATION OF CO-WORKERS AS TRAINERS

Work at the University of Washington (Fraser et al., 1990) and the recommendations by Curl et al. (1990) and Shafer (1986) emphasize that the co-workers chosen should be experienced and have a good understanding of their own position's activities within the context of the company's larger work output. They should be above average or "master" workers who are well-liked by peers and management. They must make a commitment to learn training and troubleshooting strategies, in addition to ongoing observation and evaluation strategies. Finally, there needs to be a commitment to understand the client's assets and deficits and effectively advocate for him or her within the work place. In some cases, the co-worker's desire to advocate and commit to the training regimen is based upon a prior relationship with a brain-injured client as a pre-injury co-worker or friend, or a family experience with a disabled loved one.

COMMITMENT OF MANAGERS AND SUPERVISORS

Curl et al. (1990) indicated that management must agree to provide training periods for disabled workers that will be longer than for the nondisabled. Management must also accept that co-workers will have training responsibilities and have the appropriate work schedule to train the employee with a disability. Co-worker recording of trainee performance data and periodic visits from rehabilitation agency personnel need to be accepted and supported. Any financial arrangements with the company for co-worker payment, on-the-job training funds, etc. also need to be clearly understood. Any reinforcers to be received by the co-worker for the training function also need to be approved by management (e.g., salary, vacation days, job redesign, or employer recognition) if these reinforcers are factors in the co-worker's commitment.

OTHER GENERAL TRAINING ISSUES

There are a number of continuing concerns related to the establishment of a co-worker training program. We have addressed the selection of co-workers as trainers and issues that require clarification with management to include co-worker pay and reinforcement issues. It is recommended that job trainers, coaches, and rehabilitation counselors who are to be involved in co-worker training receive formal training sessions themselves and share perspectives and strategies since this is such a new field. Curl et al. (1990) indicated that prior research supports a number of factors that are facilitative of effective co-worker training:

a. Co-workers need training scripts prepared ahead of time to facilitate optimally helpful instructions.

b. Co-workers may need to be taught a training sequence with more than one rehabilitation client because their experience with only one client does not generalize to others.

c. The use of one-minute reminders given to new trainees by co-workers before they begin each workday seemed to be the most single effective strategy to improving work performance after receiving general job training by the co-worker.

These and other issues will emerge as co-worker training becomes a standard practice and is applied more extensively with all rehabilitation clients and, specifically with those having TBI. The reader is referred to the manual by Curl et al. (1990), *Guidelines for Implementing the Co-worker Transition Model* for review of other salient training issues.

Co-worker Training: Anticipated Issues with Clients Having TBI

In contrast to co-worker training programs for developmentally disabled workers, the training of co-workers as on-site work trainers of clients having TBI presents a wider array of issues. These clients' residual skills may actually facilitate task training while injury-related cognitive deficits such as problem solving, diverse memory impairments, or visual-perceptual or sensory deficits can present other training and adjustment concerns. In a similar manner, residual social skills can initially facilitate acceptance of workers with TBI, but in other cases new workers will find themselves in situations where they become socially inappropriate due to impulsiveness, disinhibition, or lack of judgement.

Areas of both cognitive training and social management, therefore, can require a greater range of understanding than for the developmentally disabled population. The client with TBI can often present well initially, which can disarm both the co-worker trainer and others in the work environment. Particularly early in the training process, there may be an imposition on those in the work place to accept certain inconsistencies and inappropriateness.

The co-worker trainer will most definitely have to understand that each client with TBI is an individual with different residual levels and patterns of cognitive and behavioral performance. The roles of trainer, observer, and advocate will vary across the different new workers to be trained. Currently, the use of the co-worker as a trainer for clients with TBI is in its infancy. As more data is collected, a clearer picture will emerge as to which co-worker roles are most often assumed and the types of activities most frequently engaged in within each of these required roles.

Conclusion

This chapter has reviewed some of the concerns related to the standard application of traditional supported employment models, specifically as applied to workers with severe TBI. Recent research and demonstration projects have drawn attention to alternative community-based models and the use of natural supports within the work place. These models include forms of job modification, co-worker assistance, the employer/supervisor as training mentor, and the use of a community training consultant. A substantial part of this chapter was devoted to issues in implementing the co-worker training model. All community-based job mentors (co-workers, supervisors, training consultants) will require at least some structured training.

Although materials have become available for training developmentally disabled groups (Curl et al., 1987, 1990), these materials and training models are not yet readily available or refined for the training of clients with TBI. On a more basic level, there is currently a shortage of rehabilitation personnel nationally to engage in these community training activities. Our challenge for the next decade is to develop a cadre of rehabilitation personnel who can implement and refine these types of training models and be available as established community resources.

References

Curl, R. M., McConaughy, E. K., Pawley, J. M., & Salzberg, C. L. (1987). *Put That Person to Work!*. Logan, Utah: Outreach, Development, and Dissemination Division, Developmental Center for Handicapped Persons, Utah State University.

Curl, R. M., McConaughy, E. K., Pawley, J. M., & Salzberg, C. L. (1990). *Guidelines for Implementing the Co-worker Transition Model*. Logan, Utah: Outreach, Development, and Dissemination Division, Developmental Center for Handicapped Persons, Utah State University.

Fraser, R. T., Wehman, P., & Bennett, P. (November, 1990). Vocational re-entry of the traumatic brain injured: A demonstration project. In R. T. Fraser, Chair, *Summary of NIDRR Studies in the Vocational Rehabilitation of the Traumatic Brain Injured*. Symposium presented at the National Head Injury Foundation, Ninth Annual Symposium, New Orleans, Louisiana.

Fraser, R. T., Dikmen, S., McLean, A., & Temkin, N. (1988). Employability of head injured survivors: The first year post-injury. *Rehabilitation Counseling Bulletin, 31*, 278-288.

Haffey, W., & Lewis, F. (1989). Programming for occupational outcomes following traumatic brain injury. *Rehabilitation Psychology, 34*, 117-130.

Lagomarcino, T. (1986). Community services: Using the supported work model within an adult service agency. In F. Rusch (Ed.), *Competitive Employment Issues and Strategies*, (pp. 65-76). Baltimore: Paul H. Brookes.

Moss, J., Dineen, J., & Ford, L. (1986). University of Washington employment training program. In F. Rusch (Ed.), *Competitive Employment Issues and Strategies*, (pp. 77-88). Baltimore: Paul H. Brookes.

Nisbet, J., & Hagner, D. (1988). Natural supports in the work place: A reexamination of supported employment. *Journal of the Association for Persons with Severe Handicaps, 13*, 260-267.

Shafer, M. (1986). Utilizing co-workers as change agents. In F. Rusch (Ed.), *Competitive Employment Issues and Strategies* (pp. 215-244). Baltimore: Paul H. Brookes.

Sowers, J. (1989). Supported employment models and approaches for persons with physical and multiple disabilities. In J. Sowers & L. Powers (Eds.), *Vocational Preparation and Employment of Students with Physical and Multiple Disabilities*. Portland, Oregon: Oregon Research Institute.

Sowers, J., & Powers, L. (1989). Job design strategies for persons with physical and multiple disabilities. In J. Sowers & L. Powers (Eds.), *Vocational Preparation and Employment of Students with Physical and Multiple Disabilities*. Portland, Oregon: Oregon Research Institute.

Vogelsberg, R. (1986). Competitive employment in Vermont. In F. Rusch (Ed.), *Competitive Employment Issues and Strategies* (pp. 23-25). Baltimore: Paul H. Brookes.

Wehman, P. (1986). Competitive employment in Virginia. In F. Rusch (Ed.), *Competitive Employment Issues and Strategies* (pp. 23-35). Baltimore: Paul H. Brookes.

Wehman, P. (1990). Supported employment model implementation and evaluation. In J. S. Kreutzer & P. Wehman (Eds.), *Community Integration Following Traumatic Brain Injury* (pp. 185-204). Baltimore: Paul H. Brookes.

Wehman, P., Kreutzer, J., West, M., Sherron, P., Zasler, N., Gorah, C., Stonnington, H., Burns, C., & Sale, P. (1990). Return to work for persons with traumatic brain injury: A supported employment approach. *Archives of Physical Medicine and Rehabilitation*, *71*, 1047-1042.

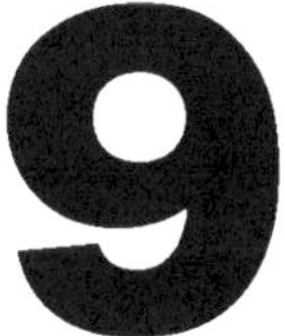

Blueprint for Success in Vocational Restoration: The Work Re-entry Program

Deborah L. Abrams
William J. Haffey

9

Blueprint for Success in Vocational Restoration: The Work Re-entry Program

Deborah L. Abrams
William J. Haffey

The ultimate goal of rehabilitation is returning the injured person to productive living. In our society, work is central to the identity and well-being of many people. Despite advances in medical and vocational rehabilitation service delivery, the majority of persons with severe and moderate traumatic brain injury TBI remained unemployed (Jacobs, 1988; Haffey & Lewis, 1989).

This chapter discusses the evolution of vocational rehabilitation programs for persons with TBI; describes the Work Re-entry program, as an example of a model TBI vocational rehabilitation program; describes program components and processes; discusses how persons with TBI access the program and provides examples of what actually occurs using selected case examples; reports the program's outcomes; and discusses directions for future development.

The Evolution of TBI Vocational Rehabilitation

EARLY EXPERIENCES

In the late '70s and early '80s, medical and vocational rehabilitation providers struggled with how to best serve the growing number of persons surviving severe and moderate TBI. Medical rehabilitative personnel became increasingly skilled at identifying the range of physical, cognitive, social/behavioral, and emotional deficits following severe and moderate TBI (McKinlay, Brooks, Bond, Martinage, & Marshall, 1981; Brooks, 1984; Dikeman, Reitan, & Temkin, 1983). They also began to develop rehabilitative techniques designed to return maximal levels of independence to the person with TBI (Udin-Aronow, 1987; Fryer & Haffey, 1987). In some programs, vocational counselors were introduced into the medical rehabilitative process in an effort to help restore the person with TBI to some level of productivity. This led to vocational counselors developing a much greater awareness of the range of deficits which characterized this disabled population and which presented formidable barriers to vocational rehabilitation.

Even in areas where medical and vocational personnel were cooperating in their rehabilitative efforts, there was general dissatisfaction with the available options. More often than not, the person with TBI would be placed in a sheltered workshop which was accustomed to serving persons with developmental disabilities. Rarely did such placements succeed. The person with TBI did not behave like those with developmental disabilities. Both supervisors and line workers found persons with TBI noncompliant, disruptive, or inconsistent. Consequently, the person with TBI was typically perceived as a "problem," and generally did not benefit from the experience. More often than not, the person with TBI had little awareness or acceptance of his or her contribution to the job-related problems.

LATER EXPERIENCES

As expertise in TBI rehabilitation evolved, vocational intervention became more heavily influenced by results of a traditional vocational evaluation and neuropsychological assessment data. There was a growing use of specific findings regarding neurobehavioral deficits as they pertained to work behaviors and attitudes and job requirements. Despite the increased use of vocational skill and aptitude data and neuropsychological information in predicting jobs that would be feasible for individuals with TBI, employment rates did not improve substantially from previous levels. This may have been partially due to the fact that neuropsychological testing is often very structured and conducted in low stimulus environments (Hart & Hayden, 1986). An individual may perform well in such circumstances, but in a less structured, highly interactive work environment, job performance and social behavior may fail to meet minimal requirements. Without testing circumstances which more closely approximate the demands of the work environment, critical information about capacities and limitations tends to remain undiscovered prior to the person actually being placed on the job. Leland, Lewis, Hinman, and Carrillo (1988) noted that many traditional work samples and psychometric vocational assessment instruments are not as well-suited for use with persons with TBI as they are for persons with other disabilities.

Even when specialized brain injury rehabilitation programs emerged to train persons with TBI to compensate for their residual deficits, there was little formal assistance provided in actually obtaining a job. Vocational counselors tended to become involved only after the individual completed a course of neuropsychological rehabilitation and was deemed "job ready." The counselors would then work with the person with TBI to secure employment, but specific job development and placement services were either unavailable or ineffective. Alternatively, the person with TBI may have found a job, but it was not a job suited to the person's residual strengths and so was short-lived. In both cases, the goal of the vocational rehabilitation process – competitive employment – was either not achieved or sustained.

Continued high levels of unemployment among persons with TBI led to a recognition that a different approach was needed. It was apparent that vocational rehabilitation professionals needed to do more than assess and counsel. More in-depth information concerning a client's work potential was needed. It also became apparent that it was necessary to create situations which would replicate the work environment and would reveal the more subtle, yet potentially devastating, barriers to employment. Most important, it was recognized that assistance in obtaining employment and adjusting to the new environment was necessary for success.

The Work Re-entry Program

The Sharp Work Re-entry Program in San Diego, California was developed in direct response to the California Department of Rehabilitation's request for a model program which would substantially increase the return-to-work rate for persons with TBI. The Work Re-entry process is based on the belief that there is more than one blueprint for returning to work. The keys to success are: discovering the individual's occupational potential, identifying and developing the right job environment to match his or her potential; and actualizing potential by securing and maintaining employment.

Over the past two and one-half years, 130 persons with severe and moderate TBI have been served in the Work Re-entry program. Based on Glasgow Outcome Scale ratings at discharge from acute rehabilitation, 57% of the clients were classified as severely disabled, 41% as moderately disabled, and only 2% were in the good recovery category. Eighty-eight (68%) have returned to gainful employment, while another 19 persons (14%) are still engaged in the Work Re-entry program. Only 23 persons (18%) have proven to be chronically unemployable. Such outcomes are promising and lend credence to this systematic approach to developing and securing paid employment for persons with severe and moderate TBI.

Work Re-entry Components

The Work Re-entry program emerged as a means of improving vocational outcomes for persons with TBI. Program components include:

- **Intake** to determine job history; social history; injury history and treatment course; post-injury social and work history; and to assess whether the individual is ready for return to prior employment or employment assistance.
- **Vocational assessment** to identify work skills, abilities, aptitudes and potential, as well as the interventions needed to achieve employment.
- **Work hardening** using real and simulated work activities to develop required stamina, work competencies, work behaviors, and/or target productivity levels.
- **Job development** to identify potential placement opportunities for Work Re-entry participants.
- **Job analysis** to determine job performance requirements; the potential for modifications to an available job; and to assess the "goodness of fit" between these and the client's competencies and support needs.
- **Transitional Employment Program (TEP)** in which a person with TBI is placed in a paid position at Sharp Memorial Hospital with a job coach for three to four months to improve stamina, productivity, and work behaviors.

- **Job placement** in which Work Re-entry counselors manage the process of job procurement by working collaboratively with the person with TBI and the employer.
- **Short-term support and long-term follow-up** in which Work Re-entry staff give limited on-the-job support for the first 60 days following placement and in which research assistants conduct formal follow-ups every six months to assess employment status.

A review of the success of the Work Re-entry program yielded several "critical processes" which have contributed to returning persons with TBI to the labor force. These include: (1) intake and evaluation; (2) counseling and guidance; (3) development of a range of employment options; (4) initial on-the-job support; and (5) follow-up.

Work Re-entry Processes

INTAKE AND EVALUATION

A critical dimension of the return-to-work process is the initial intake interview and a comprehensive evaluation of the individual's existing skills and occupational potential. The intake interview is conducted to determine whether the client is ready for employment assistance or if a referral to other services, prior to Work Re-entry, is more appropriate. At times, problems interfering with the pursuit of a job are readily apparent. For example, an active substance abuser may require an alcohol or drug treatment program prior to being ready to seek employment. In another case, a person may need neuropsychological or neurobehavioral programming to be better prepared for return to work. Such individuals receive counseling, are referred to the appropriate services, and are encouraged to return when they are more prepared for employment services. Approximately one-fourth of the individuals who were initially referred to Work Re-entry needed additional pre-employment intervention through either the Day Treatment Program, a community college program, or some form of psychotherapy/counseling support for substance abuse, personality disorders, or emotional issues. The majority of these individuals eventually returned to the Work Re-entry program.

The purpose of the intake and evaluation process is to identify work aptitudes and attitudes rather than the individual's deficits. The focus on ability rather than disability is a key characteristic of the Work Re-entry program. An initial determination of feasibility to return to a previously-held job is made. The evaluation develops a portrait of the individual's work potential and the vocational options that would maximize that potential. As mentioned earlier, a traditional vocational evaluation comprised of intelligence tests, psychometric aptitude tests, and isolated trait and factor work samples is insufficient to provide an adequate picture of work potential for clients with TBI. Investigation must go beyond this to fully explore a client's ability to cluster activities, to follow multiple steps, to perform a task in varied settings, to discriminate among competing stimuli, to respond to supervision, to interact appropriately with those in the environment, and to satisfy multiple other demands necessary for successful employment.

The Work Re-entry evaluation process is highly interactive and is customized based on the person's response to the assessment circumstances and demands. Whenever possible, it is performed in a real work environment. If actual work tasks are not available, they are closely simulated. The activities and interaction involved in this type of evaluation not only evaluate vocational skills and aptitudes, but also provide insight about the client's executive functioning, frustration tolerance, endurance, social behavior, and so forth. Consequently, the profile of the client's work potential is comprehensive and can be used to determine an appropriate occupational "match."

The evaluation is carried out over a two-week period with approximately seven full days of assessment. During the first week, the client spends four consecutive days in a variety of assessment activities. Traditional work samples (such as those developed by VALPAR, JEVS, and TOWER) are supplemented by the Singer New Concepts simulated work trials and by situational work trials in the Rehabilitation Center's greenhouse or other work activities elsewhere in the Center (e.g., office and receptionist work, central supply inventory, and so forth). These integrated activities provide valuable information about the individual's aptitudes, existing vocational skills, personality and temperament, ability to generalize, ability to use compensatory strategies, and responses to different environments. This information is compiled into a report that is shared at a final evaluation conference. This conference usually involves the work evaluator, client, Work Re-entry counselor, and state rehabilitation counselor. At this point, the client's strengths are identified and potential employment areas are targeted to guide the job development activities.

COUNSELING AND GUIDANCE

Throughout the Work Re-entry process, the vocational counselor's overriding responsibility is that of vocational exploration, counseling, and guidance. Engaging the client in the process is essential. Many of these individuals have unsuccessfully attempted to return to work and are in great need of specific vocational guidance and support. Some individuals have been isolated and idle and they really do not know where to start. The medical rehabilitation process itself causes the individual to be removed from the mainstream, often for long periods of time during which life as the individual knew it changes. Once familiar activities become major challenges. Doubt becomes firmly embedded in self perceptions. Consequently, the thought of entering the competitive work environment may be overwhelming and anxiety-provoking. Anticipation, fear, and unrealistic expectations can be major barriers to successful employment re-entry. Accurate self-awareness requires a complex interaction of many brain centers that may be compromised months and even years post-injury (Prigatano, Fordyce, Zeiner, Roueche, Pepping, & Wood, 1986; Kreutzer, Leininger, Sherron, & Groath, 1990).

The Work Re-entry counselor explores the individual's fears and dreams. During this process it is also imperative that expectations of both the client and counselor are discussed and modified, if necessary, so that they are achievable. The counselor's engagement with and honest feedback to the client is imperative. The evaluation report and work trials are important tools to clarify a client's ability and potential and to assist in the recognition and adjustment of unrealistic expectations. The counselor and client use this information to identify employment options and the supports needed for employment stability. This is accomplished by empowering the client, by encouraging independent action toward vocational and personal goals, and by developing an alliance that promotes ownership of the return-to-work plan (Condeluci, 1990). Ideally, the vocational counselor and the client arrive at a consensus about the targeted employment direction.

PRE-EMPLOYMENT AND JOB DEVELOPMENT ACTIVITIES

Due to the diversity of pre-injury histories and post-injury functioning in this population, a broad range of employment and pre-employment options must be available. Some individuals may be able, with assistance, to immediately pursue competitive employment. For others, a more extended evaluation or an occupational trial period may be necessary to determine the person's actual capacity and to provide an opportunity for self-assessment. Some individuals may be able to perform the tasks required in a job, but they need some transitional support to "smooth out the rough edges" while experiencing the demands, requirements, and rewards of work. Others will need a more traditional supported employment situation to ensure work performance and stability. The key here is providing options that lead ultimately to the "right match."

When the initial evaluation identifies the need for work hardening or work adjustment activities, a plan to meet these needs is developed. Work hardening activities, designed to increase endurance, are carried out at the greenhouse when appropriate. Other work hardening or work readiness issues of a behavioral or interpersonal nature (such as responding to supervision or working around others) are addressed through work adjustment training in carefully selected job settings. In the latter case, one key to success is choosing a job which is consistent with the type of work in which the individual eventually will be employed. The second critical condition is selecting a work environment which is tailored to meet the specific objectives of the work hardening plan. This is in contrast to the approach commonly used in post-acute TBI rehabilitation programs of placing the person in any job or work activity for work hardening purposes.

A component of the Work Re-entry program, the Transitional Employment Program (TEP), has been developed to provide an intermediate step leading to successful competitive employment. TEP is not a final employment outcome nor do all clients participate in TEP. The purpose of the program is to provide a time-limited (two to three months) employment experience with on-the-job support to develop or refine appropriate work habits and to address other work-related issues on an individual basis.

Job development, the next step in the process, is dictated by the client's specific needs, functioning levels, and occupational potential. This requires staff expertise in the areas of market and environmental analysis. The staff explore the specific job requirements, with particular attention paid to the total work environment as well as to job-related tasks and performance requirements. Important considerations include factors such as the level and style of supervision, distractions, pace and performance requirements in the workplace, tenor and level of interaction with fellow employees, and tolerance for, or acceptance of, individual differences. The challenge is to ensure that a person has the opportunity to become a viable part of that workplace (Condeluci, 1990).

EMPLOYER INVOLVEMENT

Employer involvement and education are also vital aspects of the job development phase. An individual with a TBI is often re-entering the job market with pre-injury hopes, dreams, and abilities; and post-injury alterations in skills and abilities. Additionally, there may be a significant level of frustration and grieving about lost function and status. Initially, the person with TBI may present very well to an employer, but once hired, performance may not meet the employer's expectations. The opposite may also be true, the person with TBI may appear more impaired than is actually true, and consequently is not given the opportunity to demonstrate actual work skills. A general explanation to the employer concerning the consequences of TBI and a brief education about its residual effects can increase both the employer and the client's understanding and comfort level.

ON-THE-JOB SUPPORT

When a job has been secured, the client moves into the on-the-job training or support phase. The Work Re-entry program philosophy is driven by an awareness that when serving such a diverse population the supports provided must be individualized and creative. To produce successful employment outcomes the program cannot be locked into one technique such as the use of (dependance on) a job coach. It is not cost-effective, nor is it appropriate for all clients. Natural integration is the key to success in this step. Job supports need to be as unobtrusive as possible. Such interventions often involve customized compensatory strategies, worksite modification, and transportation assistance. Using natural supports is preferred, such as employee/peer coaching, flexible schedules, or written/printed cues to guide task performance. In some circumstances, an experienced job coach is necessary for training purposes and can be an extremely valuable means of breaking down attitudinal barriers in the work environment. In such an instance, the job coach is both an advocate and a trainer. When a job coach is used, there is a concerted effort to provide only the minimal level of support which is absolutely required to ensure satisfactory client performance. As soon as possible, the level of support is systematically reduced.

FOLLOW-UP

Active follow-up is provided through periodic on-the-job and/or phone contact by both Work Re-entry staff and the state rehabilitation counselor until closure. The primary purpose of such follow-up is to identify initial problems in adjustment and to ensure a solidification of the placement. Ongoing follow-up support is provided through monthly employment support group meetings facilitated by the Work Re-entry staff. Additionally, research assistants contact the person with TBI every six months to determine employment status. Longer term follow-up is designed to ascertain employment stability and to measure program effectiveness. It also provides the opportunity to reintervene if the person with TBI has lost a job or is at risk of becoming unemployed.

Program Access

Originally, the Work Re-entry program was developed to serve persons with TBI who had received acute medical rehabilitative and/or day treatment programming at Sharp. The program was designed as the final stage in the brain injury continuum from trauma to community reintegration and return-to-work. Once ready for the Work Re-entry program, the person would be referred to the California Department of Rehabilitation, unless the client was funded under the workers' compensation program. However, there were many persons with TBI in the community who were not served at Sharp, yet desired Work Re-entry program assistance. Program access was expanded. In almost all instances, a case would be opened by a Department of Rehabilitation counselor who would refer the client to the Work Re-entry program. Eligibility is a function of having a vocational handicap as a consequence of disability following a TBI and the potential for employment.

Case Illustrations

Three cases are presented to illustrate the type of person served, their course prior to coming to the Work Re-entry program, and the processes involved in their path to employment.

The client in the first case is one for whom the Work Re-entry program was initially developed, namely someone who had received both acute medical rehabilitation and day treatment programming at Sharp immediately preceding his referral to Work Re-entry. The second individual received little formal rehabilitation after his neurosurgical care and had nearly two years of vocational failure experiences prior to coming to the Work Re-entry program. In this case, the Work Re-entry evaluation indicated that a course of day treatment was required prior to exploring employment options. Finally, the third individual was chronically unemployed after his TBI and lacked the financial support to participate in post-acute brain injury rehabilitation despite having both the need and the capacity to benefit from such intervention.

CASE 1: EDDIE

> Eddie was a 19-year-old male who was living life in the "fast lane" prior to his injury. His family and teachers described him as bright and inquisitive, but argumentative. He had not applied himself in school nor focused on any specific

goals. He had dropped out of school and became more involved with drugs and alcohol. He had a number of traffic violations involving alcohol before he was injured. At the time of his accident Eddie was working at a home repair store as a cashier. He reported that he was satisfied with his job because he earned enough money to "party" and keep his car running.

Eddie was involved in an automobile accident while driving intoxicated. He sustained severe internal, orthopedic, and head injuries. He was comatose for approximately two weeks. Eddie received acute medical rehabilitation and day treatment programming at Sharp. The Work Re-entry evaluation was conducted while he was still in the day treatment program. Eddie believed that he could return-to-work without any assistance, a belief not shared by either the day treatment or work re-entry staff. He blamed others in his surroundings for failures associated with his shortcomings. The vocational counselor determined that consistent, immediate feedback about job performance or work behavior deficiencies was the most likely means of penetrating his bravado and non-ownership of his deficiencies. The TEP was identified as the most likely means of promoting the awareness, attitude, and compensatory behaviors which Eddie needed to secure and sustain employment.

The TEP provided the structure Eddie needed. The job coach helped him become more aware of his verbosity and distractibility and its negative impact on performance. The work situation enabled him to increase his endurance. He had the opportunity to both fail and succeed in his work, and to learn from it through the job coach's direct feedback. He could no longer ignore the fact that he was responsible for both conditions. During this time Eddie worked with the vocational counselor on issues associated with his drug and alcohol use, his adjustment to life as a person with disability, and his self-expectations.

Eddie worked in the environmental services department as an environmental aide and made significant gains in this transitional work program. Even though he was headstrong, he was eager and soon became capable of performing his job duties. He used strategies developed in the day treatment program to compensate for his memory and other cognitive deficits. He developed internal controls to stay on task and to reduce his inappropriate interactions with others. During this time, with assistance from the vocational counselor, he completed his GED, maintained a sober lifestyle, and was able to reobtain his driver's license.

The next step for Eddie and his vocational counselor was to identify appropriate employment opportunities in the community. Eddie was encouraged to explore employment openings and initiate the application process with the counselor's assistance. After Eddie made the first contacts, it was agreed that the counselor would make a follow-up contact with potential employers to provide reference and background information concerning his head injury.

The Work Re-entry staff encourage clients to tell the employer about their head injury. It is not necessary to provide great detail, but some general information about how it affects functioning often helps to avoid uncomfortable situations when the head-injured person's performance is challenged or the use of compensatory strategies is questioned. In most circumstances the employer will be more understanding and tolerant of an individual's difference if the employer has some explanatory information. This job-seeking approach is used with many clients to encourage independence and increase confidence in interacting with those in the work world.

Eddie is now successfully employed as a housekeeper at another hospital in the community. Initial on-the-job support was provided by the Work Re-entry staff to assist him in organizing his daily work tasks and in establishing environmental cues to promote optimal job performance.

CASE 2: KEN

One morning in June 1988, two weeks before his high school graduation, Ken fell asleep while driving and his car plunged off a bridge. He was transported by helicopter to a county hospital north of San Diego where he underwent emergency surgery for injuries including an open head injury, facial lacerations, and a fractured orbit. Ken was comatose for approximately nine days. Three weeks later he was discharged home. He was subsequently admitted a week later to another hospital for further neurosurgery and again was discharged home. Ken did not receive any rehabilitation services following his injury.

Just prior to his accident Ken had been promoted to a position as Assistant Manager of reservations at a luxury resort. He planned to pursue a career in hotel management following high school graduation. Even though he received his diploma, Ken lost his job a few months after the accident. For two years following the accident, Ken was not able to keep a job for any significant time due to difficulties related to the brain injury. Ken and his family started to seek professional help. Ken's parents contacted the Work Re-entry program. After the initial assessment it was determined Ken would benefit from the day treatment program before attempting to secure employment.

After approximately 10 weeks in the day treatment program, Ken was reevaluated by the Work Re-entry staff. Although the day treatment staff had addressed Ken's lack of self-confidence and initiative in the course of their programming, it wasn't until he was placed in a variety of work activities and environments in the Work Re-entry evaluation that the magnitude of these problems became apparent. Ken exhibited an extreme level of helplessness in these situations. Novel or stressful experiences (such as a car breakdown) revealed a virtual absence of practical problem solving abilities. Over the course of his post-injury experience, repeated failures had intensified his dependency on his parents and few remaining friends.

The TEP was selected as the best option to address the barriers to work for Ken. Like Eddie, Ken began the TEP in an environmental aide position. Although both Eddie and Ken were involved in the same TEP experience for the purpose of refining work-related behaviors, the targeted issues and outcomes were very different. Ken's major areas of concern were related to endurance and his strong sense of inadequacy and helplessness. The job coach's approach to training and support on the job differed dramatically. Ken needed constant reinforcement and gentle introduction to new, potentially overwhelming tasks. During the paid employment experience, Ken's endurance continued to build along with his confidence. He learned to be independent in his day-to-day needs rather than relying on his parents and others. While Ken was in TEP, he also received outpatient physical therapy. He learned about biomechanics and how to use this knowledge on the job to reduce his pain, increase his stamina, and reduce the risk of injury.

During TEP, Ken and his Work Re-entry counselor began to explore his vocational interests and identify sensible options. Using this information the counselor developed a job for Ken as courier for a large business in his community. The employer was impressed with the effort Ken made to increase his abilities and endurance. The employer was well-informed about the supports Ken needed to perform his duties (e.g., instructions given from only one person, regularly scheduled breaks). He began working part-time, and has gradually increased his hours to full-time status. The employer is satisfied with Ken's performance and Ken is gaining in confidence and the degree of control over his life.

CASE 3: CHARLIE

In 1983, Charlie was a proud, healthy 18-year-old Marine. His dream was to be a career Marine like his father. Charlie was involved in a motorcycle accident with a hit-and-run automobile, that left him unconscious on the side of the road. He was transported to a trauma center where a brainstem contusion was diagnosed. He remained in a coma for 11 days. After regaining consciousness, Charlie received two months of acute medical rehabilitation at Sharp.

After discharge from the Rehabilitation Center, Charlie was determined to return to the Marine Corps. The military did allow him to return as a reservist. He put forth great effort to realize his dream despite the challenges that resulted from his head injury, but Charlie's commander recognized that he was no longer able to withstand the physical and mental demands of the Marines and recommended medical discharge.

Charlie then attempted to go to college. He enrolled in a community college program to pursue an A.A. degree in Hospitality and Travel Services. He was driven and tenacious, but the courses were difficult for him and he became discouraged. While still trying to keep up with his classes, he also wanted to work to earn money. His first attempt was as a delicatessen delivery person. This job lasted about six weeks. He frequently became confused about the deliveries and got lost. Consequently, the employer fired him, another disappointment for Charlie. Charlie had a series of other unsuccessful job experiences for the next five years ranging from a shoe salesman to a fork lift driver.

Charlie became involved with the Work Re-entry program when his state rehabilitation counselor contacted the program. The counselor wanted the Work Re-entry staff to intervene at the job site where Charlie was working as a kitchen helper as he was having a very difficult time performing his duties. A Work Re-entry job coach attempted to "rescue" the situation, but the damage had been done and the employer fired Charlie.

The Work Re-entry counselor and Charlie spent many hours talking about his frustration and sense of failure. Given his continued interest in working with people and his desire to complete his degree, he was encouraged to access student services at the college. At the same time a thorough vocational evaluation was conducted to determine his skills and abilities in addition to the specific deficits for which he would need to compensate.

The evaluation revealed that because of his cognitive deficits Charlie would require an environment in which a large part of his job would be routinized and on-the-job training could be provided. Since he performed best when task completion involved only a few steps, his job tasks had to be relatively simple. He had excellent initial socialization skills and was a very hard worker, but he was exceptionally reticent about telling a potential employer that he had been injured in a traffic accident. Since Charlie had no obvious physical limitations and since he was an attractive, naturally friendly person, he found it very easy to get a job. However, employers and supervisors could not understand why he acted so confused and was unable to perform his job responsibilities. As a result, he had been fired repeatedly.

The biggest challenge for the Work Re-entry counselor was helping Charlie to develop the emotional ability to confront his disability and to share the facts of his TBI with potential employers. This was made even more difficult due to Charlie's poor self-image and lack of confidence. The keys were to (1) develop a job which would satisfy Charlie's desire to be with people and which he could learn despite his cognitive deficits and (2) to encourage him to take the risk of telling the employer and his supervisor about his injury and its effects.

Charlie and his Work Re-entry counselor reviewed his self-initiated post-injury employment experiences focusing on the probabilities of success given his cognitive deficits and on what might have occurred if his employer had information about his brain injury. Together they concluded that pursuing a job as a hotel bellman might be better suited to his work skills and preferences. Charlie also came to the point where he was willing to tell his employer about his injury given that fact that his efforts in the past to withhold such information had proven detrimental.

The Work Re-entry counselor developed a job opportunity at a small, yet elegant, hotel in downtown San Diego. Armed with new strategies to compensate for his cognitive deficits and support from the Work Re-entry counselor and an informed employer, Charlie started his job with renewed confidence. During the first month, his Work Re-entry counselor provided occasional on-the-job support to adapt certain strategies to the new environment. On-the-job support was gradually eliminated and replaced by Charlie's periodic participation in the Work Re-entry monthly support group. This group meets to provide a forum for Work Re-entry participants who are employed but who are experiencing ongoing job and personal adjustment issues, or who have lost their jobs and are seeking another. Participation is self-initiated resulting in a different group of individuals each month as contrasted with a psychotherapy or group counseling experience.

These cases are intended to give the reader a feel for the Work Re-entry experience. They represent several different pre- and post-injury experiences Work Re-entry clients encounter. They reveal the different issues which the staff confront in job development and placement, as well as the various approaches used to overcome barriers to return-to-work. They are, however, only three cases of the 130 persons who were served since the program's inception in 1987. To systematically evaluate the program's effectiveness, a research study was undertaken. The study was funded by the Social Security Administration (Grant #13-P-10041-901). Based upon the preliminary findings, which have been submitted for publication (Haffey & Abrams, 1990), it would appear that the Work Re-entry program is achieving its primary purpose – returning persons with severe and moderate TBI to productive lives as wage earners.

Program Outcomes

SUBJECTS

The authors investigated vocational outcomes for 267 persons with severe and moderate TBI. The majority received trauma care in the San Diego Trauma System followed by inpatient medical rehabilitation at Sharp or other southern California rehabilitation centers. The subjects include all consecutive TBI discharges from Sharp Rehabilitation Center from September 1987 to August 1990, and all persons enrolled in Sharp's Day Treatment or Work Re-entry program from October 1987 to August 1990. The subjects represent three groups: (1) Work Re-entry participants who may have also received day treatment services (n=130); (2) persons with TBI whose post-acute experience was limited to day treatment (n=49); and (3) persons with TBI who received no formal post-acute rehabilitative programming (n=88). The first two groups are treatment groups and the last is a comparison group.

The subjects are primarily white (80%) males (71%) with an average age of 32. Pre-injury education was 13 years, with 82% having at least a high school education. Over three-fourths were employed in a stable situation at the time of injury. Sixty-five percent had worked for at least three years.

Almost a third had premorbid substance abuse histories, 16% had significant pre-injury medical problems, 10% had documented pre-injury behavioral control difficulties, and 5% had significant psychiatric problems which required treatment prior to the TBI. Eight percent had a previous TBI.

The average coma duration was 12 days, with 78% in coma for at least 24 hours according to the following distribution: less than a week, 30%; 7-14 days, 22%; 15-29 days, 11%; and 30 or more days, 14%. As previously noted, discharge Glasgow Outcome scores indicated 57% in the severe disability category, 41% in the moderate disability category, and only 2% in the good recovery category at the time of discharge from inpatient medical rehabilitation.

In sum, as a group these individuals are representative of the TBI population who require trauma care and inpatient rehabilitation. In other words, there are very few minor head injury cases, and the sample excludes those who remain in coma or near-coma states.

These preliminary descriptive data have yet to be analyzed for between group differences which could potentially explain differential return-to-work outcomes. Visual inspection of the data indicate that the Work Re-entry participants are slightly better educated than the other two groups, and both treatment groups have a slightly higher percentage of persons with stable pre-injury work histories. The Work Re-entry program has fewer persons with prior TBI and a higher percentage of persons with moderate versus severe disability ratings.

PLACEMENT

The Work Re-entry program assisted 88 of the 130 persons served to secure competitive employment. This nearly 68% return-to-work rate is impressive given the rather discouraging vocational outcomes yielded to date for this population (Haffey & Lewis, 1989). Moreover, only 23 persons (18%) are considered inactive and chronically unemployed. As of October 1990, 19 persons (14%) were still active program participants and considered eventual prospects for return-to-work. These outcomes are twice as good as the vocational outcomes of the no-treatment group, in which only 34% reported having *ever* worked for pay since their injury. This lower rate of return-to-work is consistent with the naturally-occurring rate for the TBI population (Prigatano, Klonoff, & Bailey, 1987; Brooks, McKinlay, Symington, Beattie, & Campsie, 1987; Haffey & Lewis, 1989).

The day treatment-only cases had a 39% return-to-work rate, only slightly better than the natural history rate. This is consistent with prior reports of disappointing vocational outcomes from even those day treatment programs which specialize in serving those with TBI and which seek to return these persons to the work force (Prigatano, Fordyce, Zeiner, Roueche, Pepping, & Wood, 1984). It also lends support to the initial hypothesis that the philosophy and methods of the Work Re-entry program would yield substantially improved return-to-work rates for persons with severe and moderate TBI.

For the Work Re-entry group, approximately 22% returned to prior jobs (many with some work site modification or with alterations in job conditions), whereas the greater number (78%) returned to work in new positions. Over 70% were employed for more than 20 hours, with 43% full-time and 28% between half-time and full-time. Average hourly earnings were $7, with half between minimum wage and $7, 21% between $7 and $10, and 10% above $10.

Employment support during the first 30 days was quite modest, with 53% requiring little or no support, a third receiving minimal support, and only 12% requiring substantial or even constant support. One-third received some sort of job accommodation. Work Re-entry support was reduced during the second month, with no on-the-job support provided after 60 days.

Detailed comparison with other published vocational outcomes for persons with severe and moderate TBI is available elsewhere (Haffey & Abrams, 1990; Haffey & Lewis, 1989). Ben-Yishay's landmark program at NYU reported a 76% return-to-work rate (Ben-Yishay, Silver, Piasetsky, & Rattok, 1987), but only 53% were competitively employed, and replication of such outcomes has not been achieved by similar specialized programs (Prigatano et al., 1984). Preliminary data from programs which use the supported employment approach for persons with severe and moderate TBI have yet to report greater than a 50% return to paid employment even given the levels of on-the-job support inherent in such an approach (Wehman et al., 1988a; Wehman, Kreutzer, Wood, Morton, & Sherron, 1988b; Ellerd, 1990).

RETENTION

Returning persons with severe and moderate TBI to the labor force is a noteworthy accomplishment. Nonetheless, this outcome is of limited benefit if those placed do not sustain employment. The research design involved completing a job placement form once the person had been employed 30 days. Systematic follow-up occurred every six months from the date of *admittance* to the Work Re-entry program. This is in contrast to the more common practice of conducting follow-ups every six months after obtaining a job. Consequently, a person might be called one month to six months after initial placement depending on his or her Work Re-entry *admitting* anniversary date.

The data on retention reflect findings in the most recent follow-up, which was conducted during the period from April to October 1990. Figure 1 depicts employment status at most recent follow-up. The data are presented to indicate time from initial placement. In all but one time period, there were substantially more persons with TBI still working than were currently unemployed. The overall retention rate was 71% (62/88), and 71% of those placed at least one year prior to most recent follow-up were employed.

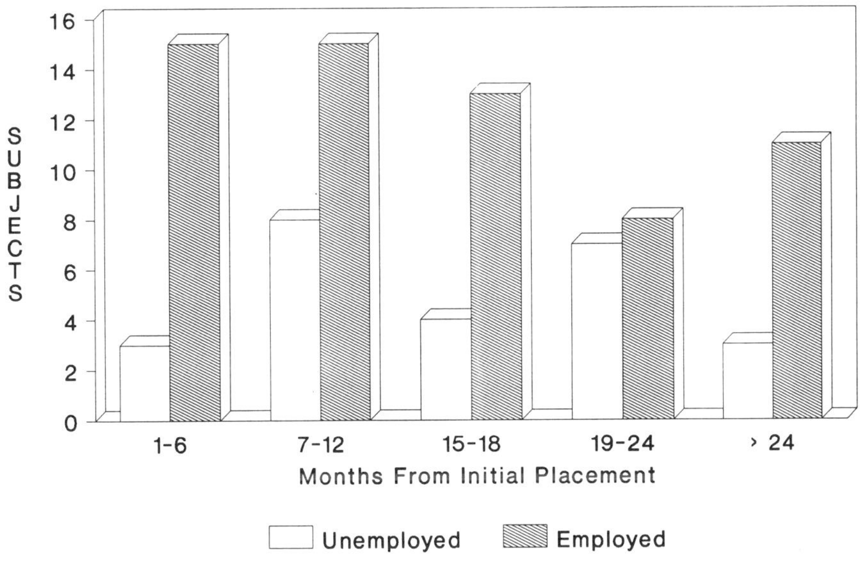

Fig 1. Employment Outcomes and Time From Initial Placement

These data reflect employment status at one point in time. An even more pertinent statistic, however, is the total time actually worked from the time of initial placement. This reflects the disabled person's post-Work Re-entry employment experience. The findings are displayed in Figure 2. The 62 persons who were employed at most recent follow-up worked an average of 12.4 months of a possible 13.7 months. In other words, as a group they worked 90% of the time since being placed. By contrast, for the 25 (one case was lost in follow-up) who were employed, they worked only half as much as the employed group. As a group, they averaged 7.1 months of employment of the possible 15.7 months (45%).

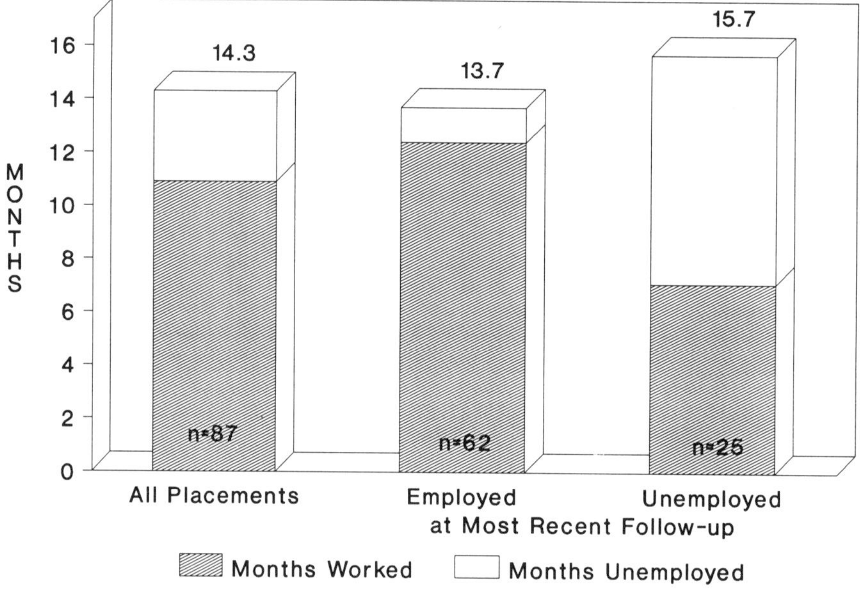

Fig 2. Relationship of Actual Employment to Possible Employment

Job stability was also investigated. Half of the Work Re-entry participants did not remain in the job they initially secured, irrespective of whether they were working or unemployed at most recent follow-up. There is little that can be said regarding the factors influencing job stability until the data reflecting reasons for job loss/change, duration of unemployment between jobs, and differences between subjects are analyzed.

Based on these preliminary data, it seems reasonable to assume that participation in the Work Re-entry program was a primary determinant of return-to-work for these persons with severe and moderate TBI. Moreover, preliminary findings reveal that this effect is more than temporary, and is robust for at least 70% of those who obtained jobs.

Future Development

The data collected on all 267 persons in the Social Security Administration funded research is currently being prepared for analysis and interpretation by project personnel at Berkeley Planning Associates of Oakland, California. The main focus is to delineate those factors which contribute to successful return-to-work. Dissemination of these findings is a high priority because of our conviction that the Work Re-entry program is highly replicable. Were this belief to be validated, there could be a substantial reduction in the long-term morbidity associated with severe and moderate TBI.

Dissemination of these findings is very important for another reason. The experience of the Work Re-entry program has caused us to examine our own beliefs about employment of persons with TBI. As we reflected on our own actions in the late '70s and early '80s, we concluded that despite our commitment to the rehabilitation of persons with TBI, we were quite pessimistic about the potential for return to paid employment in the "normal" work force. Our own negative beliefs helped create the reality. Cases which we now routinely expect to return to the labor force would have rarely been referred for vocational services, nor would return-to-work ever have become the targeted outcome for our rehabilitative efforts. Indeed, persons with TBI who expressed such intentions were considered unrealistic. Our rehabilitative efforts were often directed at helping them adopt "more attainable" goals or avocational activities and at helping them adjust to these changed realities. In short, the Work Re-entry experience has convinced us that return-to-work is feasible for many severely disabled persons *under the right circumstances*. We have come to believe that it is our professional responsibility to create the circumstances necessary to achieve employment instead of contributing to a climate in which return-to-work is precluded from the start.

Once preliminary analyses are concluded, the focus will shift to examining factors which impact on employment retention and job stability. The preliminary data appear to support the conclusion that there are two subgroups among those who obtain employment following participation in the Work Re-entry program — one which stays employed most of the time, and one whose employment is less well-sustained. We have considered investing in a job retention specialist to improve employment retention, but until the data reveal the factors which are associated with employment retention and/or attrition, it is difficult to assess whether such an approach is the best solution or exactly what specific factors such a person would attempt to address and solve.

Alcohol and illicit drug use is a principal barrier to both placement and employment retention (Ben-Yishay et al., 1987). Discovering better ways to curtail the negative impact of drinking and drug use in the TBI population is a widespread need, but it is especially critical in the area of obtaining and sustaining employment.

Conclusion

This chapter described an approach to vocational rehabilitation which has proven very promising. It is founded on the belief that work is possible for many persons with severe and moderate TBI. A tailored intake and assessment process which seeks to discover vocational potential (as contrasted to chronicling the deficits which would preclude return to paid employment) is one key to success. Another is a job development and placement process which creates the circumstances essential for achieving a "goodness of fit" between the person's competencies and the specific environmental demands of a job. Central to job development and placement success is an honest, ongoing relationship with the business community, especially with key persons in organizations who can influence hiring practices. Another key element is having a range of employment and pre-employment options in which employees permit targeted interventions and individualized means of overcoming barriers to employment. Finally, a strong commitment to accountability (in which we are willing to forego payment for services rendered unless placement for at least 60 days occurs) is another fundamental cornerstone of program success.

More detailed results and interpretation of the findings will be forthcoming. Nonetheless, the preliminary data strongly suggest the validity of the approach. Persons who may be interested in replicating the service and/or participating in informational exchanges are always welcome to visit and participate in ongoing program development.

References

Ben-Yishay, Y., Silver, S. M., Piasetsky, E., & Rattok, J. (1987). Relationship between employability and vocational outcome after intensive holistic cognitive rehabilitation. *Journal of Head Trauma Rehabilitation*, *2*, 35-48.

Brooks, D. N. (Ed.) (1984). *Closed head injury: Psychological, social, and family consequences.* Oxford: Oxford University Press.

Brooks, D. N., McKinlay, W., Symington, C., Beattie, A., & Campsie, L. (1987). Return to work within the first seven years of severe head injury. *Brain Injury*, *1*(1), 5-19.

Condeluci, A. (1990). Community factors and successful work re-entry. In P. Wehman & J. S. Kreutzer (Eds.), *Vocational rehabilitation for persons with traumatic brain injury* (pp. 307-321). Rockville, MD: Aspen.

Dikeman, S., Reitan, R. M., & Temkin, N. R. (1983). Neuropsychological recovery in head injury. *Archives of Neurology*, *40*, 333-338.

Ellerd, D. (1990). Development of a work re-entry program. In P. Wehman & J. S. Kreutzer (Eds.), *Vocational rehabilitation for persons with traumatic brain injury* (pp. 105-118). Rockville, MD: Aspen.

Fryer, J., & Haffey, W. (1987). Cognitive rehabilitation and community readaptation: Outcomes from two program models. *Journal of Head Trauma Rehabilitation*, *2*, 51-63.

Haffey, W. J., & Abrams, D. L. (1990). Employment outcomes for participants in a brain injury work re-entry program: Preliminary findings. In editorial review.

Haffey, W. J., & Lewis, F. D. (1989). Programming for occupational outcomes following traumatic brain injury. *Rehabilitation Psychology*, *34*(2), 147-158.

Hart, T., & Hayden, M. E. (1986). The ecological validity of neuropsychological assessment and remediation. In B. Uzzell & Y. Gross (Eds.), *Clinical neuropsychology of intervention* (pp. 21-50). Boston: Martinus Nijhoff.

Jacobs, H. E. (1988). The Los Angeles Head Injury Survey: Procedures and preliminary findings. *Archives of Physical Medicine and Rehabilitation*, *69*, 425-431.

Kreutzer, J. S., Leininger, B. E., Sherron, P. D., & Groath, C. H. (1990). Managing psychosocial dysfunction. In P. Wehman & J. S. Kreutzer (Eds.), *Vocational rehabilitation for persons with traumatic brain injury* (pp. 35-69). Rockville, MD: Aspen.

Leland, M., Lewis, F. D., Hinman, S., & Carrillo, R. (1988). Functional retraining of traumatic brain injured adults in a transdisciplinary environment. *Rehabilitation Counseling Bulletin*, *31*(4), 289-297.

McKinlay, W. W., Brooks, D. N., Bond, M. R., Martinage, D., & Marshall, M. M. (1981). The short-term outcome of severe blunt head injury as reported by relatives of the injured persons. *Journal of Neurology, Neurosurgery, and Psychiatry*, *44*, 527-533.

Prigatano, G. P., Fordyce, D. J., Zeiner, H. K., Roueche, J. R., Pepping, M., & Wood, B. C. (1984). Neuropsychological rehabilitation after closed head injury in young adults. *Journal of Neurology, Neurosurgery, and Psychiatry*, *47*, 505-513.

Prigatano, G. P., Fordyce, D. J., Zeiner, H. K., Roueche, J. R., Pepping, M., & Wood, B. (1986). *Neuropsychological rehabilitation after brain injury*. Baltimore: Johns Hopkins University Press.

Prigatano, G. P., Klonoff, P. S., & Bailey, I. (1987). Psychosocial adjustment associated with traumatic brain injury: Statistics BNI neurorehabilitation must beat. *BNI Quarterly*, 3, 10-17.

Udin-Aronow, H. (1987). Rehabilitation effectiveness with severe brain injury: Translating research into policy. *Journal of Head Trauma Rehabilitation*, 2(3), 24-36.

Wehman, P., Kreutzer, J., Stonnington, H., Wood, W., Sherron, P., Diambra, J., Fry, R., & Groah, C. (1988a). Supported employment for persons with TBI: A preliminary report. *Journal of Head Trauma Rehabilitation*, *3*, 82-93.

Wehman, P., Kreutzer, J., Wood, W., Morton, M. V., & Sherron, P. (1988b). Supported work model for persons with traumatic brain injury: Toward job placement and retention. *Rehabilitation Counseling Bulletin*, *31*, 298-312.

3

Community Re-entry

10

Preventing Post-injury Alcohol-related Problems: A Behavioral Approach

Mervin J. Langley

10

Preventing Post-injury Alcohol-related Problems: A Behavioral Approach

Mervin J. Langley

Introduction

Not only is alcohol use involved in the acquisition of 35 to 66 percent of all traumatic brain injuries (TBI's) (Rimel, Giordani, Barth, Boll, & Jane, 1981; Brismar, Engstrom, & Rydberg, 1983; Kreutzer, Leininger, & Harris, 1989), it is also a key factor in the failure of community reintegration efforts for many clients (Burke, Weselowski, & Guth, 1988). Alcohol detrimentally affects functions associated with the pre-frontal and temporal lobes including memory, planning, verbal fluency, complex motor control, and the modulation of emotionality (Ryan & Butters, 1983; Peterson, Rothfleisch, Zelazo, & Pihl, 1990). For those clients who have compromised prefrontal-temporal functioning due to TBI, ingestion of alcohol may further reduce the capacity for behavioral self-regulation.

Behavioral deregulation is manifested in a variety of forms. Alcohol use aggravates depression in TBI clients (Gualtieri, 1990), and is a risk factor in suicides occurring late after injury (Lishman, 1978). The potential for aggressive behavior is increased by alcohol intake (Maletzky, 1973), and this may be especially true for those clients with temporolimbic epilepsy syndrome (Haffey & Scibak, 1989). In addition to directly retarding the cortical recovery process (Hillbom & Holm, 1986), drinking may also counteract compensatory skills learned in rehabilitation. Clients may quickly habituate to the kind of unsophisticated information processing strategies consistent with intoxication as these require much less mental effort (Hasher & Zacks, 1979).

Other drugs, notably marijuana and cocaine, pose similar problems for survivors of TBI. Marijuana tends to concentrate in fatty tissue from which it is released gradually impairing attention, motivation, and short-term memory for up to four weeks after the last dose (Cox, Jacobs, LeBlanc, & Marshman, 1983). Although alcohol use will be the main focus of this chapter, the principles described apply to addictive behaviors in general.

Despite widespread recognition of the negative effects of drinking after TBI, few interventions have been proposed which specifically address this aspect during rehabilitation (Langley, Lindsey, Lam, & Priddy, 1990). Educational methods are frequently ineffective due to deficits in arousal, attention, and memory which prevent the retention of information considered necessary for decision making (Sanchez-Craig & Walker, 1982; Alterman, Holahan, Baughman, & Michels, 1989). Similarly, psychotherapy and support group interventions may fail due to the impairment of concept formation abilities. Hence, clients may be unable to apply solutions discussed in treatment to new situations. While they attend and appear to understand, they are often unable to profit from group psychotherapy which requires the capacity to maintain a self-reflective pose (Vannicelli, 1982). "Organic insightlessness" rather than denial may characterize these clients (Wood, 1987), preventing recognition of the need for change.

Even if a decision to abstain from alcohol use is made, maintaining such a decision will be very difficult. Impaired impulse control, together with a sense of being overwhelmed by the consequences of TBI, may contrast sharply with the easy availability, reinforcement value, and coping functions of alcohol.

A primary goal of rehabilitation is to help clients develop a lifestyle incompatible with drinking. As Vuchinich and Tucker (1988) indicate, preference for alcohol use (a) varies inversely with constraints on drinking and (b) varies inversely with the availability of alternative reinforcers and directly with constraints on access to them. Although there is an intuitive logic in assuming that clients who were alcohol dependent may continue substance abuse after injury, the typical "at-risk" client appears not to be the pre-injury "alcoholic." Instead the nonaddicted person for whom alcohol was a central lifestyle component before the injury, and who now has fewer alternative reinforcers or coping responses, may represent the typical at-risk client.

FUNCTIONAL ANALYSIS

The effectiveness of interventions addressing problems of alcohol use among persons with TBI will be enhanced by conducting a preliminary functional analysis of drinking. This includes an examination of the functional utility of alcohol for the individual with TBI (i.e., the ways in which the individual with TBI may perceive alcohol as helpful to him in various aspects of "coping"). The functional analysis also includes an examination of ingredients of a decision to abstain, as well as the impact of TBI upon the process of making robust decisions.

FUNCTIONAL UTILITY OF DRINKING

By the time they enter into community re-entry programs most TBI survivors have not used alcohol for weeks or months. Because alcohol-related situational cues are not present in the rehabilitation setting, craving for alcohol is seldom seen (Langley et al., 1990). The picture may change quickly once the client returns home.

Marlatt and Gordon (1985) used a social learning framework to develop a model of psychological processes governing a return to drinking. According to this model clients will, after a period of abstinence, encounter high-risk situations for drinking. The lack of appropriate coping responses in these situations leads to a reduction in self-efficacy (Bandura, 1986) and the triggering of positive expectations for the effects of alcohol. Self-efficacy refers to one's sense of mastery in a given situation and has been shown to be a good predictor of drinking behavior (Rist & Watzl, 1983). Low personal mastery coupled with compelling memories of alcohol's coping functions, form a backdrop for the resumption of drinking.

High-risk situations typically include contexts in which alcohol has become a preferred coping response or reinforcer. Annis and Davis (1989) identified categories of high-risk situations including unpleasant emotions, physical discomfort, pleasant emotions, testing personal control, urges/temptations to drink, conflict with others, social pressure to drink, and pleasant times with others.

Within any of these categories the reinforcement or coping value of alcohol may be enhanced for people with TBI. Positive expectations for the effects of alcohol are ingrained in long-term memory storage, having been acquired through modeling over many years (Christiansen &

Goldman, 1983). However, clients with TBI may be unable to evaluate the current (negative) effects of consumption due to their impairment of self-monitoring capacity (Vogenthaler, 1987).

In some cases, cognitive and vocational adjustment may precede the ability to initiate and perform everyday leisure and social activities (Oddy & Humphrey, 1980; Weddell, Oddy, & Jenkins, 1980). For such individuals, alcohol consumption may serve to structure time, organize interpersonal relationships, overcome isolation, and alter mood (Chaney, 1989). Undoubtedly, this could develop into a problematic coping mechanism, increase impulsivity, reduce problem solving, and prevent the client from acquiring adaptive social skills.

Closely linked to social isolation are the problems of anxiety and depression during recovery from TBI. Cumulative experiences of failure can lead to a catastrophic anxiety reaction, and withdrawal from the environment (Prigatano, 1986). Drinking becomes one means of dealing with failure. Alcohol directly alters the encoding of negative social feedback, even though the feedback may be accurately identified as inherently negative (Yankofsky, Wilson, Adler, Hay, & Vrana, 1986). In this way clients may be temporarily protected from catastrophic anxiety following repeated failure.

"Alcohol helps me to think more clearly" is a statement frequently made by people with TBI. This belief may be grounded in the individual's post-injury experience with anxiety. Anxiety seriously impairs the ability to attend adequately to task cues, diverting attention to off-task cognitions such as worry and self-doubt (Mikulincer, 1989). If it has anxiolytic effects alcohol may actually improve cognitive functioning, at least in small doses (Ryan & Butters, 1983). Recent evidence has indicated, however, that in the absence of a pleasant distractor drinking fails to produce anxiolytic effects and instead narrows attention to the anxiety-related cues themselves, thereby increasing tension (Sayette, Wilson, & Carpenter, 1989). Herein lies the danger that clients with selective memory of anxiolytic effects may drink when anxious and become more focused on anxiety cues leading to further drinking, and then engage in poorly considered, high-risk behaviors. This disinhibition is exacerbated by the existence of a frontal injury.

Another feature of recovery from TBI is the denial of cognitive and other sequelae as a means of reducing threat to the sense of self (Deaton, 1986). Alcohol consumption may facilitate this denial process through a self-handicapping mechanism (Jones & Berglas, 1978). Consider the predicament of a person who, because he processes information very slowly, cannot keep up with a conversation. Denial of his impairment prevents him from asking questions and requesting others to restate key points – strategies which have been suggested by his counselor. Instead, by consuming alcohol in advance of situations in which he is uncertain about his competence, he can attribute poor performance to his intoxicated state and not the brain injury. In this sense the client is drinking not only in spite of a cognitive impairment but, indeed, because of it.

Specific problems associated with prefrontal lobe injury may restrict a person's coping in the high-risk situations described. Impairment in the capacity to utilize feedback and to exercise flexibility in the face of changing situations is often seen. This may be reflected as a reduced ability to plan or to shift from one conceptual set to another. Hence, individuals may be unable to generate a new coping response, persisting instead with ineffective responses (Grimm & Filskov, 1986). Despite being able to state the necessary steps for dealing with a situation, the individual may be unable to carry out the steps due to behavioral deregulation (Luria, 1973). Consequently, this person might be more likely to fall back upon a habitual (automatic) response, such as drinking, in a high-risk situation.

To compensate for these impairments it is necessary to use a skill acquisition sequence in which clients are first trained to recognize specific high-risk situations related to their pre-injury lifestyle or TBI. This is followed by teaching strategies to improve problem solving and response flexibility in each high-risk situation. The client is trained to monitor and utilize feedback and to apply skills automatically, with little disruption by external influences, in a variety of contexts. Finally, family and support group members are trained to understand the specific high-risk situations, to anticipate problems, and to reinforce effective responses.

DECISION MAKING PROCESSES

Coping skill training is only likely to succeed when clients have made a decision to abstain. However, people are unlikely to relinquish so powerful a coping resource as alcohol without first gaining meaningful alternative strategies. For this reason skill training and motivational enhancement should be carried out concurrently.

How does change in addictive behavior occur? Saunders and Allsop (1987) suggest that spontaneous remission is initiated by a gradual recognition that the costs of continued drinking exceed the benefits. The person takes a "leap of faith" to eliminate these threats, and learns the coping skills needed as he goes. Positive outcome expectancies for the effects of alcohol (such as an expectation of relaxation) are meanwhile kept in check by the balancing influence of negative outcome expectancies (such as a fear of losing a job). Chick (1985) expresses this tension as follows:

> *Motivation is not about admitting being an alcoholic; It means believing that the good things about drinking are now outweighed by the adverse consequences and deciding to do something about it.* (p. 643)

Clearly, motivation is a fluid rather than a static condition. The strength of a decision to avoid alcohol will depend on current awareness of costs versus benefits of drinking. For TBI clients, however, an accurate appraisal of the harmfulness of drinking may be difficult due to damage to those areas of the brain which subtend perception and understanding. The client seems unable to call to mind any negative consequences. Positive expectancies for the benefits of alcohol are often more resilient, and in the face of failure to cope with high-risk situations, could reduce motivation to abstain.

We would probably be wise to expect fluctuations in motivation, particularly in those individuals with (organic) disorders of hedonic responsiveness. These disorders, related to damaged frontal or septal regions or their connections, can leave clients "out of touch" with the hedonic impact of their environment (Wood, 1987), such that they seem unable to perceive new rewards. Habitual, overlearned reinforcers like alcohol may then replace multiple, more subtle reinforcers in the environment.

A technique frequently encountered in the addictions field is that of directly confronting the denial of drinking behavior. This author, however, believes that confrontational strategies have questionable value for clients with TBI. Instead of promoting decision making, such techniques may increase anxiety and mental inflexibility, and damage the essential collaborative relationship with the clinician (Miller, 1989). It is necessary to go beyond influencing the content of decisions to facilitating the process of decision making itself.

Viewed in this light, each high-risk situation is a stimulus for decision making regarding alcohol use, and may confirm or disconfirm previous decisions. Robust decision making will depend upon the extent to which the client learns to accurately weigh the costs versus the benefits of drinking in response to each high-risk situation. "Cognitive vigilance," an awareness of and sensitivity to high-risk situations, is critical in this regard (Litman, Stapleton, Oppenheim, Peleg, & Jackson, 1983).

Stages of Treatment

The close relationship between alcohol use and TBI dictates that an integrated, multidisciplinary rehabilitation approach be adopted. This section will describe a multidisciplinary intervention for the alcohol-related problems of TBI survivors, within the context of the overall rehabilitation program.

The interventions utilized in addressing such alcohol-related issues are highly structured. Clinicians are directive and active, setting out an agenda for each meeting. A collaborative, empathic relationship is established as early as possible. This is especially important for TBI clients who may be dependent on the coping functions of alcohol. These individuals might perceive the clinician as taking something vital away from them.

Although the procedures described in this chapter can be conducted in a group context, in the early stages this often provokes excessive defensiveness. Group therapy in traditional substance abuse treatment is frequently seen as a means of confronting denial. As this author has argued, direct confrontation is best avoided in favor of a more Socratic approach conducted in dyadic sessions. Subsequent skill training sessions may, indeed, be conducted in group contexts, wherein powerful group forces (such as the availability of multiple sources of feedback), can be harnessed.

Miller (1989) suggested a number of approaches which are valuable in sustaining the collaborative relationship between therapist and client. These include:

1. The avoidance of labels such as "alcoholic";
2. Meeting resistance with reflection and empathy rather than confrontation;
3. Not imposing conclusions on the client;
4. Eliciting the client's own concerns as well as goals for the future.

These standards are continuously invoked as the assessment proceeds.

The intervention sequence is comprised of four stages:

1. Comprehensive Evaluation;
2. Motivational Enhancement;
3. Coping Skill Training;
4. Structured Generalization.

At each stage techniques are implemented by a multidisciplinary team under the direction of a TBI Addictions Specialist.

COMPREHENSIVE EVALUATION

Who should receive specialized TBI/substance abuse treatment? Langley et al. (1990) suggest that all clients be exposed to a prevention program. In this chapter, however, the emphasis is specifically upon those at risk for developing problematic substance use patterns after injury.

SCREENING

A screening process aimed at assessment of risk should be completed as soon as possible after admission. At a minimum screening should include:

1. An interview with family members;
2. A review of psychosocial/medical history;
3. A review of blood alcohol level at the time of injury;
4. A review of biomedical markers of alcohol dependence such as the hematological marker mean cellular volume (MCV), or the Gamma-glutamyl transferase (GGT) liver enzyme test (Heather, 1989);
5. Pre- or post-injury alcohol dependence as established through a structured interview utilizing the 25-item Alcohol Dependence Scale (Skinner & Horn, 1984) or a similar instrument.

The assessment of risk for future alcohol use, however, requires a still more encompassing investigation. Risk is also associated with such factors as the extent to which drinking has previously been established as a pervasive feature of social functioning. Pre-injury reliance on alcohol as a means of facilitating interaction would be included in this factor if socialization abilities are now impaired even when the individual was not perceived to be a "problem drinker" premorbidly.

ASSESSING LIFESTYLE FACTORS

A number of standardized instruments have value in assessing the centrality of alcohol use in the client's lifestyle. The Alcohol Use Inventory (Horn, Wanberg, & Foster, 1987), a 228-item self-report inventory, is written at a sixth-grade reading level. Its 24 scales provide detailed information about drinking styles, benefits, consequences, and acknowledgements/concerns.

The centrality of alcohol to pre-injury social functioning is revealed by the style, perceived benefits, and consequences of drinking. For example, a rigidly structured style of drinking might be exacerbated by TBI, particularly if the impairment results in a constricted behavioral repertoire. Alcohol may have been used in anticipation of tension reduction benefits. To the degree that the client now experiences increased tension, drinking may be more likely to follow. In addition, people who have experienced few serious consequences of drinking prior to injury might be less inclined to accept abstinence as a treatment goal.

An inability to monitor current negative consequences may contribute further to this reluctance.

If a client presents with a compulsive style of drinking, high perceived benefits, and few negative consequences, coupled with reduced abstract reasoning, any attempt to convince such an individual about the dangers of drinking could prove fruitless. It might be more useful to focus upon developing robust alternative behaviors which are incompatible with drinking. Positive addictions, such as physical exercise, are good examples.

Drinking may have short-term adaptive consequences for family functioning (Steinglass, Bennett, Wolin, & Reiss, 1987) after head injury. A family denying the extent of cognitive impairments might attribute a client's uncontrolled behavior to drinking. In this case drinking could be indirectly reinforced, serving to protect the family from overwhelming anxiety about the brain injury which is perceived to threaten its existence. Such families require intensive counseling to understand both the head injury and the drinking issues and to deal with the consequences.

The Family Assessment Device (FAD) (Epstein, Baldwin, & Bishop, 1983) measures seven dimensions of family functioning including problem solving, communication, roles, affective responsiveness, affective involvement, behavior control, and general functioning. The FAD, used in conjunction with a family interview, could help to pinpoint family adjustment problems after the TBI. These adjustment problems could diminish the family's ability to prevent or cope with drinking episodes.

It is essential to conduct an assessment of the roles and activities in which the client typically engages within his community. Roles and activities which are associated with the presence of alcohol (e.g., bartender, pool player), should be the focus of cue exposure/response prevention interventions. This involves extinction of conditioned craving responses which are elicited by situational cues (e.g., the sight or smell of alcohol). For example, procedures could be conducted in a tavern, allowing for the elicitation of craving not followed by consumption, thereby extinguishing craving over multiple trials (Blakey & Baker, 1980). At the same time, clients could be taught to request and consume soft drinks and to refuse offers of alcohol in a naturalistic setting.

For other clients, notably those with significantly reduced impulse control, it might be wiser to structure alternative roles and activities, and to teach avoidance strategies. A reinforcement survey is essential, but careful attention should be paid to access to these reinforcers. The ability of the community to restrict the availability of alcohol and to respond to drinking episodes may then be assessed.

ASSESSING HIGH-RISK SITUATIONS

The heart of the evaluation process is the anticipation of high-risk situations which, due to the client's impairments and/or drinking history, may precipitate alcohol use. Decision making training and coping skill training will be focused on the rehearsal of resilient responses to these situations.

Careful analysis of the projected discharge environment including social relationships, expected roles, recreational activities, vocational pursuits, and living arrangements, coupled with a review of the client's strengths and deficits, will often reveal a variety of high-risk situations. An individual returning to a peer group comprised of heavy drinkers may be expected to experience direct or indirect social pressures to drink. Likewise, the client working with hard-drinking co-workers on a construction site may experience temptations to join them for drinks after work. TBI survivors with social skill deficits resulting in social isolation will be especially vulnerable to "giving in" to the ambience of such situations.

The Inventory Of Drinking Situations (IDS-100) and the Situational Confidence Questionnaire (SCQ) are useful adjunctive tools for identifying high-risk situations and establishing baseline data. The first tool evaluates the extent of previous alcohol use in specific situations, and the second measures current self-efficacy in each situation (Annis & Davis, 1989). As indicated previously, self-efficacy is well-established as a predictor of drinking behavior (Rist & Watzl, 1983). A history of excessive drinking in particular situations, combined with low self-efficacy and cognitive impairments which limit the client's ability to cope, suggest the need for skill training in those contexts.

Having completed the process of identifying high-risk situations, a hierarchy of scenarios in order of difficulty can be established. A scenario may be presented in a brief, concrete form, to ease recognition. For example:

Level of Difficulty #7

> You forgot to pay an important bill last month and now you have to pay two installments. The more you think about it the more angry you feel with yourself. You are thinking about having a few drinks to help you get over it.

By having clients role-play or describe their responses to each situation, their social competence can be measured (Chaney, O'Leary, & Marlatt, 1978) using a simple five-point scale of adequacy. At first clients may find this difficult because it requires responding "as if" in the situation. Nevertheless, once clients are accustomed to the strategy, valid information about the impact of cognitive deficits in real-life situations can be obtained.

ASSESSING COGNITIVE ABILITIES IN HIGH-RISK SITUATIONS

Evaluation of cognitive strengths and deficits seeks to determine the client's ability to make decisions in high-risk situations, to generate effective coping responses, and to apply knowledge gained in treatment. Cognitive abilities needed for decision making include the abilities to perceive and understand the risks of drinking, to generate alternative behaviors, and to weigh the alternatives. It may be necessary to mobilize external sources of decision making (e.g., family) for clients who have severe deficits in these areas.

The ability to generate effective coping responses is reliant on the capacity to utilize feedback in the face of changing situations, to shift conceptual sets, to make plans, and to transcend the immediate context and consider the demands of the entire situation. In addition to experiencing difficulty in these areas, clients may have difficulty in executing the plans they have formulated (Grimm & Filskov, 1986). Extensive impairment of these abilities would suggest the need for instruction in automatic avoidance responses in high-risk situations instead of flexible coping responses.

Retaining and using treatment information depends upon attention and memory abilities and the extent to which the client is capable of self-regulation. The client's abilities in these areas determine which methods will be used. Cognitive-behavioral methods rely on self-generated thought processes as opposed to the use of external structure and reinforcement, which are the hallmark of traditional behavior modification (Horton & Barret, 1988). Accordingly, someone with reasonably intact problem solving abilities might benefit from self-instructional training (Meichenbaum & Jaremko, 1983) to maintain a task focus in high-risk situations. Alternatively, another client with severely impaired executive abilities might benefit more from contingency contracts specifying rewards for attending support group meetings.

Attention to the site of localized pathology provides additional guidelines. A client with extensive left hemisphere injury and language impairments will benefit from techniques which are less verbal in nature (Horton & Barret, 1988). Some examples are discussed in the next sections.

MOTIVATIONAL ENHANCEMENT

One of the primary tasks in brain injury/addictive behavior rehabilitation is to prevent premature closure in decision making. If the goal is to produce robust decisions, capable of weathering a variety of high-risk situations, then the client must learn to weigh the costs of drinking against the benefits most likely to result. Rather than simply making decisions, new decision making skills are needed. Therefore, throughout the motivational enhancement stage of treatment, it is wise to provide concurrent decision making training. This will include considering short- versus long-term consequences of actions in particular situations. During initial treatment sessions, clients are also encouraged to postpone decisions until they have considered all the information. Restraining change is a paradoxical strategy which may include encouraging the client to change more slowly or to consider the benefits of his present condition (Dowd & Milne, 1986). This strategy has the effect of producing more deliberate change decisions, especially among ambivalent yet defiant clients.

Recreational therapists have an important role to play in facilitating decision making through the expansion of the behavioral repertoire. Indeed, the perception of having choices and alternatives has been shown to reduce resistance to change (Parker, Winstead, & Willi, 1979). For example, one client found new sources of reinforcement at a local zoo and was soon accepted by a group of animal enthusiasts, despite his speech and language difficulties. Only then did he begin to participate in motivational interviewing regarding his alcohol use, which had previously occurred mainly in convivial group contexts.

MOTIVATIONAL INTERVIEWING

The goal of motivational interviewing is to create dissonance (i.e., a discrepancy between the person's drinking behavior and the achievement of important personal goals) (Miller, 1989). Instead of giving general information about alcohol, which is unlikely to be remembered or utilized, specific feedback is given. This kind of personal feedback about how alcohol is harming the person has been found to have a strong motivational effect (Kristenson, 1983).

Generally speaking, motivational interviewing, should be spread over several brief sessions. Note-taking should be encouraged when memory problems impinge. Comprehension of the information can be evaluated by asking the person to explain the information in his own words, asking for an example that demonstrates the point, or asking what the information means to him (Gorski & Miller, 1982). A successive approximations approach is adopted in which any approximation of the desired response is reinforced. Hence, a client who adamantly refuses to stop drinking but will agree to cut down is initially given praise and support.

Two or three feedback sessions scheduled soon after completing the evaluation are devoted to sharing evaluation findings in a concrete and nonjudgemental way. The objective of these sessions is to have the client gain an understanding about how alcohol will interact with specific impairments, and so reduce the ability to achieve important personal goals. Naturally this means that the clinician must relate evaluation findings to deficits which the client recognizes as legitimate. For example, a client who displays episodic aggression due to a temporolimbic epileptic syndrome might be given information about how alcohol, in lowering the seizure threshold, could contribute to violent outbursts , thereby endangering his job (see Haffey and Scibak [1989] for review of aggressive disorders). However, if the client denies aggression, this approach will not be meaningful and a different "hook" must be sought. It is obviously important to deal with denial (of brain injury sequelae) in concurrent sessions (see Deaton [1986] for relevant techniques).

At this stage, feedback is simply offered and the client is asked what he makes of the information. Resistance is met with reflection. By containing client defensiveness, more of the personally relevant information is likely to be absorbed.

The next step is to have the client express his or her own concerns about drinking and to express a willingness for change. As Miller (1989) points out, the principle is that "As I hear myself talk, I learn what I believe." Instead of imposing conclusions on the person, the clinician may say, "I have described some effects that alcohol is likely to have for you, tell me what things about your drinking you think might become problems." Usually some ambivalence is heard. The clinician's task is then to reflect both sides, but to place greater stress on the perceived problems. For example, "On the one hand you don't feel that drinking has caused problems in the past, but on the other hand you are really nervous about losing your temper because of the effects of alcohol and your brain injury."

Mildly challenging the client's statements has a beneficial, somewhat paradoxical effect. By forcing the person to defend his views, it is possible to increase the client's understanding and commitment to those views. For example, the clinician may argue, "How can you be sure that alcohol will have harmful effects?"

A likely outcome of this process is a tentative decision to cut down or quit for a period of time. For those individuals with compromised frontal or temporal functioning, abstinence is strongly desirable, and this creates a dilemma for the clinician. Should the client be pushed to extend the decision to one of abstinence? In most cases it is probably more important to proceed with skill training at this point, enabling the person to gain a sense of mastery. An expectation of being able to cope without drinking strengthens decisions in favor of abstinence. Subsequently, a return to motivational interviewing may produce abstinence decisions.

A less hopeful outcome will be that the client fails to gain any appreciation of the potential hazards of drinking. Diminished insight is frequently a consequence of frontal lobe injury (Wood, 1987), such that the person is unable to monitor behavior or to predict the consequences of a chosen behavior (Grimm & Filskov, 1986). Two possibilities then remain: to resort to the use of external contingencies to control drinking (e.g., behavioral contracts, supervised living arrangements); or to proceed with coping skill training with the objective of engineering a new pattern of daily living despite insight deficits.

Cue exposure/response prevention is a technique based upon a conditioning model of drinking behavior which does not rely on insight formation (Rankin, Hodgson, & Stockwell, 1983). Conditioned craving responses emerge when drinking repeatedly occurs in specific settings. Hence, a community re-entry variation of this technique would involve gradually exposing a client to individualized situational cues for alcohol consumption, while consuming soft drinks. Blakey and Baker (1980) and Cooney, Baker, Pomerleau, and Josephy, (1984) found that with sufficient trials of exposure, the desire to drink was sharply reduced.

"Cognitive vigilance" (Litman et al., 1983) is the end product of successful motivational interviewing. This involves an awareness of and sensitivity to high-risk situations, as well as the capacity to "stop and think" about the costs of drinking. After TBI a person may have difficulty monitoring environmental cues, or recognizing the high-risk situations discussed in the rehabilitation setting. Hesitation about abstaining from alcohol in a given situation provides grist for the mill, and an opportunity to make decision making contextually relevant. When this occurs, motivational interviewing should be undertaken specifically in regard to that situation.

COPING SKILLS TRAINING

The assessment of high-risk situations, discussed earlier, usually produces 10 to 15 "scenarios." Beginning with the least difficult of these, skill training involves the following components: problem solving training, instructions, modeling, behavioral rehearsal, feedback, and homework tasks (Chaney, 1989; Hawkins, Catalano, Gillmore, & Wells, 1989; Rose, 1990). When mastery is achieved in a particular situation the clinician moves to the next, until all scenarios have been addressed.

The content of skill training will depend on the client's unique strengths and deficits. For example, verbal learning deficits will require the application of nonverbal techniques such as differential relaxation. Coping skill training is ideally conducted in groups which allow for multiple models, feedback sources, and peer support (Rose, 1989). In a group context, clients with frontal lobe injuries are better able to learn such skills as attending to the perceptions of others.

PROBLEM SOLVING TRAINING

Problem solving training seeks to improve the client's ability to recognize high-risk situations, inhibit impulsive responding, generate a variety of possible responses, and adapt responses in the light of feedback (D'Zurilla & Goldfried, 1971). Self-monitoring can be used to facilitate recognition of high-risk situations in the environment. Given examples of personalized high-risk situations, the client can record occurrences of these conditions in both the community and rehabilitation setting. In this way, the client is sensitized to drinking-related cues, which subsequently become cues to begin problem solving. Whenever a survivor of TBI presents with a lack of self-awareness in relation to the immediate environment (Wood, 1987), sensitization is essential. Self-monitoring also provides opportunities to evaluate coping responses and for feedback.

It is not necessary for people to be able to recall the steps of problem solving in order to adopt a problem solving style of thinking which is characterized by planfulness. Nevertheless, it is useful to teach self-instructions for each stage of problem solving. Self-instructions provide a means of attentional control, enabling people to stay on-task despite distracting environmental influences (Meichenbaum & Jaremko, 1983).

Modeled after the approach of D'Zurilla and Goldfried (1971), the following self-instructions have proved helpful:

> Stop and think (problem sensitivity and orientation);
> What is the problem? (problem identification and formulation);
> What can I do to solve the problem? (generation of solutions);
> Which is the best solution? (decision making);
> What is my plan of action? (implementation).

After demonstrating this approach to clients, cue cards can be used to strengthen skill acquisition (Foxx, Martella, & Merchand-Martella, 1989). Initially these cards should provide response guidelines which are subsequently faded, along with verbal prompts as the client learns the technique. For example, "What can I do to solve the problem?" Remember to think of as many solutions as possible — brainstorm.

INSTRUCTIONS, MODELING, REHEARSAL, FEEDBACK, AND HOMEWORK

Having completed problem solving in relation to a given scenario, the client will have generated a preliminary plan of action. However, many survivors of TBI experience great difficulty in carrying out plans due to executive deficits (Grimm & Filskov, 1986). As Wood (1987) points out, skills need to be practiced before they can be used automatically and without disruption by external influences.

Coping skill training is predicated on the assumption that survivors of TBI may be using alcohol rather than other, more effective coping skills in response to stressors. Alcohol consumption produces feelings of power and control (Marlatt & Gordon, 1985), perhaps compensating partially for the feelings of powerlessness resulting from a TBI. Problem solving may be ineffective if the client does not have a repertoire of specific coping responses to draw upon in planning.

Task-relevant instructions and prompts are used to enhance the client's coping repertoire. In many cases these instructions may refer to verbal and nonverbal social skills or to self-instructions. Hall and Rose (1980) propose such criteria as eye contact, volume of voice, interpersonal distance, use of empathy, humor, and personal expressions, among others. These responses should be modeled by clinicians, before the client rehearses them in role-plays or by other methods (Foxx et al., 1989).

Learning to modify responses in the light of feedback is an important skill. In group interventions, participants may be trained to consistently provide a balance of positive and negative feedback to each other. At the same time, those receiving feedback should be reinforced for modifying their responses accordingly. Feedback is most effective when it is specific rather than global (Rose, 1989), and when it is perceived by the client to be personally relevant.

Finally, homework tasks provide a link between clinical intervention and the client's world, thereby promoting generalization of change. A stress inoculation approach (Meichenbaum & Jaremko, 1983), incorporates the notion that learning will be facilitated if the client is guided in implementing newly acquired skills in such a way that success is assured, particularly in the early stages. Each homework task should challenge but not overwhelm coping abilities, thereby creating the effect of "inoculation to stressors."

OTHER SKILL-TRAINING TECHNIQUES

A number of additional interventions have been shown to be effective in the treatment of addictive problems (Hester & Miller, 1989; Marlatt & Gordon, 1985). Each technique should be modified to "fit" the client's unique cognitive and neurobehavioral profile. No single intervention is likely to be effective for all clients. Instead, treatment matching on the basis of the client's cognitive functioning and history of alcohol use should be undertaken. Two interventions will be briefly described.

Covert sensitization is an imagery-based aversion technique (Rimmele, Miller, & Dougher, 1989) which has been found to be effective in reducing drinking behavior. The treatment goal is to develop an avoidance response by repeatedly pairing drinking cues (images of the sight, taste, and smell of alcohol) with aversive imagery (death of loved ones, pain, and vomit). Elicitation of aversive imagery is followed by an escape response (pleasant images, relaxation) which, in turn, is paired with the removal of drinking cues (e.g., running from a tavern). Sensory aspects of each scene are emphasized. Clients who have good visualization and sensory perception abilities could benefit from covert sensitization, particularly if they are highly cue-reactive (Kaplan, Cooney, & Baker, 1985). Cue reactivity refers to the tendency to produce strong physiological responses to the presentation of drinking stimuli, subjectively experienced as craving.

It is likely that the individual will be unaware of the antecedent events which elicit craving. An attentional capacity disorder may also limit the initial processing of information, rendering the person unable to generate avoidance responses. Both covert sensitization and cue exposure/response prevention (discussed previously) are based on a classical conditioning paradigm. As such they are useful for individuals who lack insight due to bifrontal or extensive right hemisphere injury (Wood, 1987). Some inoculation against craving might be achieved despite the client's inability to deliberately implement coping strategies.

Azrin's Community Reinforcement Approach (CRA) is consistent with a community re-entry model of TBI rehabilitation and is perhaps one of the most commonly tried and tested approaches (Sisson & Azrin, 1989). The purpose of CRA is to "rearrange the vocational, family, and social reinforcers of the client such that time out from these reinforcers would occur if he began to drink" (Hunt & Azrin, 1973, p. 93). Typically, this includes providing an alcohol-free social environment in which there is access to many social and recreational activities, vocational opportunities including support if needed, and family enrichment. Reinforcers are promptly suspended in the event that drinking resumes.

Usually, CRA includes an antidipsotropic pharmacological component, such as disulfiram (antabuse) which produces an unpleasant physiological reaction if alcohol is consumed. Reactions might include flushing, irregular heartbeat, dizziness, nausea, vomiting, and breathing difficulty (Fuller, 1989). However, the use of antabuse is seldom advisable for those clients with TBI who are unable to fully perceive the potentially dangerous consequences of the disulfiram-ethanol reaction (DER). Drinking may have powerful coping functions as discussed, and it is possible that these individuals may drink despite the negative effects. Moreover, as Fuller (1989, p. 125) observes, "Poor compliance with the drug regimen is the Achilles' heel of conventional disulfiram treatment." The very high level of supervision required in the use of the medication is prohibitive.

STRUCTURED GENERALIZATION

It is a common observation that clients with TBI often do not generalize strategies beyond the context of training (Foxx et al., 1989). The approach advocated in this chapter is one in which generalization is programmed from the outset by conducting training in community settings, and by prescribing homework tasks. A number of additional components are offered in this section.

Historically, addictions treatment has been virtually synonymous with support groups, notably Alcoholics Anonymous (AA). Although there is sparse scientific evidence of the effectiveness of AA (McCrady & Irvine, 1989), there is little doubt that many benefit from the support it provides. Involvement with AA may enable a person to begin developing a new support group early in the rehabilitation process. However, many individuals, particularly those without an extensive drinking history, are unwilling to attend AA. Additionally, the abstract nature of the material, the inability of some clients to assume a self-reflective pose, or deficient insight formation abilities may prevent the success of this approach for survivors of TBI.

An unfortunate tendency in TBI rehabilitation has been to separate the brain injury and addictions problems, and to provide only AA-based treatment to those clients with drinking histories. This overlooks the fact that many, if not most clients, do not have histories of dependence but are, nevertheless, at risk for alcohol abuse due to a breakdown of coping. In addition, brain injury and alcohol use are often interrelated such that drinking may serve to facilitate denial of TBI sequelae. For example, by attributing disinhibited behavior to drinking, the client can avoid having to confront his neurological deficits. Keeping the focus on both brain injury and alcohol use will help to prevent such traps.

Variations of the AA model which emphasize skill-based peer support are needed for clients with TBI. Working with existing brain injury support groups to provide specialized support, reinforcement, and even skill training for clients at-risk might prove to be a useful strategy. As indicated earlier, the goal of rehabilitation is to promote a lifestyle which is incompatible with drinking. Brain injury support groups are ideally situated to carry out this objective. One possibility might be for the support group to provide clients with reinforcers (e.g., activities and vocational resources) which are suspended following drinking episodes, as part of a Community Reinforcement Approach (addressed earlier).

Relapse is a common phenomenon with addictive behaviors. Brownell, Marlatt, Lichtenstein, and Wilson (1986) note that change seldom occurs without the client proceeding through several cycles of contemplation, determination, action, maintenance, and relapse (Prochaska & DiClemente, 1982). Both support groups and families need training to anticipate and cope effectively with relapses. This includes an analysis of the antecedents and consequences of each episode to modify controlling factors. Functional analysis could, by way of illustration, reveal that drinking leads to an increase in the frequency of visits from concerned support group members, and is thus reinforced.

Behavioral family therapy (O'Farrell & Cowles, 1989) is a powerful generalization tool. Marital or family problems may stimulate drinking behavior. Moreover, drinking may provide subtle adaptive consequences for the family, such as increasing the expression of emotion or closeness between family members (Steinglass et al., 1987). Mood changes in depressed clients, brought about by drinking, are often welcomed by the family, despite subsequent negative consequences.

In some cases, family denial of TBI consequences may be associated with a tendency to attribute the client's cognitive and behavior control problems to drinking. In the shared denial system, alcohol abuse may be perceived as less permanent or pervasive than TBI, and accordingly less threatening to family stability. Consequently, family homeostasis might be contingent upon subtle reinforcement for drinking.

For these reasons, family education about TBI consequences is essential if generalization is to be achieved. The balance between hope and realism is seldom achieved without some degree of agonizing. If alcohol use is to be avoided as a factor of family denial, its potential role must be made explicit. More importantly, the family will have to achieve a new family identity, which incorporates the reality of the injury.

Behavioral marital therapy includes strategies for structuring the family's role in the recovery process; for behavioral contracting between family members regarding the consequences of drinking; and for improving marital and family relationships. Conflict management skills are a primary component of these interventions (McCrady, Moreau, Paolino, & Longabaugh, 1982). In addition, specific training in the reinforcement and maintenance of skill training interventions is enormously helpful. For example, family members could be trained to provide unobtrusive cues to clients regarding appropriate social skills, or to administer relaxation procedures in stressful situations.

Throughout this chapter we have emphasized the need to increase the client's self-efficacy, or sense of mastery over high-risk situations. One way of doing so is to focus continually upon situational antecedents, and to teach skills specifically in response to these situations instead of global strategies. Consequently, an association between daily stress situations and coping skills is learned.

However, some clients may have difficulty monitoring their behaviors as a result of prefrontal lobe damage. Self-monitoring training is one means to facilitate recall of successes and failures with skill-training techniques. A self-monitoring form, reviewed weekly, will provide opportunities for ongoing skill-training as well as reinforcement. By attributing improvement to personal efforts, personal mastery is greatly enhanced.

Summary and Conclusions

Brain injury and alcohol use are closely related. Each may exacerbate the problems of the other. Each problem in turn may have origins in both sources. For these reasons TBI and substance abuse rehabilitation efforts must be carefully and deliberately integrated.

The rehabilitation process described in this chapter is founded upon observations that alcohol is a powerful coping resource and reinforcer. Accordingly, TBI/substance abuse rehabilitation is designed to structure an alternative lifestyle in which drinking is less central. Four stages of treatment are proposed: comprehensive evaluation, motivational enhancement, coping skill training, and structured generalization. In each stage a multidisciplinary approach is adapted and behavioral techniques are described. These techniques are specifically adapted to "fit" the client's neuropsychological profile.

Brain injury rehabilitation can no longer claim to be an embryonic field. Great strides have been made in developing intervention technology. Many TBI rehabilitationists, however, remain skeptical about their ability to effectively deal with addictive disorders. In this chapter an attempt has been made to show that addiction behaviors are often not only associated with TBI, but are, in fact, one of the consequences of brain injury. The time for integration of brain injury and addictive behavior technologies has arrived and treatment models, however preliminary, are now available.

References

Alterman, A. I., Holahan, J. M., Baughman, T. G., & Michels, S. (1989). Predictors of alcoholic's acquisition of treatment-related knowledge. *Journal of Substance Abuse Treatment, 6*, 49-53.

Annis, H. M., & Davis, C. S. (1989). Relapse prevention. In R. K. Hester & W. R. Miller (Eds.) *Handbook of alcoholism treatment approaches.* New York: Pergamon Press.

Bandura, A. (1986). *Social foundations of thought and action: A social cognitive theory.* Englewood Cliffs, NJ: Prentice-Hall.

Blakey, R., & Baker, R. (1980). An exposure approach to alcohol abuse. *Behavior Research and Therapy, 18*, 319-325.

Brismar, B., Engstrom, A., & Rydberg, V. (1983). Head injury and intoxication: A diagnostic and therapeutic dilemma. *Acta Chirurgica Scandanavica, 149*, 11-14.

Brownell, K. D., Marlatt, G. A., Lichtenstein, E., & Wilson, G. T. (1986). Understanding and preventing relapse. *American Psychologist, 41*, 765-783.

Burke, W. H., Weselowski, M. D., & Guth, W. L. (1988). Comprehensive head injury rehabilitation: An outcome evaluation. *Brain Injury, 2*, 313-322.

Chaney, E. F., O'Leary, M. R., & Marlatt, G. A. (1978). Skill training with alcoholics. *Journal of Consulting and Clinical Psychology, 46*, 1092-1104.

Chaney, E. F. (1989). Social skills training. In R. K. Hester & W. R. Miller (Eds.), *Handbook of alcoholism treatment approaches.* New York: Pergamon Press.

Chick, J. (1985). Management of the problem drinker. *Medicine International, 2*, 641-644.

Christiansen, B. A., & Goldman, M. S. (1983). Alcohol-related expectancies versus demographic background variables in the prediction of adolescent drinking. *Journal of Consulting and Clinical Psychology, 5*, 249-257.

Cooney, N. L., Baker, L. H., Pomerleau, O. F., & Josephy, B. (1984). Salivation to drinking cues in alcohol abuse: Toward the validation of a physiological measure of craving. *Addictive Behaviors, 9*, 91-94.

Cox, T. C., Jacobs, M. R., LeBlanc, A. E., & Marshman, J. A. (1983). *Drugs and drug abuse: A reference text.* Toronto: Addiction Research Foundation.

D'Zurilla, T. J., & Goldfried, M. R. (1971). Problem solving and behavior modification. *Journal of Abnormal Psychology, 78*, 197-226.

Deaton, A. V. (1986). Denial in the aftermath of traumatic head injury: Its manifestations, measurement, and treatment. *Rehabilitation Psychology, 31*, 231-240.

Dowd, E. T., & Milne, C. R. (1986). Paradoxical interventions in counseling psychology. *The Counseling Psychologist, 14*, 237-282.

Epstein, N., Baldwin, L., & Bishop, S. (1983). The McMaster Family Assessment Device. *Journal of Marital and Family Therapy*, *9*, 171-180.

Foxx, R. M., Martella, R. C., & Merchand-Martella, N. E. (1989). The acquisition, maintenance, and generalization of problem solving skills by closed head-injured adults. *Behavior Therapy*, *20*, 61-76.

Fuller, R. K. (1989). Antidipsotropic medications. In R. K. Hester & W. R. Miller (Eds.), *Handbook of alcoholism treatment approaches* (pp. 117-127). New York: Pergamon Press.

Gorski, T. T.., & Miller, M. (1982). *Counseling for relapse prevention*. Independence, Missouri: Independence Press.

Grimm, B. H., & Filskov, S. B. (1986). Neuropsychological assessment. In A. R. Ciminero, K. S. Calhoun, H. E. Adams (Eds.), *Handbook of behavioral assessment* (pp. 722-750). New York: John Wiley & Sons.

Gualtieri, T. (1990). The neuropharmacology of inadvertent drug effects in patients with traumatic brain injuries. *Journal of Head Trauma Rehabilitation*, *5*, 32-40.

Haffey, W. J., & Scibak, J. W. (1989). Management of aggressive behavior following traumatic brain injury. In D. W. Ellis, & A. L. Christensen (Eds.), *Neuropsychological treatment after brain injury* (pp. 317-360). Norwell: Kluwer Academic Publishers.

Hall, J. A., & Rose, S. D. (1980). Assertion training in a group. In S. D. Rose (Ed). *A casebook in group therapy* (pp. 19-65). Englewood Cliffs, New Jersey: Prentice Hall.

Hasher, L., & Zacks, R. T. (1979). Automatic and effortful processes in memory. *Journal of Experimental Psychology Gen.*, *108*, 356-388.

Hawkins, J. D., Catalano, R. F., Gillmore, M. R., & Wells, E. A. (1989). Skills training for drug abusers: Generalization, maintenance, and effects on drug use. *Journal of Consulting and Clinical Psychology*, *57*, 559-563.

Heather, N. (1989). Brief intervention strategies. In R. K. Hester, & W. R. Miller (Eds.), *Handbook of alcoholism treatment approaches* (pp. 93-116). New York: Pergamon Press.

Hester, R. K., & Miller, W. R. (1989). *Handbook of alcoholism treatment approaches*. New York: Pergamon Press.

Hillbom, M., & Holm, L. (1986). Contribution of traumatic brain injury to neuropsychological deficits in alcoholics. *Journal of Neurological & Neurosurgical Psychiatry*, *49*, 1348-1353.

Horn, J. L., Wanberg, K. W., & Foster, F. M. (1987). *Guide to the Alcohol Use Inventory*. Minneapolis, MN: National Computer Systems.

Horton, A. M., & Barret, D. (1988). Neuropsychological assessment and behavior therapy: New directions in head trauma rehabilitation. *Journal of Head Trauma Rehabilitation*, *3*, 57-64.

Hunt, G. M., & Azrin, N. H. (1973). A community reinforcement approach to alcoholism. *Behavior Research and Therapy*, *11*, 91-104.

Jones, E. E., & Berglas, S. (1978). Control of attributions about the self through self-handicapping strategies: The appeal of alcohol and the role of underachievement. *Personality and Social Psychology Bulletin, 4*, 200-206.

Kaplan, R. F., Cooney, N. L., & Baker, L. H. (1985). Reactivity to alcohol-related cues: Physiological and subjective responses in alcoholics and non-problem drinkers. *Journal of Studies on Alcohol, 46*, 267-272.

Kreutzer, J. S., Leininger, B. E., & Harris, J. A. (1989). The evolving role of neuropsychology in community integration. In J. S. Kreutzer & P. Wehman (Eds.), *Community integration following traumatic brain injury* (pp. 49-66). Baltimore: Paul H. Brookes Publishing Co.

Kristenson, H. (1983). *Studies on alcohol related disabilities in a medical intervention (2nd Ed.)*, Malmo, Sweden: University of Lund.

Langley, M. J., Lindsey, W. P., Lam, C. S., & Priddy, D. A. (1990). A comprehensive alcohol abuse treatment programme for persons with traumatic brain injury. *Brain Injury, 4*, 77-86.

Lishman, W. A. (1978). *Organic psychiatry*. Oxford, England: Blackwell.

Litman, G. K., Stapleton, J., Oppenheim, A. N., Peleg, M., & Jackson, P. (1983). An instrument for measuring coping behaviors in hospitalized alcoholics: Implications for relapse prevention treatment. *British Journal of Addiction, 78*, 269-276.

Luria, A. R. (1973). *The working brain*. New York: Basic.

Maletzky, B. M. (1973). The episodic dyscontrol syndrome. *Disorders of the Nervous System, 34*, 178-185.

Marlatt, G. A., & Gordon, J. R. (1985). *Relapse prevention: Maintenance strategies in the treatment of addictive behaviors*. New York: Guilford Press.

McCrady, B. S., & Irvine, S. (1989). Self-help groups. In R. K. Hester & W. R. Miller (Eds.), *Handbook of alcoholism treatment approaches* (pp. 153-169). New York: Pergamon Press.

McCrady, B. S., Moreau, J., Paolino, T. J., & Longabaugh, R. (1982). Joint hospitalization and couples therapy for alcoholism: A four-year follow-up. *Journal of Studies on Alcohol, 43*, 1244-1250.

Meichenbaum, D., & Jaremko, M. E. (1983). *Stress reduction and prevention*. New York: Plenum Press

Mikulincer, M. (1989). Cognitive interference and learned helplessness: The effects of off-task cognitions on performance following unsolvable problems. *Journal of Personality and Social Psychology, 57*, 129-135.

Miller, W. R. (1989). Increasing motivation for change. In R. K. Hester & W. R. Miller (Eds.), *Handbook of alcoholism treatment approaches* (pp. 67-80). New York: Pergamon Press.

O'Farrell, T. J., & Cowles, K. S. (1989). Marital and family therapy. In R. K. Hester & W. R. Miller (Eds.), *Handbook of alcoholism treatment approaches* (pp. 183-205). New York: Pergamon Press.

Oddy, M., & Humphrey, M. (1980). Social recovery during the year following severe head injury. *Journal of Neurological and Neurosurgical Psychiatry, 43*, 798-802.

Parker, M. W., Winstead, D. K., & Willi, F. J. P. (1979). Patient autonomy in alcohol rehabilitation: 1. Literature review. *International Journal of the Addictions, 14*, 1015-1022.

Peterson, J. B., Rothfleisch, J., Zelazo, P. D., & Pihl, R. O. (1990). Acute alcohol intoxication and cognitive functioning. *Journal of Studies on Alcohol, 51*, 114-122.

Prigatano, G. P. (1986). Personality and psychosocial consequences after brain injury. In M. J. Meier, A. L. Benton, & L. Diller (Eds.), *Neuropsychological rehabilitation* (pp. 355-378). New York: Guilford Press.

Prochaska, J. O., & DiClemente, C. C. (1982). Transtheoretical therapy: Toward a more integrative model of change. *Psychotherapy: Theory, Research, & Practice, Vol. 19*, 276-288.

Rankin, H., Hodgson, R. I., & Stockwell, T. (1983). Cue exposure and response prevention with alcoholics: A controlled trial. *Behavior Research and Therapy, 21*, 435-446.

Rimel, R. W., Giordani, B. G., Barth, J. T., Boll, T. J., & Jane, J. A. (1981). Disability caused by minor head injury. *Neurosurgery, 9*, 221-228.

Rimmele, C. T., Miller, W. R., & Dougher, M. J. (1989). Aversion therapies. In R. K. Hester & W. R. Miller (Eds.), *Handbook of Alcoholism Treatment Approaches* (pp. 128-140). New York: Pergamon Press.

Rist, F., & Watzl, H. (1983). Self-assessment of relapse risk and assertiveness in relation to treatment outcome of female alcoholics. *Addictive Behaviors, 8*, 121-127.

Rose, S. D. (1989). Coping skill training in groups. *International Journal of Group Psychotherapy, 39*, 59-78.

Ryan, C., & Butters, N. (1983). Cognitive deficits in alcoholics. In B. Kissin & H. Begleiter (Eds.), *The pathogenesis of alcoholism: Biological factors*. New York: Plenum Press.

Sanchez-Craig, M., & Walker, K. (1982). Teaching coping skills to alcoholics in a co-educational halfway house: 1. Assessment of programme effects. *British Journal of Addiction, 77*, 35-50.

Saunders, B., & Allsop, S. (1987). Relapse: A psychological perspective. *British Journal of Addiction, 82*, 417-429.

Sayette, M. A., Wilson, G. T., & Carpenter, J. A. (1989). Cognitive moderators of alcohol's effects on anxiety. *Behavior Research and Therapy, 27*, 685-690.

Sisson, R., & Azrin, N. (1989). The community reinforcement approach. In R. K. Hester & W. R. Miller (Eds.), *Handbook of alcoholism treatment approaches* (pp. 242-258). New York: Pergamon Press.

Skinner, H. A., & Horn, J. L. (1984). *Alcohol Dependence Scale (ADS) users guide*. Toronto, Ontario: Addiction Research Foundation.

Steinglass, P., Bennett, L. A., Wolin, S. J., & Reiss, D. (1987). *The alcoholic family*. New York: Basic.

Vannicelli, M. (1982). Group psychotherapy with alcoholics: Special techniques. *Journal of Studies on Alcohol*, *43*, 17-37.

Vogenthaler, D. R. (1987). An overview of head injury: Its consequences and rehabilitation. *Brain Injury*, *1*, 113-127.

Vuchinich, R. E., & Tucker, J. A. (1988). Contributions from behavioral theories of choice to an analysis of alcohol abuse. *Journal of Abnormal Psychology*, *97*, 181-195.

Weddell, R., Oddy, M., & Jenkins, D. (1980). Social adjustment after rehabilitation: A two-year follow-up of patients with severe head injury. *Psychological Medicine*, *10*, 257-263.

Wood, R. (1987). *Brain injury rehabilitation: A neurobehavioral approach*. Rockville, Maryland: Aspen Publishers.

Yankofsky, L., Wilson, G. T., Adler, J., Hay, W., & Vrana, S. (1986). The effect of alcohol on self-evaluation, awareness of negative interpersonal feedback, and perceptions of control and power. *Journal of Studies on Alcohol*, *47*, 26-33.

11

The Life Coach Model of Community Re-entry

Michael L. Jones
Peter D. Patrick
Randall W. Evans
J. Jepson Wulff

11

The Life Coach Model of Community Re-entry

Michael L. Jones
Peter D. Patrick
Randall W. Evans
J. Jepson Wulff

Introduction

The 1980s witnessed tremendous growth in the field of head injury rehabilitation, particularly in the "post-acute" stage of rehabilitation. Post-acute rehabilitation refers to services provided after acute hospitalization (including inpatient rehabilitation programs). Post-acute models include residential community re-entry or transitional living programs (Boake, 1990), integrated day treatment programs (Evans and Preston, 1990), outpatient services, and home-health services (Ozga, 1978). The goal shared by all such programs is successful community reintegration of individuals with acquired brain injury.

The proliferation of post-acute services for persons with acquired brain injury has been prompted by several clinical and market (i.e., reimbursement) issues. Clinically, post-acute programs have emerged to address deficits in functioning that cannot be adequately addressed during acute-stage rehabilitation. Traditionally, the goal of acute rehabilitation has been to preserve life, prevent further loss of functioning (e.g., prevention of contractures), and restore basic functions (e.g., sensorimotor and basic cognitive functions). But after often heroic rehabilitation efforts at the acute stage, many individuals with acquired brain injury are discharged from hospital settings with continued, significant deficits in functioning. Although the nature and extent of deficits exhibited by these individuals may vary significantly, a common result of these deficits is the inability to perform everyday activities of community living.

Experience from applications of the community re-entry model in head injury rehabilitation (Cope, Cole, Hall, & Barkan, 1990; Evans, 1991) and from other fields (e.g., treatment of chronic mental illness and developmental disabilities) suggests that a different treatment approach may be necessary to address deficits seen by head-injured individuals after acute rehabilitation. Once restorative therapy has derived maximum benefit, amelioration of remaining deficits in everyday functioning requires the acquisition of new skills. The necessary approach becomes one of *skills training and application*. Post-acute rehabilitation is characterized by the application of learning technology to the development of adaptive skills which allow the head-injured individual to successfully cope with community living.

Experience also suggests that acute hospital settings are not ideal for training the skills necessary for successful community living. While many acute settings attempt to simulate community settings, this typically is not adequate to ensure generalization of necessary skills to the home community. A community-referenced treatment context is required to achieve adequate generalization and maintenance of skills.

Because of market pressures to shorten lengths of stay in acute hospitalization, head-injured individuals are leaving acute settings with more "acute" deficits, furthering the need for post-acute services. These pressures notwithstanding, financial providers are insisting that service providers take more accountability for achieving significant, functional outcomes from rehabilitation. While maintenance of life and basic functions — the purview of acute rehabilitation — are certainly significant outcomes, the need to lessen the long-term cost of care by returning head-injured individuals to optimal independent functioning is a major market force shaping post-acute services.

The challenge for post-acute programs is to achieve functional outcomes in returning head-injured individuals to community life and to do so at a reasonable cost. In response to this challenge, post-acute rehabilitation models continue to evolve. This chapter describes a home-based, post-acute rehabilitation model called Life Coaching. Initiated in the Spring of 1990, the Life Coach program provides rehabilitation services in a client's home and community settings. The Life Coach program is intended to complement existing community re-entry services (e.g., residential, day treatment) and provides an option for clients and families who, for a variety of reasons, may be more suitable candidates for home-based treatment.

Theoretical Foundation for the Life Coach Model

The Life Coach model is based in part on principles of behavioral learning technology and their application to community-based instruction (Flynn & Nitsch, 1980; Horner, Dunlap, & Koegel, 1988). A wealth of technology exists outside of traditional medical rehabilitation which focuses on skills training to achieve functional and durable outcomes in community integration of persons who are severely disabled. Key components of an integrated, community-based instructional model include context relevance, treatment integration, and use of behavioral-based learning technology.

CONTEXT RELEVANCE

Skills training is most successful when skills are taught in the variety of settings in which they must be used. Context-relevant instruction incorporates the following characteristics:

1. The skills being taught have *immediate utility* (i.e., use of the skill will produce something useful for the trainee);
2. Skills are taught in the *actual, physical context* in which they will be used;
3. Skills are *adaptable* or *generalizable* (i.e., they enable the trainee to respond to different situations with appropriate adaptations) (Sailor, Goetz, Anderson, Hunt, & Gee, 1988).

INTEGRATED TREATMENT APPROACH

An important distinction should be made between delivery of services and an *integrated* treatment approach. An integrated approach requires comprehensive and consistent application and this is the result of detailed coordination through case management. The following example highlights this difference. Traditionally, speech therapy takes place in a "pull-out" fashion. The client joins a speech therapist in a treatment room and receives repeated trials on linguistic content that may be arbitrary and irrelevant for the client's future functioning in his or her home community. In an integrated approach, the speech therapist would work with the client, other clinicians, and family members in a consultative fashion to examine the client's communication needs in a variety of natural settings, including interactions with different individuals. Based on this analysis, client- and context-relevant instructional materials and activities would be developed. A variety of individuals, including family members and other clinicians, would be enlisted to assist the client in conducting these activities.

USE OF BEHAVIORAL-BASED LEARNING TECHNOLOGY

The instructional technology used in Life Coaching is based on the "Direct Instruction" approach developed by Engelmann and Carnine (1982) and elaborated on by Horner and colleagues (Horner & Albin, 1988) to teach community living skills to persons who are severely disabled. Direct Instruction is a systematic approach for establishing stimulus control. Stimulus control refers to the functional relationship between an antecedent stimulus and changes in the probability that a desired response will occur following this stimulus (Terrace, 1966). The purpose of Direct Instruction is to ensure the appropriate generalization of skills. By establishing stimulus control, Direct Instruction promotes response precision (i.e., both the generalization of skills to appropriate situations and the discrimination of occasions when responsing is not appropriate).

The Direct Instruction literature includes numerous applications to teaching appropriate community skills, such as street crossing (Horner, Jones, & Williams, 1985), use of public transportation (Horner & Albin, 1988), shopping (Horner, Albin, & Ralph, 1986), and vocational tasks (Horner, Eberhard, & Sheehan, 1986). Direct Instruction techniques have also been applied to teaching of higher level skills, such as academic skills (Carnine & Silbert, 1979; Silbert, Carnine, & Stein, 1981), identification of safe and unsafe home and community situations (Madigan, 1989), appropriate social skills (Walker, 1986, 1988), and memory retraining with head-injured individuals (Madigan, 1987).

Factors Contributing to Development of Life Coaching Model

Life Coaching was developed in response to several factors. First, the program was developed in response to the need to provide rehabilitation services to a largely underserved population of head-injured individuals – those with minor head injuries. It is estimated that there are over 400,000 new head injuries annually. Of those who seek medical attention, over 95% are classified as minor head injuries. Kay (1988) points out that if only five percent of individuals with minor head injuries suffer significant functional disabilities, their number would equal those with moderate to severe injuries.

Minor head injury is most often the result of trauma where there is no or brief loss of consciousness. Immediately after the accident, there is usually confusion, headaches, dizziness, and short-term memory loss. Hospitalization may be brief or nonexistent. Neurological examination typically identifies no gross abnormalities. There is usually discharge home without any referral or follow-up into the rehabilitation system. The explicit or implicit message to the patient is that there should be no long-term complications.

For most individuals who have suffered a minor head injury, recovery occurs over a period of days with few residual difficulties. But a significant number of individuals begin to experience difficulties, especially when they attempt to resume their previous life activities at home, school, or work. Such individuals are not able to function as they did before. Memory problems persist. They make frequent mistakes and find that more concentrated effort is required to complete activities that used to be automatic. Physical ailments, such as headache and vertigo, may persist.

Kay (1988) describes a set of cognitive deficits that are commonly seen in minor head injury. He refers to these as *complex attentional deficits* which produce problems with sustained attention and concentrated mental effort. Problems with new learning, memory, and information processing are also typical.

Behavioral deficits resulting from minor head injury may include irritability, anger outbursts, personality changes, anxiety, and depression. A general lack of confidence is also observed, as the individual begins to lose faith in his or her ability to function in the everyday world. As the individual's inability to function takes its toll psychologically, cognitive performance worsens, and a downward spiral ensues.

Kay (1988) describes four stages in the rehabilitation of minor head injury, all of which are fully compatible with the Life Coach approach. The first stage, involves thorough evaluation of deficits to give clients a description of "what is wrong." The second stage is support, both personal and professional, in the sense of rebuilding self-esteem. The third stage is treatment with a general cognitive and behavioral approach that involves identifying cognitive deficits and developing alternative strategies for functioning (i.e., learning new skills to compensate for deficits). The final stage is internal change on the part of the injured individual through the process of accommodation and redefinition of self. This involves assessing one's capabilities, establishing new goals, and getting on with life.

In addition to persons with minor head injuries, Life Coaching also appears to be an alternative vehicle for the community reintegration of more severely disabled clients who have undergone extensive rehabilitation such that any remaining deficits are mild to moderate. An example is the client who has gone through a residential post-acute program and is ready to make the transition home.

In addition to reaching underserved populations, a second factor leading to development of the Life Coach program is the potential for improved clinical effectiveness. The Life Coach model represents an opportunity to incorporate critical success factors for community integration that were described previously (i.e., context relevance, treatment integration, and applications of behavioral-based learning technology). Context relevance is ensured by providing treatment in the client's home and community. Consequently, greater generalization and maintenance of necessary living skills may be expected. Treatment integration and consistency are ensured through the 1:1 relationship between Life Coach and client. Opportunities for learning are maximized by incorporating treatment goals and activities into virtually all of the client's daily activities.

A third factor which prompted development of the Life Coach program is the increasing demand for more *cost-effective* solutions to meeting the rehabilitation needs of persons with acquired brain injury. Because treatment focuses on successful integration of the client into his or her permanent living environment, it may be assumed that treatment goals can be achieved in less time (and at less initial expense) than with other treatment options. For example, problems with the transfer of training from the treatment setting to the home setting are eliminated. Further, Life Coaching is presumed to be more clinically effective because more "durable" or lasting outcomes can be achieved. If the outcomes achieved in Life Coaching are indeed more durable, the need for further expenditures on continued rehabilitation is reduced or eliminated.

Distinguishing Features of the Life Coach Model

Although other home-based treatment models exist (e.g., outpatient services and home-health models), the approach in these models is often to provide discrete, fragmented rehabilitation therapies with no mechanism for coordination among services. Most home-based services have little or no emphasis on overall client accountability. In fact, accountability is often implicitly given to the client and his or her family, parties who have no training or experience managing comprehensive clinical services.

This is the primary disadvantage of traditional home-based services – they are not sensitive to the need for managing comprehensive services. Traditional home-based approaches may be acceptable for the client who can manage his or her own "program" or when only one or two clinical services are needed. But in cases where treatment needs are more diverse and the community is seen as an integral part of treatment, a more systematic approach to service management is required.

The Life Coach model incorporates a well-defined, systematized accountability system, wherein a single Clinical Case Manager has responsibility for managing a client's rehabilitation. The Case Manager is held accountable both for achieving specified clinical outcomes and for managing the cost of rehabilitation services. Five additional features distinguish the Life Coach model from other service delivery options.

THE CONTEXT OF TREATMENT

Virtually all treatment is provided in the "real world" – the client's home, workplace, school, and other community settings where the client conducts his or her daily affairs. Unlike outpatient services, which are typically provided in a clinical setting, and traditional home-health services, which rarely are provided outside of the client's living environment, Life Coaching involves training in all of the community settings in which the client is expected to use community living skills.

THE PROVIDER OF TREATMENT

Rather than using different therapists to provide different, often fragmented therapies, most treatment in the Life Coach program is provided to a client by a single Life Coach. The Life Coach is a licensed or certified clinician (e.g., Occupational Therapist, Speech Pathologist,

Vocational Specialist, Education Specialist) who has received additional training as a "Generalist," which permits the Life Coach to address most, if not all, of the client's treatment needs. A major focus of this generalist training is the application of behavioral-based learning technologies to teach the skills essential to successful community living.

A related distinction is the clinical relationship between Life Coach and client. As the name implies, the Life Coach takes on more of a management or coaching role than that of a direct change agent. Initially, the Life Coach may play a more directive role, but over time, as the client begins to acquire more skills and self-confidence, the Life Coach assumes the role of consultant. As treatment progresses, the client takes increasing responsibility for achieving targeted outcomes. The Life Coach remains involved to advise, support, and assist the client as needed to achieve the highest level of autonomy possible. The ultimate goal of treatment is to assist the client in acquiring the *self-management* skills he or she will need for successful community living.

THE FOCUS OF TREATMENT

Perhaps the best way to describe the difference in treatment focus is as follows: In traditional post-acute programs, the primary focus is on the *acquisition* of skills which the client will need when he or she returns home. In the Life Coach program, the primary focus is on the *application* of skills as the client performs everyday activities at home and in the community. The client and Life Coach identify specific situations in which skill deficits occur and focus treatment efforts on training necessary skills in those situations.

INCREASED SYSTEMS EMPHASIS

Rather than focus only on the client and correcting his or her deficits, the Life Coach program permits a *systems* approach. This approach involves an assessment of "ecological variables" which will influence the client's outcome. These "ecological variables" include factors such as the client's family and the dynamics between different family members, the client's job and work setting, and the client's social support network. Treatment efforts are focused both on improving client competencies and arranging an "ecosystem" that promotes client progress and ensures durable outcomes. For example, because the family plays a pivotal role in supporting treatment, part of the treatment program may involve teaching family members ways to interact with the client to promote his or her acquisition and use of appropriate skills.

INDIVIDUALIZED TREATMENT

While most rehabilitation services are tailored to clients' individual needs, the Life Coach program ensures that each client receives comprehensive treatment that is tailored to the client and his or her unique living situation. The 1:1 approach provides the client with a single, lead clinician whose primary focus is the treatment needs of that particular client.

Client Selection Factors

Our preliminary findings suggest that the Life Coach program has great promise as a clinically effective and cost-effective service delivery model. It should be emphasized, however, that the Life Coach program is not appropriate for *all* head-injured individuals. It has been developed for a specific subpopulation of individuals with acquired brain injury. The ideal client for Life Coaching is an adult who has a safe and stable home environment, with a supportive family. This client's needs are primarily for assistance in returning to work, learning to manage his or her own affairs, and resuming a normalized social life. While the clinical innovations derived from the Life Coach program may ultimately benefit a much larger cross section of head-injured individuals, the program in its present configuration is intended for individuals and situations that meet certain eligibility criteria. These criteria are detailed below:

1. **Client safety**. The services will be provided in the client's home and community, and since the client will not be under 24-hour supervision of treatment staff, it must be expected that the client will be safe living at home while he or she participates in the Life Coach program. Variables to consider in making a determination of client safety include the client's safety awareness, the amount of supervision that is required, and whether adequate supervision can be provided if needed. Several additional risk factors are weighed, such as history of drug/alcohol dependency or depression (e.g., Is the client at risk for drug/alcohol abuse, suicide?); "appropriateness" of the client's relationship with other family members (e.g., Is the relationship counterproductive to treatment goals?); and safety of the home and community (i.e., Will the client or the Life Coach be placed at risk in providing services in the client's home?).

2. **Severity of deficits.** Generally speaking, the Life Coach program is most appropriate for the person who has realistic potential for a successful return to community living. This may be an individual who has sustained only a minor head injury or who has undergone rehabilitation to the point that any deficits in functioning which remain from the injury are mild to moderate. It is noted that although currently mild, the client's deficits may, without treatment, present a major impediment to successful community living.

3. **Client motivation.** The Life Coach model places increasing responsibility on the client to achieve desired outcomes. Rather than a passive participant in therapy, the client is an active learner, who has specific responsibilities in all phases of treatment, including assessment of skill deficits (e.g., use of self-monitoring), treatment planning (e.g., behavioral contracting), treatment delivery (e.g., personalized self-instruction, self-directed behavior change strategies), and follow-up (e.g., accessing community resources). Because the client plays a very active role in treatment, motivation to improve is essential.

4. **Type and amount of required treatment.** A key distinction between Life Coaching and other service models is the range of services required by the client and the corresponding variety of clinicians who must deliver these services. As noted, Life Coach services are typically delivered to a single client by a single Life Coach. Clients who require extensive, individual therapies (e.g., physical therapy) may be better suited for a program employing a complete clinical team. From a practical and financial standpoint, it is often not feasible to provide substantial hours of specialized therapy at home.

5. **Proximity to a Life Coach module.** Life Coach services are typically provided from "modules" located in major population centers. Because of the transportation "down time" created by serving clients at great distance from each other, clients should live within 45 minutes' driving time of the module.

Structure and Staffing of the Life Coach Program

A Life Coach module is intended to serve three to four clients. Table 1 illustrates the configuration of a Life Coach module. The module includes a Clinical Case Manager and two to three Clinical Life Coaches. The Clinical Case Manager is a senior, licensed clinician with extensive background in the rehabilitation of acquired brain injury. The Case Manager has total accountability for both the clinical and business excellence of the module. He or she is responsible for delivering agreed-upon client outcomes according to agreed-upon timelines, and with judicious use of the client's financial resources.

Table 1

The Life Coach Module

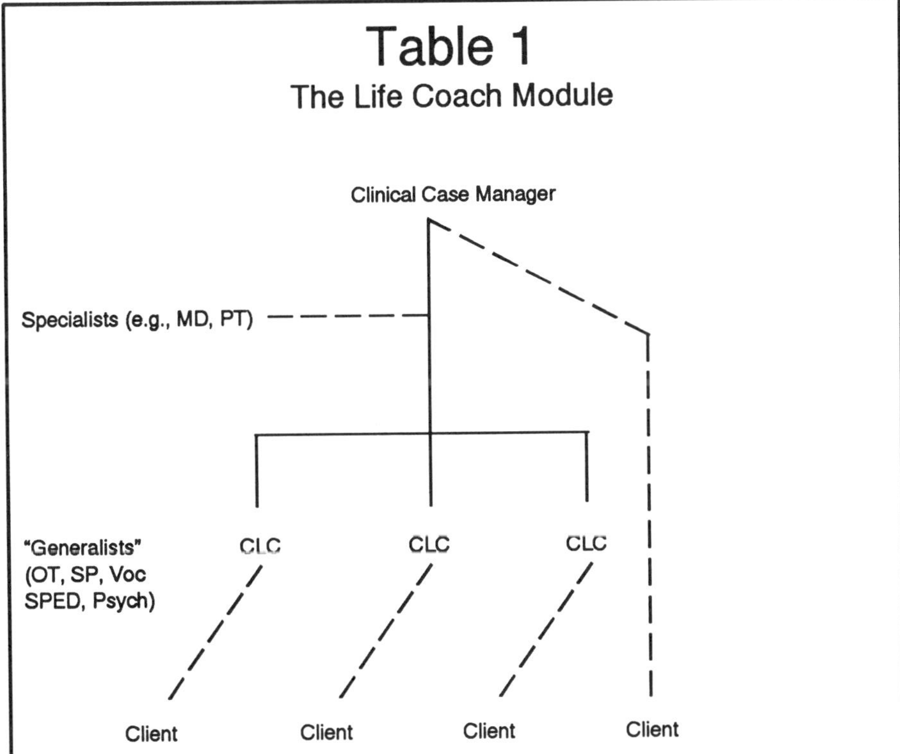

Clinical Life Coaches (CLCs) function as "generalists" and have training in allied health (OR, SP) or learning fields (psych, SpEd). Specialists are employed as needed to support the CLC clinical expertise.

Although all CLCs may provide some treatment to all clients, one CLC has primary responsibility for one client. When the census is four, the Clinical Case Manager takes primary responsibility for the fourth client. Primary responsibility involves designing the client's treatment plan and coordinating its implementation.

As noted, Life Coaches are licensed or certified clinicians. Each Life Coach has only one principal client and is paired with that client from enrollment to program completion. Although the primary pairing is 1:1, treatment for a particular client may be provided by other members of the Life Coach team, depending on the client's needs and staff's areas of expertise.

Life Coaches confer with each other and the Case Manager to design a treatment program that meets each client's individual rehabilitation needs. When additional expertise is needed, the Case Manager contracts for consultation from outside specialists. These outside specialists may provide service directly to the client and/or family. Alternately, the specialist may work with the Life Coach to design a treatment procedure that will be carried out by the Life Coach, with consultation from the specialist.

Progression of Treatment in the Life Coach Program

Perhaps the best picture of the Life Coach model can be provided by describing a typical client "pathway" through the Life Coach program. Stages in the pathway include assessment, treatment planning, treatment delivery, and follow-up.

1. **Assessment**. Client assessment occurs in two stages. A *pre-enrollment* assessment is conducted to:

1) make a basic determination of the nature and extent of a potential client's skill deficits;
2) determine if the potential client is appropriate for the Life Coach program or another treatment program (e.g., residential, day treatment); and
3) generate a preliminary list of treatment goals. This pre-enrollment assessment is conducted with all clients referred, however more attention is given to assessment of risk factors for potential Life Coach clients. In particular, we attempt to determine if the client can be safely and effectively treated in his or her home environment.

After acceptance into the Life Coach program, a *post-enrollment* assessment is completed to more thoroughly delineate client deficits and provide information necessary for treatment planning. Unique to the Life Coach program is the use of a broad-based screening instrument to assess client functioning in areas of community living. Content areas of the instrument are based in part on the Rehabilitation Status Indicators (Diller, Fordyce, Jacobs, & Brown, 1982). Table 2 provides a complete listing of the areas assessed.

Table 2
Assessment Categories

I. MEDICAL AND HEALTH STATUS

- Physical Health
- Dental Health
- Diet
- Medications
- Health Risks

II. PSYCHOSOCIAL HISTORY AND RESOURCES

- Family Adjustment and Expectations
- Home and Community Supports
- Financial Resources

III. BASIC FUNCTIONS

- Sensory and Perceptual Functions
- Motor Functions
- Functional Mobility
- Fitness and Endurance
- Cognitive and Learning Functions
- Executive Functions
- Communicative Functions
- Academic Skills
- Social and Interpersonal Skills
- Motivational Factors

IV. AREAS OF NEED SATISFACTION

- Self-care and Health Maintenance
- Mental Health
    - Counterproductive behavior
    - Psychiatric disorders
    - Emotional stability
- Nutritional Maintenance
- Housing and Household Management
- Accessing Community Resources
- Productive Activity
    - Employment
    - Productive use of leisure time
    - Time management

The assessment is a comprehensive screening. General problem areas are identified first, then a more detailed, functional assessment is performed only in those areas where problems are noted. This functional assessment operationally defines the nature and extent of deficits. Professional evaluations by licensed or certified clinicians are performed, if warranted, to validate problem identification and to provide the Life Coach with a prescription for client treatment.

The post-enrollment assessment is also rooted in real-world activities. It entails completing a carefully scripted protocol over a four-day evaluation period, wherein the Life Coach accompanies the client through a series of home and community-based exercises. For example, one of the exercises involves planning and preparing lunch for the client and Life Coach. This entails planning a menu, determining necessary grocery items, preparing a grocery list, giving directions to the grocery store, orienting within the store, locating necessary grocery items, comparison shopping, calculating costs, purchasing groceries, and preparing and serving the meal. Throughout this activity, the Life Coach is also assessing client proficiency in other areas such as social behavior, distractibility (e.g., carrying out a conversation while driving to the store), and adaptability and frustration tolerance (responding to the Life Coach taking a wrong turn). This and similar exercises provide occasions to evaluate the client's ability to carry out daily activities in various contexts.

2. **Treatment Planning**. Evaluation results are reviewed by the Clinical Case Manager and all Life Coaches in the module to generate treatment goals. Findings and proposed goals are then presented by the Case Manager and Life Coach to the client, family, and financial provider for review and input. Goals (stated in terms of measurable outcomes) are negotiated and agreed to by all parties and a formal treatment plan is drafted. The treatment plan is developed in the form of a behavioral contract (DeRisi & Butz, 1975), which states the responsibilities of all parties – the Life Coach, client, participating family members, and the financial provider). The behavioral contract specifies desired outcomes and provides "checkpoints" (intermediate outcomes) by which treatment progress can be gauged.

3. **Treatment**. The Life Coach program incorporates several treatment principles derived from behavioral-based learning technology, most notably the use of Direct Instruction methodology. Additional features of the treatment approach that warrant further discussion include:

1) the importance of maximizing learning opportunities;
2) the changing relationship between client and Life Coach;
3) the focus on training of self-management skills.

The *focus on maximizing learning opportunities* is founded on the principle that active behavioral engagement with the environment promotes learning. Behavioral engagement refers to the amount of time an individual spends interacting with the environment in an appropriate, adaptive manner (McWilliams, Trivette, & Dunst, 1985). Engagement may consist of simply attending to events in the environment, actively manipulating and exploring the environment, or interacting with others in the environment. Ideally, engagement is initiated independently and results in feedback from the environment (i.e., feedback that a response has affected the environment).

In whatever form, engagement is important for a number of reasons. First, it is the basis for learning adaptive behavior. Adaptation occurs in response to interaction with the environment. More frequent interaction with the environment has a practice effect and leads to fluency in responding. Ample experimental research exists to illustrate the importance of environmental engagement to development and the impact of limited engagement on delayed development (Bower, 1977; McCall, 1974; Yarrow, Rubenstein, & Pederson, 1975).

Second, appropriate engagement provides a context for teaching. A learner is more responsive to new learning when he or she is engaged with the subject matter. The concept of "incidental teaching" (Hart & Risley, 1975) capitalizes on learner-initiated opportunities for teaching. The technique involves the instructor responding to a learner-initiated response by prompting a second, more elaborate response. High levels of engagement result in more opportunities for incidental teaching to occur.

Third, appropriate engagement is important because it is inversely related to undesirable behavior. When individuals are not engaged in appropriate behaviors, they are either doing nothing or engaged in undesirable behaviors. Conversely, appropriate engagement is preventative in the sense that high levels of engagement preclude inappropriate or nonresponding.

There is ample evidence to suggest that engagement is largely a function of the opportunities provided by the environment for engagement. In the behavioral-instructional literature, the concept of maximizing opportunities to respond is well-established. (Delquadri, Greenwood, & Hall, 1979; Hall, Delquadri, & Harris, 1977).

To maximize learning, the Life Coach looks for a variety of opportunities for the client to apply newly acquired skills. One advantage of the 1:1 approach is that the Life Coach can work with the client to "script" a day's activities to incorporate opportunities to respond. The Life Coach reviews the client's daily schedule with respect to specific treatment goals. Together, the Life Coach and client identify situations where skills can be applied. Role-playing exercises permit the client to practice correct responding with the Life Coach and receive feedback on performance before venturing into the "real world."

An example is provided by the client who has difficulty with the pragmatics of conversational speech. Good conversation skills involve making a number of subtle discriminations and responding appropriately to discrete social cues from others in conversation (e.g., body "language," eye contact, voice tone, gestures, changes in topic). Training might consist of:

1. working with the client to identify subtle social cues in conversation and appropriate responses to these cues;
2. teaching the client how to monitor conversation to identify social cues;
3. role-playing conversations in which the Life Coach presents subtle social cues and provides feedback to the client on his or her responses;
4. identifying with the client various opportunities in everyday activities to practice monitoring and responding to subtle social cues (e.g., interactions with bank tellers, waiters, sales clerks, co-workers, friends, and business associates); and
5. making an assignment for the client to monitor everyday conversations, documenting occurrences of targeted social cues, appropriate responses, and subsequent reactions of the conversational partner.

As noted previously, the *relationship between the client and Life Coach* must necessarily evolve over time. As the client's performance level improves, the Life Coach must assume a less directive role in managing treatment. This is important to promote greater client autonomy and to ensure that the client does not become too dependent upon the Life Coach for direction and support. Ultimately, the client must be able to manage his or her own affairs without the assistance of a Life Coach.

The varying roles assumed by the Life Coach over the course of treatment are based on theories of management style developed by Hersey and Blanchard (1977). This theory maintains that a manager's style must change in response to changes in the performance level of his or her subordinates. Hersey and Blanchard (1977) describe four distinct management styles that vary along two coordinates: the extent to which the manager is task-oriented and the extent to which the manager is personally affiliated with his or her subordinates. A high task orientation is one in which most interactions focus on the job to be done. A high affiliation style is one in which the manager assumes a more collegial relationship with subordinates. Figure 1 illustrates the four management styles as a function of high/low task orientation and high/low affiliation. It also illustrates which management style is most effective at different performance levels of subordinates.

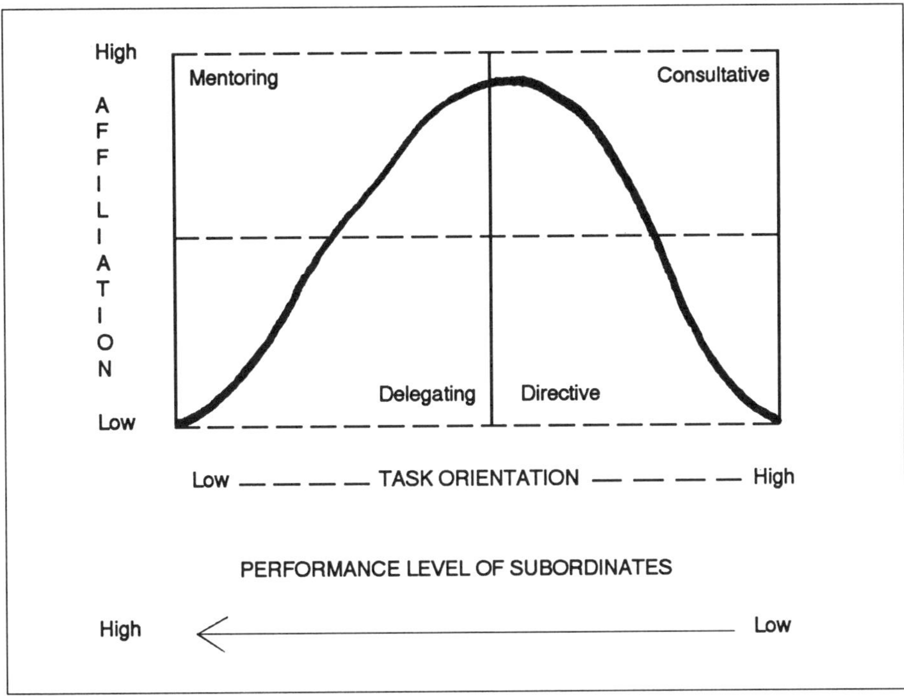

Fig. 1. Hersey and Blanchard's Dynamic Management Style Model (1977)

When performance is low, the preferred management style is more *directive* or high in task orientation and low in affiliation. As performance improves, the preferred management style is *consultative*, somewhat lower in task orientation and higher in affiliation. With continued improvements in performance, the style becomes more participatory as in *mentoring*, lower in task orientation but still high in affiliation. As performance reaches optimal levels, the preferred style is *delegation*, low in both task orientation and affiliation. It should be noted that the Life Coach's management style will vary over the course of treatment and as the client's performance level in all areas improves. For purposes of explanation, an example of varying management styles as applied to a specific skill area (money management) is provided.

Regardless of the client's level of performance, the client and Life Coach would discuss the desired outcome of good money management practices – ensuring that one's living expenses do not exceed financial resources. For the client with limited deficits in this area (i.e., high performance level), the Life Coach may simply delegate to the client the responsibility for planning a monthly budget that achieves the desired outcome. If the client has difficulty with the assignment, the Life Coach may assume a *mentoring* role, offer advice on financial planning, and share those money management strategies which the Life Coach has found useful. Still, however, responsibility for achieving the desired outcome – a workable monthly budget – would remain with the client. If the client's performance level is lower, the Life Coach might provide specific guidelines and recommendations about areas such as budgeting techniques and resources. Finally, for the client with limited money management skills, the Life Coach would take a more directive role by, for example, designing specific exercises for the client to carry out, assigning responsibility to the client for completing the exercises, and monitoring closely the client's performance on these exercises.

A final feature of the Life Coach treatment approach is an emphasis on *self-management*. Once treatment is completed, the client should ideally be able to manage his or her own affairs with minimal assistance from others. By acquiring self-management skills the client is better equipped to deal with new problems that emerge after the completion of treatment.

Self-management procedures have evolved from two areas of applied behavior analysis – special education and behavior therapy. Self-management has been used effectively in special education to promote learning and generalization of new skills by autistic and developmentally delayed children (Fowler, 1984; Koegel, Koegel, & Ingham, 1986). In behavior therapy, the effectiveness of self-management procedures is well-founded in self-control techniques applied to problems such as weight control and smoking. Self-management varies from more traditional self-control strategies because the emphasis is on teaching a set of self-management skills that can be generalized to new target behaviors.

Self-management procedures involve two basic processes – self-monitoring and self-reinforcement. In the Life Coach program, clients begin to learn self-monitoring procedures during the assessment process. One assignment during the four-day post-enrollment assessment period is for the client to maintain a time diary – the client records what he or she is doing during time sampling observations taken over a 12-hour period. As treatment progresses, the client is taught additional self-monitoring techniques including defining target behaviors, selecting valid measurements, using different observation techniques, and summarizing self-monitoring information.

Self-reinforcement refers to the delivery of predetermined consequences when targeted behavior change occurs. Self-reinforcement in this context also includes the process of specifying consequences for desired performance and developing a behavioral contract which spells out the contingency arrangement. Clients begin learning self-reinforcement techniques during treatment planning when behavioral contracting is initiated. The treatment plan – which typically evolves as treatment progresses – comprises a succession of behavioral contracts. In the later stages of treatment, the client takes responsibility for developing his or her own behavioral contracts.

An added dimension to self-management procedures used in Life Coaching is teaching the client how to access continuing support services in his or her community. While the goal of Life Coaching is to maximize independent functioning, many clients will require ongoing supports — both formal and informal — to maintain optimal community living. For example, many of our clients have long-standing histories of drug or alcohol dependency. We encourage these clients to become active participants in Alcoholics Anonymous and similar programs in their community. (This often becomes the basis for self-management through behavioral contracting.) Clients are also advised in accessing other community supports such as human service agencies for persons with disabilities, adult education programs, social groups, self-help groups, and advocacy organizations that may be appropriate to the clients' needs and interests.

4. **Follow-up**. As treatment reaches its end stages, the Case Manager, Life Coach, and client develop a document called the Long-Term Living Plan (LTLP). This document specifies in some detail the client's most optimal outcome with respect to successful community living after the conclusion of treatment. The LTLP includes a description of the client's optimal level of functioning in all areas of community life (e.g., vocational, leisure, social); the optimal living situation for the client, including any environmental supports that may be required; financial resources necessary and available to live successfully in the community; a description of continuing supports (e.g., formal and informal psychosocial supports) which the client may need to live successfully; and a schedule of follow-up by the Life Coach and Case Manager to monitor outcome durability.

The final objective of treatment is to implement the Long-Term Living Plan. Part of this effort is solidifying the client's involvement with formal and informal supports that will help maintain success.

Beyond program completion, a formal follow-up protocol, that involves a graduated schedule of follow-up visits with the client and his or her family is desirable. Follow-up contacts are made weekly for the first month after treatment completion, monthly for three additional months, quarterly for the next nine months, and then at six-month intervals for the next year. At the 6-, 12-, and 18-month intervals, the Life Coach reviews the Long-Term Living Plan with the client and family to identify areas where "slippage" has occurred. Problem areas are reported to the Case Manager and, when appropriate, to the financial provider. Whenever possible, problems are corrected without re-initiating treatment.

Conclusions

Since initiating the Life Coach program, the authors have observed 17 clients who have successfully completed treatment. Although our sample to date is too small to draw any definitive conclusions about the program's overall success, we have determined that the program works exceedingly well for certain clients. There are also clients who have experienced less success with the Life Coach model and every case results in continued refinements in our approach.

This is not to say that Life Coaching is only successful with the "easy" clients. In fact, many of the clients who have participated in the program did so as a last resort. Success appears to be a function of the type of deficits exhibited by the client. We appear to be most successful with clients who exhibit problems in psychosocial adjustment and executive functions, and who are motivated to learn new skills for adjusting to community life. Clients who exhibit motivation and compliance problems – especially those who lack insight into their deficits – have been less successful. A program with more externally imposed structure appears to be necessary for these individuals.

Our experience has also taught us a lot about the type of staff who are best-suited for the Life Coach role. Key characteristics of the successful Life Coach appear to be flexibility, high motivation, self-confidence, autonomy, and creativity. As with our clients, we have found that staff who require a lot of externally imposed structure do not fare well as Life Coaches. To be sure, it is a demanding job but those clinicians who are suited for it would have it no other way.

Even for ideally prepared staff, the demands of treatment are rigorous. The intensity of the 1:1 relationship between client and Life Coach and the isolated working conditions are legitimate concerns. Typically, the duration of treatment in the Life Coach program is short enough (average is 90 days) to avoid overtaxing the 1:1 relationship in a particular case. Variety in the types of clinical problems addressed from client to client also appears to be an effective prevention against burnout. We have offered short "respites" for Life Coaches between cases, during which they work on program development as a break from the constant clinical "grind." We have also taken steps to alleviate the clinical isolation by conducting weekly resource meetings, during which Life Coaches share clinical problems and strategies, and by requiring daily phone contact between the Life Coach and Case Manager.

As noted, there is not yet sufficient data to determine the overall clinical and cost-effectiveness of the Life Coach model, especially in comparison with other programs serving similar clients (e.g., outpatient services, day treatment programs, and traditional home-health services). Longitudinal outcome verification studies are needed to determine if the

Life Coach program lives up to its promise of more durable and substantial outcomes. Given the highly successful applications of community-based instructional strategies to community integration of other populations and the documented effectiveness of integrated rehabilitation management strategies for community re-entry of persons with acquired brain injury, the Life Coach program has the ingredients for success. Time and experience will prove whether this is true.

References

Boake, C. (1990). Transitional living centers in head injury rehabilitation. In J. Kreutzer and P. Wehman (Eds.), *Community integration following traumatic brain injury* (pp. 115-124). Baltimore: Paul H. Brookes Publishing Co.

Bower, T. (1977). *A primer of infant development.* San Francisco: W. H. Freeman and Company.

Carnine, D., & Silbert, J. (1979). *Direct instruction reading.* Columbus, OH: Charles E. Merril Publishing Co.

Cope, N., Cole, J., Hall, K., & Barkan, H. (1990). *Brain injury: Analysis of outcome in a post-acute rehabilitation system.* Manuscript submitted for publication.

Delquadri, J., Greenwood, C., & Hall, V. (1979, June). *Opportunity to respond: An update.* Invited address at the fifth annual meeting of the Association for Behavior Analysis, Dearborn, MI.

Derisi, W. J., & Butz, G. (1975). *Writing behavioral contracts: A case simulation practice manual.* Champaign, IL: Research Press.

Diller, L., Fordyce, W., Jacobs, D., & Brown, M. (1982). *Rehabilitation indicators project.* New York: New York University Medical Center.

Engelmann, S., & Carnine, D. (1982). *Theory of instruction: Principles and applications.* New York: Irvington.

Evans, R., & Preston, B. (1990). Day rehabilitation programming: A theoretical model. In J. Kreutzer and P. Wehman (Eds.), *Community integration following traumatic brain injury* (pp. 125-138). Baltimore: Paul H. Brookes Publishing Co.

Evans, R. (1991). Personal communication.

Flynn, R. J., & Nitsch, K. E. (1980). *Normalization, social integration, and community services.* Baltimore: University Park Press.

Fowler, S. (1984). Introductory comments: The pragmatics of self-management for the developmentally disabled. *Analysis and Intervention in Developmental Disabilities, 4*, 85-89.

Hall, R. V., Delquadri, J., & Harris, J. (1977, May). *Opportunities to respond: A new focus in the field of applied behavior analysis.* Invited address at the third annual meeting of the Association for Behavior Analysis, Chicago, IL.

Hart, B. M., & Risley, T. R. (1975). Incidential teaching of language in the preschool. *Journal of Applied Behavior Analysis, 8*, 411-420.

Hersey, P., & Blanchard, K. (1977). *Management of organizational behavior.* Englewood Cliffs, New Jersey: Prentice-Hall.

Horner, R. H., & Albin, R. W. (1988). Research on general-case procedures for learners with severe disabilities. *Education and Treatment of Children, 11*(4), 375-388.

Horner, R. H., Jones, D., & Williams, J. A. (1985). A functional approach to teaching generalized street crossing. *Journal of the Association for Persons with Severe Handicaps, 10*, 71-78.

Horner, R. H., Eberhard, J., & Sheehan, M. R. (1986). Teaching generalized table bussing: The importance of negative teaching examples. *Behavior Modification, 10*, 457-471.

Horner, R. H., Albin, R. W., & Ralph, G. (1986). Generalization with precision: The role of negative teaching examples in the instruction of generalized grocery item selection. *Journal of the Association for Persons with Severe Handicaps, 11*, 300-308.

Horner, R. H., Dunlap, G., & Koegel, R. L. (1988). *Generalization and maintenance: Life-style changes in applied settings*. Baltimore: Paul H. Brookes Publishing Co.

Kay, T. (1988). Mild head injury: An overview of clinical manifestations and research agenda. *Trends in Rehabilitation, 3*(3), 10-17.

Koegel, R. L., Koegel, L. K., & Ingham, J. C. (1986). Programming rapid generalization of correct articulation through self-monitoring procedures. *Journal of Speech and Hearing Disorders, 51*, 24-32.

Madigan, K. (1987). *Memory retraining for the head injured: A direct instruction approach.* Paper presented at the Annual Conference of the Association for Behavior Analysis, Nashville, TN.

Madigan, K. (1989). *Walking around your community: A mobility training program.* Workshop presented at the Special Education Local Planning Agency, Monterey, CA.

McCall, R. (1974). Exploratory manipulation and play in the human infant. *Monographs of the Society for Research in Child Development, 39*(2), 208-215.

McWilliams, R. A., Trivette, C. M., & Dunst, C. J. (1985). Behavior engagement as a measure of the efficacy of early intervention. *Analysis and Intervention in Developmental Disabilities, 5*, 33-45.

Ozga, A. (1978). Home follow-up for the brain injured patient. *Journal of the Association of Rehabilitation Nurses, 3*(3), 17-20.

Sailor, W., Goetz, L., Anderson, J., Hunt, P., & Gee, K. (1988). Research on community intensive instruction as a model for building functional, generalized skills. In R. Horner, G. Dunlap, & R. Koegel (Eds.), *Generalization and maintenance: Life-style changes in applied settings*, (pp. 67-98). Baltimore: Paul H. Brookes Publishing Co.

Silbert, J., Carnine, D., & Stein, M. (1981). *Direct instruction mathematics.* Columbus, OH: Charles E. Merrill Publishing Co.

Terrace, H. (1966). Stimulus control. In W. Honig (Ed.), *Operant behavior: Areas of research and application*, (pp. 271-344). New York: Appleton-Century-Crofts.

Walker, H. M. (1986). *The Walker social skills curriculum: The ACCESS program (Adolescent Curriculum for Communication and Effective Social Skills).* Austin, TX: Pro-Ed Publishing.

Walker, H. M. (1988). The assessment of integration in mainstream settings (AIMS) assessment system: Rationale, instruments, procedures, and outcomes. *Journal of Clinical Child Psychology, 15*(1), 55-63.

Yarrow, L., Rubenstein, J., & Pederson, F. (1975). *Infant and environment: Early cognitive and motivational development.* New York: John Wiley and Sons.

12

Community Skills Training

Lynn P. Cullity
Jodi D. Jackson
Linda R. Shaw

12

Community Skills Training

Lynn P. Cullity
Jodi D. Jackson
Linda R. Shaw

Within the past decade, brain injury rehabilitation has matured beyond its early infancy stage, when clinicians attempted to apply traditional strategies in traditional settings to the brain injury population. Through trial and error and utilization of an ever-increasing body of research, brain injury rehabilitation professionals have begun to adapt traditional approaches and develop novel strategies to meet the unique needs of this population. For example, multidisciplinary treatment approaches have given way to interdisciplinary and, in some cases, transdisciplinary treatment approaches (Eames, 1989). Traditional standardized assessment instruments have been modified, used in nontraditional ways, and, in some cases, have been supplanted by other assessment approaches (Fraser, Clemmons, & McMahon, 1990).

The Case for Community-Based Community Skills Training

As treatment providers have become more experienced, some have begun to advocate for moving treatment out of the rehabilitation facility into the community (Cervelli, 1990) ("Community" is referred to here as the external community outside or separate from the client's home or rehabilitation facility). This approach has been advocated for several reasons. First, while most treatment providers advocate specific training in community skills, it would appear that our traditional facility-based treatment methods have not yielded optimal results. Brooks, Campsie, Symington, Beattie, and McKinlay (1987) found that even seven years post-injury, relatives of head-injured individuals reported significant concerns about their head-injured relatives' ability to function independently in the community with 36% reporting that the head-injured individual still needed "looking after" and 24% reporting worries about the patient going out alone.

Second, while generalization of treatment effects is always a concern for clinicians, generalization tends to be particularly difficult for persons with brain injuries (Parente & Anderson-Parente, 1990). Because of difficulties in generalization, several researchers have emphasized the importance of teaching functional skills within the actual environment in which the skills will eventually be utilized (Patrick, 1990; Wood, 1987). Not only is treatment considered more effective when provided "in situ," but evaluation of community skills may also yield more accurate results when performed within the community. Formalized testing has repeatedly been found to inadequately assess functional skills (Brooks, 1990). Vocational specialists, noting the serious limitations of traditional vocational evaluation tools with the head injury population, advocate the use of on-the-job evaluation techniques (Fraser, McMahon, & Vogenthaler, 1988). Perhaps those assessing independent living or community skills might find "in-the-community" evaluation techniques to be more valid indicators of performance in this area as well.

Despite such evidence supporting the need for developing community-based, functional programming, the shift has been slow to occur. This may be due to a perceived threat to the medical model and, by extension, to the physician's role in directing treatment. Condeluci and Gretz-Lasky (1987) note that "the transition from a medical model to a community service philosophy may be particularly challenging to rehabilitation practitioners" (p. 50). They theorize that this may be due to the relative newness of the independent living model within brain injury rehabilitation as well as to the inexperience of treatment providers with community-based programming. Clearly, a need exists to provide practitioners with models and specific techniques for the development of community skills programs which are community-based. Toward this end the authors recommend several guidelines for the development of community skills training programs.

Program Guidelines

1. **The program should be community-based.** The benefits of incorporating functional activities from clients' daily lives into their rehabilitation programs have been well documented (Gordon, Hibbard, & Kreutzer, 1989; Leland, Lewis, Hinman, & Carillo, 1988). When access to the client's community is not feasible, providers should attempt to simulate elements of that community setting whenever possible (Parente & Anderson-Parente, 1990).

2. **The program should be behaviorally based.** Numerous studies have demonstrated the efficacy of behavioral strategies in head injury rehabilitation (Howard, 1988; Wood, 1987). Behavioral principles and techniques can be easily and effectively utilized in teaching community skills (Neistadt & Marques, 1984).

3. **The program should be comprehensive in scope.** A wide range of critical community re-entry skills should be addressed. Minimally, the following areas should be included:

   Safety
   Environmental Orientation
   Driving and/or Use of Public Transportation
   Social Behavior
   Time Management
   Banking and Shopping
   Accessing Community Resources
   Recreation

4. **The program should stress the "dignity of risk"** (see Chapter 1). Treatment providers continuously struggle between the need to assure client safety and the need to encourage client autonomy and independent decision making. Particularly in today's litigious society there is a tendency to err on the side of caution.

   Unfortunately, however, this stance often results in a sheltered treatment environment where clients are ill-prepared to master the demands of their environment upon discharge. In developing community skills programs providers can allow for risk-taking, provided that they also acknowledge their responsibility to teach the skills necessary for coping with "risky" situations and assess clients' readiness to handle increased levels of responsibility.

5. **The program should emphasize client self-determination and control.** There is ample documentation for the observation that clients who have acquired an internal locus of control achieve better functional rehabilitation outcomes (Dinardo, 1971; Swenson, 1976). By allowing the client some measure of control through active participation in problem-identification, goal setting, and behavioral contracting, staff may minimize power struggles, client assumption of the "sick role" and perpetuation of an external locus of control among clients.

6. **The program should utilize an interdisciplinary or transdisciplinary treatment team model.** Due to the many varied sequelae that contribute to deficits in community living skills, it is imperative that all involved rehabilitation specialists work closely together in program planning and implementation (Corthell & Tooman, 1985; McMahon, Shaw, & Mahaffey, 1988). The success of such a program is dependent on the effective functioning of an interdisciplinary or transdisciplinary team.

7. **The program should involve the family.** The client's family members often serve as a primary emotional, physical, and financial resource to the client, both before and after discharge. Families and, ultimately, the client will benefit by receiving instruction, support, and the opportunity to participate in rehabilitation (McKinlay & Hickox, 1988; Shaw & McMahon, 1990).

The remainder of this chapter presents an overview of a community skills training program which may serve as a model to practictioners wishing to develop similar programs within their treatment settings.

The Community Mobility Training Program

The Community Mobility Training Program was developed in response to the need for a consistent method by which to teach brain-injured clients the necessary skills for community reintegration. The majority of clients in the program have sustained severe closed-head injuries resulting in cognitive sequelae, including memory loss; perceptual limitations; difficulty in absorbing, interpreting, and integrating environmental and social information; the inability to process the "gestalt" of a given situation; limited insight; unrealistic self-expectations; and behavioral disinhibition. Resultant behaviors are often viewed as being socially aberrant, ineffective in meeting given objectives, and, in some cases, may be potentially dangerous to the client or others. These deficits severely restrict the client's ability to resume independent living situations, to return to employment, and to access the community safely. Because the client is often cognitively and psychologically unable to evaluate his or her own skills accurately, a consistent, highly structured, and objective training system was designed to efficiently bring about behavioral change.

PROGRAM GOALS

The purpose of the Community Mobility Training Program is to provide the brain-injured individual with the opportunity to acquire the skills needed to safely access the community with the highest degree of autonomy possible. The goals of the Community Mobility Program are:

1. To assess the client's initial performance and estimate his or her capacity for acquiring functional skills.

2. To provide the mechanism for skill development and maintenance within a defined structure, tailored to meet individual needs.

3. To provide the client with a hierarchical system of privileges and responsibilities through which the client progresses as increased competence is demonstrated.

4. To provide the means by which each client may receive feedback specifically focused on strengths and weaknesses, and to have the opportunity to practice alternate behaviors in the actual community setting.

5. To compare a client's functional performance with the demands of the projected discharge site and to establish a priority of therapy needs relative to the discharge site.

6. To promote and enhance awareness of and compensation for safety performance, cognitive skills and limitations, and social behaviors.

7. To allow the staff to communicate to the client in a nonthreatening, objective manner surrounding issues that are frequently emotionally charged for the client.

8. To provide an opportunity for the client to practice and refine compensation strategies.

9. To provide training in safety procedures, map reading, following directions, and the use of community resources, community services, telephone and other directories, and public transportation.

THE INTERDISCIPLINARY TEAM APPROACH

The Community Mobility Training Program is based on the premise that the Interdisciplinary Treatment Team model offers the most comprehensive and cohesive services to the client. To effectively implement the program, it is necessary to establish a staff member or members who act as the Coordinator(s) of the program. The Coordinator is responsble for the organization, coordination, and implementation of all aspects of the program. Community Mobility Trainers assist the Coordinator in implementing the program.

In addition to the coordinator and trainers, the other members of the rehabilitation team are involved in the development and implementation of the Community Mobility Training Program, and provide distinct contributions at various stages of the program. The disciplines represented on the interdisciplinary team include Physical Therapy, Occupational Therapy, Speech Therapy, Cognitive Rehabilitation, Neuropsychology/Psychology, Vocational Rehabilitation, Therapeutic Recreation, and Case Management. Collectively, the entire team supports the development of Community Mobility Skills as a desirable treatment goal for the client. Components of each discipline's initial assessment are utilized in the Community Mobility Assessment. Additionally, each staff member shares responsibility for understanding and supporting the client's specific Community Mobility treatment objectives and privileges.

Rehabilitation goals are often incorporated into and are reinforced by the Community Mobility Training Program. For example, the team may decide during an Interdisciplinary Meeting that one of the client's major barriers to community re-entry is his or her inappropriate social interactions. In addition to other strategies that may be implemented to address this problem, the client is also provided with specific strategies to use when in the community. The client is then given the opportunity to utilize and perfect these strategies in the Community Mobility Training Program.

PROGRAM LEVELS

The program is structured around six levels of progressively increased expectations, responsibilities, and privileges. The client is automatically moved forward from Level 1 (Evaluation) to Level 2 (Skill Development). The criteria for moving through Levels 3 through 6 are flexible so that each client's individual needs may best be addressed. The client and staff work together to negotiate an individualized Community Mobility Contract with which all parties are comfortable. The client is able to see progress in a concrete way as he or she moves through the levels systematically. Not all individuals will be able to attain the independent Levels 4 through 6. In such instances, the Community Mobility Coordinator may wish to create an individualized privilege system which capitalizes on that client's strengths in the community.

Level 1: Assessment

Level 1 of the Community Mobility Training Program is initiated following the client's admission to the facility and typically lasts for about four weeks. During this time, the client receives an initial orientation and assessment.

Orientation helps the client to understand the program, and begins the process of client investment in participation. A basic description of the program is reviewed with the client and the family during the admission interview. Effective orientation to the program can be maximized by taking into consideration the client's learning style, rate of cognitive processing, language impairments, memory deficits and ability to integrate information. Information should be presented in such a manner as to provide the appropriate degree of information while avoiding confusion. The "Client Introduction Sheet" is provided to the client during the week following admission (see Appendix A). After it has been reviewed, the client is asked to sign it, indicating that he or she understands and will comply with the program. Orientation to all facets of the program continues throughout the first several weeks of treatment until the client thoroughly understands the program structure and expectations.

It is particularly important that families also receive a thorough orientation to the program. Issues which may be pertinent to families include program liability, the decision making process relative to client risk, and projected outcome for the client's skill level in the community. Families will also require information about the structure and limitations of the program and the training principles utilized. The family's support of the program during client home visits can be an important asset in the treatment process, and their ongoing involvement should be encouraged.

The Community Mobility Assessment is performed by observing the client as he or she prepares for and participates in community outings and gathering relevant data. During the assessment period, it is recommended that the Coordinator devote as much one-to-one time with the client as possible, so that potential safety risks can be quickly identified. Behavioral Criteria (see Appendix B) are utilized to assist the Coordinator and other staff in assessing the client. Using the Behavioral Criteria, the evaluator notes which behaviors are present or absent and the degree and type of assistance the client requires to engage in the behaviors.

During the initial weeks of the client's stay at the facility, the interdisciplinary team is completing a comprehensive clinical assessment of the client. It is critically important that all disciplinary assessments be utilized and incorporated into the Community Mobility Assessment. Similarly, familiarity with the client's history is critical in obtaining an accurate assessment.

Level 2: Skill Development

Level 2 is achieved automatically by the client following the completion of the Assessment. The Level 2 client is provided the opportunity for supervised access to the community with the specific focus on developing and utilizing community skills. Repeated exposure to situations that require the performance of safety, orientation, time management, and social behavior skills is structured by the Community Mobility Coordinator and/or Trainers. Commonly, the brain-injured client sees the Community Mobility sessions only as a chance to purchase items or to meet his or her needs without taking the perspective that practical skills are gained. Level 2 may be a critical point in the client's progress as the Community Mobility Coordinator assists the client to integrate information and to reaffirm the purpose and goals of the Community Mobility Program. During Level 2, the Community Mobility Coordinator and Trainers begin to give the client more direct feedback. Areas of success as well as problems are addressed. Community Mobility outings are planned and may be organized on a one-to-one basis or in small groups of up to four persons.

Level 2 has no specific duration. Those clients who are able to learn from experience, receive and act on staff feedback and adapt to the local community generally will progress through Level 2 rapidly. The Community Mobility Trainer routinely consults with other Team Members prior to moving the client to the next level to be certain the client is ready to move forward. Often the client may believe he or she is ready for the next level before the required competencies have been demonstrated. The Community Mobility Coordinator may use the opportunity to target those specific behaviors which the client must consistently demonstrate to be promoted to Level 3.

Level 3: Developing a Contract

Level 3 is the point at which intensive efforts to establish consistent skill behaviors occur. In contrast to Levels 1 and 2, movement through the remaining levels requires focused effort by the client. By the time the client progresses to Level 3, he or she should have a working knowledge of the behaviors expected in the community associated with safety, orientation, social behavior, and time management. The Community Mobility Coordinator actively assists the client in developing a working set of personalized guidelines for use in community outings. As a dialogue between the client and Coordinator develops regarding specific Community Mobility issues that are relevant to that individual, other members of the Team become directly involved. For example, the Psychologist may be working with the client on implementing strategies for increasing pro-social behaviors. This goal may be adapted to become a community mobility objective. The more often the client is able to practice adaptive social responses in the public as well as at the facility level, the more optimistic is the functional outcome. When the client enters Level 3, Skill Area Worksheets are introduced. The Skill Area Worksheets are directly based upon the Behavioral Criteria. They consist of a set of self-directed questions asking the client, "How well do I...?", followed by the behaviors contained within the Behavioral Criteria. The client then engages in the following activities culminating in the creation of a contract to achieve Level 4:

1. The client chooses several destinations which he or she wishes to visit independently. These destinations should be familiar places where legitimate business can occur, and will help meet the client's needs (e.g., drugstore, hairdresser).

2. The Skill Area Worksheets are reviewed with the client. The client is asked to choose the items that are problematic for him or her. When the client is particularly sensitive

to the concepts of "deficits" or "problem areas" he or she may be asked to identify the items he or she feels are important, or some alternate phraseology. The Coordinator negotiates items to be included in the contract. Occasionally, it may be necessary to alter the terminology to meet specific client needs while maintaining the concepts. For example, "Wear clothes that are appropriate for the occasion/event" may be rephrased to say "Put on clothes that fit."

3. Following outings into the community, the client is asked to list the behaviors in which he or she engaged that showed safety, etc. The list is added to after each outing so that it becomes a running record for the client. Clients with severe memory deficits may need to be prompted or may be encouraged to develop the list while actually in the community.

4. The Contract Score Sheet (see Appendix C) is constructed such that 16 items can be targeted for improvement, divided among the four categories of Safety, Orientation, Time Management, and Social Behavior, not necessarily in equal numbers. On each contract it is important to include several "give away" items (i.e., behaviors that the client almost always displays, but are still important). By doing this the client is ensured some measure of success, setting a positive atmosphere within which the more critical behaviors that are substandard can be discussed. For the client who becomes easily overwhelmed, fewer than 16 scorable items may be included on the Contract Score Sheet. However, those behaviors viewed as primary obstacles to community re-integration must be included.

The client is provided with the opportunity to take Community Mobility practice outings prior to being scored on his or her performance. Practice outings are desirable in order to assist the client in making the transition to a more pressured situation in which behaviors are critically viewed. Practice outings are conducted with the level of structure and guidance the client requires, with gradually decreasing dependence upon the Community Mobility Trainer. When the client and Trainer have come to an agreement that actual contract outings are ready to be taken, the client is asked to submit for approval the Request to Begin Contract Outings for Level 4 (see Appendix D). Once the client has completed these steps and the Team has approved the request, the client enters into an agreement by filling out and signing the Client Contract (see Appendix E).

This form is designed to augment the client's increasing sense of responsibility. When the contract is completed and signed, the client may take "official" contract outings.

Contract outings are conducted with identified Trainers or other members of the Team. The client is given the responsibility for planning and initiating a contract outing. Contract outings usually require one-to-one supervision and may be videotaped for later review. A separate Contract Score Sheet is used for each contract outing. For each outing, the client and Trainer fill out the information on the top, including the date, destination, and time. The Trainer attempts to give minimal cues as the client prepares for the outing, but uses any opportunities to suggest compensation strategies that might be useful to the client. The destination of each outing is chosen from the various sites previously identified. At the scheduled time, the client and Trainer leave the facility with the client in the lead. The Trainer attempts not to provide cues, either verbal or nonverbal, unless an emergency arises. It is important to be aware of the subtle cueing that occurs easily and may be noticed by the client, such as briefly glancing in the intended direction when the client is struggling to locate landmarks for orientation.

In most cases, it is recommended that the Trainer follow the client at a distance that ensures a sense of independence and autonomy, while at the same time staying close enough to intervene should it become necessary. Those individuals who exhibit questionable safety judgement should be within speaking or even reaching distance. The well-informed and experienced Trainer will be able to use his or her own discretion in the matters such as distance, feedback style, or adaptation of the system. The Trainer should observe the client's performance in relation to the identified target behaviors and may wish to take notes discretely to provide accurate information later upon review of the outing. New behaviors that appear problematic and those positive in nature should also be noted for later discussion. The Trainer should continually compare the client's performance with the acceptable range of safety standards. If the cient does not demonstrate adequate skills or experiences significant unexpected difficulties in the community, the Coordinator may wish to alter that individual's program so that Level 4 is achieved only when an acceptable level of risk-taking is identified.

The client and Trainer meet immediately after the contract outing to review the outing. The Trainer may invite other Team Members to participate as well. This is particularly recommended if the client displays cognitive and/or psychological barriers that impede the ability to process information. The Contract Score Sheet is reviewed item by item. Five points are awarded for successful completion 100% of the time. No points are awarded for less than 100% performance. No partial points are awarded. The Trainer may at times find it difficult to determine whether the client has successfully met the criteria for successful completion. A general guide in making such decisions is that safety-related behaviors have the least degree of flexibility in terms of allotting points for the outing. For a contract with 16 items, 70 out of 80 points must be met to be considered a successful outing. For contracts with fewer items, two items (or 10 points) can be missed and still be considered to be successfully achieved. It is advisable for the Trainer to write comments directly on the score sheet so that the client may review it later. Both positive and critical comments should be included. The client continues to make contract outings until he or she has completed four consecutive successful outings.

Level 4: Defined Community Privileges

Following successful completion of four contract outings, the client has earned the privilege of going without staff supervison to the previously selected locations during daytime hours. The specific facility procedures of leaving grounds should be made clear to the client with written information provided if needed. For example, the client may be expected to use a sign-out book which includes filling in the name, destination, time leaving, and estimated time of return. Some clients may require coaching to choose a reasonable number of times per day or per week to visit a contract location.

Good communication between client, Community Mobility Coordinator, Trainers, and other Team Members is essential as the client engages in what may be the first independent community experience following the injury.

Shortly after the client has reached independent status, the Community Mobility Coordinator may accompany or observe the client discretely in the community to determine that skill performance is maintained.

Generally, the client is encouraged to exercise the Level 4 independent privileges for a specified time period (which varies according to client skills and competencies) before progressing further with the Community Mobility Program. During this time staff continue to stress the significance of becoming an integrated community citizen, one that "fits in" and is responsible for his or her behaviors. The client may discover that the public is not as understanding or supportive as family or staff members and may require assistance to gain perspective regarding those issues.

Unless the client demonstrates serious safety risk behaviors, it is uncommon for Level 4 privileges to be revoked, although the facility retains the right to do so. In that case, the client may be required to complete additional contract outings to establish consistent safety awareness and behaviors.

There are two options for further movement in the program at this stage:

1. **Expanded Level 4**: The client may have additional destinations added to the list of independent locations with additional contract outings required.

2. **Developing a Contract to Achieve Level 5**: The client who demonstrates reliable skills to utilize environmental information, use applicable compensatory strategies, and adapt to unfamiliar situations may begin working toward Level 5, Extended Community Privileges.

Level 5 is achieved by developing a new contract which reflects the added responsibilities of functioning within novel environments. The planning and information-gathering demands are greater, with reduced assistance given by the staff. The client is encouraged to utilize community resources and use public transportation as part of the contract. The destinations of contract outings can be chosen by the client or the Coordinator, but must be a place with which the client will realistically need to become familiar, and which is currently unfamiliar to the client. The Coordinator may request that the client make a contract outing to a difficult location so as to evaluate adaptability. At this level the Coordinator may set up realistic situations that require problem solving and the ability to adaptively seek out support within the community. The procedure of making contract outings to achieve Level 5 is the same as that used to attain Level 4. The Coordinator may draw up a new Contract Score Sheet, add to the existing one or continue to use the Level 4 Score Sheet if it remains pertinent.

Level 5: Extended Community Privileges

The client who reaches Level 5 has shown the ability to operate with minimal structure and adapt to new, different, and changing environments. This individual is now able to independently access any location in the community during daylight hours and is encouraged to use public transportation. The client may, however, require some supportive services to assist in the planning aspects of community outings. The type and frequency of any necessary assistance should be carefully described and documented as the information will be valuable in the discharge planning process.

The client may now begin to prepare for movement to Level 6, Nighttime Community Privileges. The client and the Coordinator, with the Team's input, decide on the number of contract outings, destinations, etc. The Coordinator must be cognizant of the potential social ramifications implied in evening privileges, particularly if the client has a history of substance abuse. The Coordinator should solicit input from the client's Psychologist or other appropriate personnel to establish the relevant issues.

The Coordinator and client draw up a contract that reflects the unique considerations in going out unaccompanied at night. This includes social behaviors and awareness of potential social risks, the visual-perceptual changes that occur in darkness or reduced lighting, and the need to establish different landmarks to ensure orientation.

Level 6: Nighttime Community Privileges

The client who achieves Level 6 has attained the most advanced Level of the Community Mobility Program. This individual is able to go independently to any location of choice during the day and evening. It should be emphasized that each client's range of privileges can be tailored to meet his or her level of ability, allowing for the highest degree of independence while assuring adequate safety, social behavior, orientation, and time management skills.

TRAINING METHODS

As the client moves through the program levels, he or she receives training in community skills through both individual and group treatment. Individual treatment takes place on a one-to-one basis with the client and the Coordinator of the program. Individual sessions may occur once every two weeks to twice a week, depending on the needs of the client and the facility. Individual treatment is utilized to review specific Community Mobility issues with the client, to provide feedback during the Assessment, and to design and implement the client's Community Mobiliity Contract. Progress through the program is discussed with the client during this time, and members of the Interdisciplinary Team may be utilized for co-treatment to meet various treatment objectives. Individual treatment provides the client with an opportunity to wrestle with issues of Community Mobility outside a group setting, and to have specific needs addressed.

Each client is also assigned to a Community Mobility Planning Group and a Community Mobility Outing Group. These groups provide an introduction to the subject of Community Mobility, training in the Skill Areas, and information and support regarding restrictions. Clients are assigned to groups consistent with their program level and abilities.

COMMUNITY MOBILITY PLANNING GROUP

Community Mobility Planning Group is a clinic-based group with a twofold purpose. First, the group is used as a mechanism for communicating information about the program and teaching skill behaviors. Second, the group is used as a time for clients to plan community outings in order to work on improving community skills or to be evaluated in preparation to being promoted to another level.

Usually, the group is held in the morning, and clients spend part of the session planning for an afternoon outing. Each client is given a Community Mobility Planning Sheet (see Appendix F) on which to organize personal errands, shopping needs, appointments, etc. Information listed includes the client's desired destination(s), estimated time the outing will take, cost, and things that need to be brought along, (e.g., money, lists, watch, logbook).

The remainder of Community Mobility Planning Group is used for teaching various topics. One standard topic focuses on helping clients learn the levels of the program using written handouts designed for client use. Also, the four skill areas are continuously reviewed using written handouts (see Appendix G). Various behaviorally based training techniques are utilized to teach these skill areas, including modeling, role-play, group exercises, etc. Community Mobility Planning Group is adapted from week-to-week, depending upon the specific needs of the cients involved at any particular point.

COMMUNITY MOBILITY OUTING GROUP

The Community Mobility Outing Group is a community-based practicum, and generally meets in the afternoon. The goal of the group is to provide the client with regular, ongoing access to the community as a mechanism for assessing and improving the skills of safety, time management, orientation, and social behavior. Due to safety issues, a minimum of a 1:4 staff/client ratio is advised. The time needed for the group varies, however, a one-hour time frame is recommended for the cognitive and physical endurance of clients just beginning the program. Destinations for the outing are determined by the needs of the clients involved and by the resources the community has to offer. Ideally, community re-entry programs are situated near downtown locations with easy access to resources such as shopping, postal services, banking, and entertainment. In some suburban or rural localities, transportation may become a restricting programming issue.

Once in the community it is each staff member's responsibility to ensure safety and dignity for the client at all times. Behaviors which place the client or others at serious risk or arc aberrant are terminated immediately through intervention by the trainer. During routine outings, when clients are learning basic community skills, the trainer may converse with the client and offer as many cues as needed. For practice Contract Outings and scored Contract Outings, the trainer refrains from conversing with the client, and acts instead as a "shadow." This allows the client to fully concentrate on performing the necessary skill behaviors. In either case, the trainer must always remain close enough so that immediate intervention can occur if necessary.

When public transportation or a taxi service is being used, the trainer accompanies the cient, but the client carries out all communications independently (e.g., purchasing a ticket, giving the destination). In the event that the client becomes disoriented to place, or loses track of the time during an outing, the trainer may choose to intervene. The trainer should allow time at the end of the outing to process the experience with the client, and provide immediate feedback regarding performance. Because of memory issues, it is not advisable to delay such processing until a later treatment session, because it is difficult for both the client and the trainer to recapture all the events that took place. Some clients with significant short-term memory loss may even require that feedback be presented immediately in the community.

Community Mobility Outing Group offers a number of challenges for both the trainer and the client. Variable factors, like inclement weather, unreceptive community members, construction detours, and traffic jams, all provide real-life obstacles to which the client must adjust. Because the group is time-consuming, physically tiring, and stressful for all parties involved, rest should be provided for the client following the group if needed. Several staff members should be trained and prepared to be called upon should increased staffing be necessary. Finally, it is important to remember that the group can also be quite fun, and may be one of the best opportunities that the client has to experience the "real world."

Administration and Implementation

The Community Mobility Training Program is suitable for adapted use in a variety of treatment settings, including residential programs, outpatient clinics, and home health agencies. Although it was designed to be employed at a post-acute residential treatment program by an interdisciplinary team, various treatment providers working individually or cooperatively could be appropriate Coordinators of the program. The professions of Occupational Therapy, Physical Therapy, Cognitive Therapy, Recreational Therapy, and Vocational Rehabilitation each include expertise relevant to the philosophy, theory, and practical training knowledge needed for implementation of the program. Most essential for providers is a thorough clinical understanding of the physical, cognitive, and perceptual issues involved in traumatic brain injury as well as a background in behavioral training techniques. Various elements of the program may need to be modified when adapting it to other treatment settings. For example, where facility rules allow and where comprehensive driving evaluations are available, clients might be provided with the opportunity to work on driving skills in addition to or in place of public transportation.

Individuals considering utilizing this program are advised to become thoroughly familiar with all training materials prior to implementation. Administrative and clinical support for the model, support from family members and direct care staff, and investment on the part of the client should all be established at the outset. Legal implications and agency/facility liabilities should be researched, and all program release forms should be completed and signed. Access to photocopying services for processing of the data sheets, client contracts, and other materials, will be needed. Also needed in the course of implementation will be the following minimal resources and materials:

Chalkboard
Telephone
Local street maps
Telephone directory
Local newspapers
Bus schedules & routes
Subway schedules
Taxi services
Train schedules

Optional materials include:

Local entertainment guides
Shopping directories
Portable video camera
Car-pool directories
VHS tapes
Maps of malls
Videocassette recorder

Each town's local Chamber of Commerce or Tourist Information Agency is an excellent and inexpensive (often free) source of information about the local community, and generally these organizations are pleased to offer their materials and assistance when told of the nature of the program.

In addition to acquiring resources, staff should become familiar with the local community, nearby commercial establishments, streets, landmarks, traffic patterns, and social climate. The treatment provider's personal knowledge is the primary resource for the client until he or she develops the skills needed to access pertinent information independently.

Conclusion

It is the authors' position that community-based community skills training should be an integral part of any head injury rehabilitation program that purports to provide community re-entry services. To encourage the development of such programs, guidelines for the development of community skills training programs have been provided. One program is described here in the hope that it might be replicated, adapted, or simply provide practitioners with the inspiration to develop their own community skills program. If a primary goal of rehabilitation is to foster independent functioning in our clients, practitioners must not shirk from the responsibility of teaching and providing opportunities for the client to function independently, outside of the cloistered world of the rehabilitation facility. While such an undertaking necessarily involves some risk, that risk can be minimized through careful planning and thorough training. As rehabilitation professionals we attempt to impress upon our clients that they must work hard to prepare themselves, and finally, take the risk of re-entering the "real world." As providers of rehabilitation we would be well-advised to heed our own advice.

Appendix A

COMMUNITY MOBILITY TRAINING PROGRAM

CLIENT INTRODUCTION

The purpose of the Community Mobility Training Program is to help clients become as independent as possible in the community.

There are six levels of Community Mobility. You are now at Level 1. Each level has challenges and privileges for you. Throughout the program, you will work on improving your safety, social behavior, orientation, and time management skills. All of the members of your team will assist you in achieving your goals in the community.

More specific information will be given to you after you have completed the evaluation period (Level 1). During this time, you will have the opportunity to plan and participate in community outings as a regular part of your treatment program. A trainer will come with you on these outings, and give you feedback about your community skills. At the end of the month, you will automatically progress to Level 2 of Community Mobility.

CLIENT AGREEMENT

I have read and understand the above statement.

I acknowledge that Community Mobility is an important part of my treatment program.

I agree to negotiate with a staff member to escort me off campus if I feel the need to go at unscheduled times.

Signed: ______________________________

Date: ________________________________

Staff: ________________________________

Appendix B

COMMUNITY MOBILITY TRAINING PROGRAM

BEHAVIORAL CRITERIA: SAFETY

1. Uses crosswalks whenever available.
2. Remains on curb while waiting to cross street.
3. Is able to accurately judge traffic for distance and speed.
4. Observes and obeys traffic lights and signals.
5. Uses sidewalks or chooses safe alternative.
6. Adapts to poor weather conditions (e.g., ice and snow).
7. Walks at a moderate pace.
8. Has adequate motor coordination for safe ambulation, or wheelchair mobility on various terrains.
9. Has adequate endurance for the scheduled trip.
10. Moves about with head up and eyes forward.
11. Recognizes traffic signs and can interpret their meaning accurately.
12. Maneuvers inside stores safely.
13. Wears appropriate footwear and clothing.
14. Navigates safely in parking lots.
15. Stays on safest route.
16. Negotiates through crowds without colliding with others.
17. Stops completely at curb before entering road.

18. Looks in all directions for traffic.

19. Compensates for physical and/or perceptual deficits (e.g., field cut).

NOTE: This is a list of baseline criteria, others may be added on an individual basis.

COMMUNITY MOBILITY TRAINING PROGRAM

BEHAVIORAL CRITERIA: ORIENTATION

1. Can describe streets in two-block area surrounding facility.
2. Can discriminate directions of right and left.
3. Can use resources (e.g., map or person) to find location in the community.
4. Can accurately recall or use compensatory strategy to follow directions.
5. Knows address and phone number of facility, or can refer to ID card with the information.
6. Can use telephone to make local, collect, and long-distance calls.
7. Can locate items in phone book, both white and yellow pages, or uses directory assistance accurately.
8. Can use problem solving to locate destinations by using street and number.
9. Notices signs, especially novel or temporary ones (e.g., "detour").
10. Scans environment for landmarks while walking.
11. Is able to generate and follow shortest safe route to destination.

NOTE: This is a list of baseline criteria, others may be added on an individual basis.

COMMUNITY MOBILITY TRAINING PROGRAM

BEHAVIORAL CRITERIA: SOCIAL BEHAVIOR

1. Dresses neatly and cleanly for outing.
2. Dresses appropriately for the weather.
3. Dresses appropriately for the occasion.
4. Does not litter.
5. Does not use profanity.
6. Keeps voice at a moderate tone/level.
7. Asks questions politely and speaks directly to vendors.
8. Uses common courtesy terms like "please" and "excuse me."
9. Makes eye contact when speaking.
10. Avoids sexual gestures (either physical or verbal).
11. Does not argue with vendors or community members.
12. Does not loiter.
13. Does not speak to strangers without specific purpose.
14. Stays on scheduled task.
15. Notices nonverbal cues from community members.
16. Waits for his or her turn patiently.
17. Avoids derogatory gestures or remarks.
18. Excuses self if neccessary.

NOTE: This is a list of baseline criteria, others may be added on an individual basis.

COMMUNITY MOBILITY TRAINING PROGRAM

BEHAVIORAL CRITERIA: TIME MANAGEMENT

1. Understands concepts of time.
2. Is able to tell time accurately using a clock.
3. Demonstrates the ability to be on time for scheduled events at the facility consistently.
4. Negotiates best time to make outings by referring to his or her schedule.
5. Signs out and back into residence accurately.
6. Arrives on time for scheduled outings.
7. Can accurately estimate time needed to reach location, complete errands, and return.
8. Plans accurate number of tasks per outing (does not plan too many).
9. Wears watch or timepiece in community.
10. Checks time while on outing.
11. Returns to facility within designated time.

NOTE: This is a list of baseline criteria, others may be added on an individual basis.

Appendix C

COMMUNITY MOBILITY TRAINING PROGRAM

CLIENT CONTRACT SCORE SHEET TO ACHIEVE LEVEL ____

CLIENT: ____________________ TRAINER: ____________________

DATE: ____________________ TIME: ____________________

DESTINATION: ____

Skill Area	Specific Item - worth 5 points each	Points Given

Total points ____________

# of points needed to pass ____________

Appendix D

COMMUNITY MOBILITY TRAINING PROGRAM

REQUEST TO BEGIN CONTRACT OUTINGS FOR LEVEL 4 COMMUNITY MOBILITY

NAME: ______________________________

DATE: ______________________________

CASE MANAGER: ________________________

I would like to begin making contract outings to achieve Level 4 Community Mobility.

1. Level 4 means:

2. The place(s) I would like to go independently are:

3. A contract outing is:

4. Level 4 Community Mobility would help my rehabilitation because:

Signed: __________________________________ Approved: ________
(Client Signature)

Denied: __________

Signed: __________________________________
(Case Manager Signature)

Appendix E

COMMUNITY MOBILITY TRAINING PROGRAM

CLIENT CONTRACT

Achievement of Community Mobility privileges means that a client has demonstrated knowledge and performance of basic safety, orientation, social behavior, and time management skills while in the community.

To attain Level ____, I agree to participate in four contract outings with a Trainer to have my performance evaluated.

I agree to follow program guidelines at all times while in the community.

My performance may be reviewed at any time by my Treatment Team. I understand that if I am unable to maintain my skills in safety, orientation, social behavior, and time management, the status of my Community Mobility privileges may be changed.

I accept full responsibility for myself and my actions while in the community.

Date: ____________________ Signature: ____________________________

Date: ____________________ Witness: ______________________________

Appendix F

COMMUNITY MOBILITY TRAINING PROGRAM
PLANNING SHEET

NAME: ______________________________

DATE: ______________________________

TIME LEAVING: __________ TIME RETURNING: ______________

THINGS I NEED TO BRING TO BE ORGANIZED AND PREPARED:

____

____

____

TASK/ACTIVITY

WHAT	WHERE	ESTIMATED COST

Appendix G

COMMUNITY MOBILITY GROUP

ORIENTATION

What is orientation?

Orientation is the ability to find your way around, know where you are, and know what is going on around you. It is the ability to become familiar to a new community or setting so that you do not get lost.

Why is orientation important?

Orientation is important in the home, work place, or in the community. A person must be oriented in order to find stores, get to work, or go out with friends. Not being oriented leads to confusion, frustration, and wasted time. It can also be unsafe for a person to be disoriented.

Why is orientation harder after a brain injury?

Orientation is more difficult after a brain injury for many reasons. First, usually after spending a lot of time in rehabilitation, it is necessary to get reacquainted with your hometown, or get to know a new place you may live after discharge. Most brain-injured persons have cognitive problems, like impaired memory, that make it harder to find one's way around. Also, perceptual deficits can make it more difficult to notice things in the environment, read signs, tell right from left, follow directions, etc. All of these problems can cause confusion in busy environments, and result in a person getting lost or being unsafe.

What are some examples of orientation skills?

1. Being able to find your way around your home or treatment facility.

2. Recognizing familiar faces, places, and your belongings.

3. Scanning the environment to pick out important information.

4. Reading signs (e.g., street signs, names of stores, aisles in a grocery store).

5. Being able to follow spoken or written directions in the community.

6. Using a map correctly to find new locations.

7. Finding your way home from a location you visited.

Are there any problems you have now which make it harder for you to be oriented in the community? Write them here:

NOTE: This is a list of baseline criteria, others may be added on an individual basis.

COMMUNITY MOBILITY GROUP

TIME MANAGEMENT

What is time management?

Time management is the ability to understand time and use it efficiently. It means being punctual, not wasting time, and noticing how long things take.

Why is time management important?

Time management is important because a person needs to be on time for many things in life, including work, appointments, or just to follow a daily schedule. People who are not efficient with time have difficulty taking care of their home and keeping commitments in the course of each busy day.

Why is time management harder after a brain injury?

Time management is frequently harder after a brain injury because physical and cognitive problems make a person slower than they used to be. Daily activities, like bathing, dressing, cooking, or just getting from place to place can all be slowed down by a brain injury. Also, it may be more difficult to get tasks organized, pay attention to time, or notice that time has passed. This happens because of changes in the brain's level of awareness of time.

What are some examples of time management skills?

1. Arriving for scheduled outings on time.

2. Signing out of and into the facility accurately.

3. Wearing a watch while in the community.

4. Accurately estimating the time needed for an outing.

5. Knowing how long it will take to complete an errand.

6. Not planning too many tasks in a limited time period.

7. Checking the time while in the community.

8. Returning to the facility at the time planned.

Are there any problems you have now which make time management more difficult? Write them here:

NOTE: This is a list of baseline criteria, others may be added on an individual basis.

COMMUNITY MOBILITY GROUP

SOCIAL BEHAVIOR

What is social behavior?

Social behavior is how a person looks, sounds, acts, and what he or she says. It is how well you get along with others.

Why is social behavior important?

Social behavior is important because it affects the way other people think of us, how comfortable they are around us, and whether or not they want to be with us. The ability to use social behavior affects all of our relationships in life, with family, friends, employers, etc.

Why is social behavior harder after a brain injury?

Most people who have suffered a brain injury are in some way different in appearance and actions than before the injury. A person may have slurred speech, problems with walking, scars which are visible, eyes which no longer focus properly, etc. All of these things are noticeable to others, and may make them wonder or feel uncomfortable. Also, frequently after a brain injury a person has difficulty in judging how others are reacting to him or her, and may need help in social situations in order to fit in.

What are some examples of good social behavior?

1. Dressing neatly and according to the weather.
2. Speaking clearly, or using a strategy so you can be understood.
3. Limiting the use of profanity when in public.
4. Using common courtesy terms.
5. Avoiding sexual comments or gestures.
6. Not littering.
7. Waiting patiently for one's turn.
8. Noticing the reactions of others and responding to them.

Are there any problems you have now which make social behavior difficult for you? Write them here:

NOTE: This is a list of baseline criteria, others may be added on an individual basis.

COMMUNITY MOBILITY GROUP

SAFETY

What is safety?

Safety is the ability to keep yourself from harm in any situation where there is a possible danger. The community is one place where there are many safety hazards.

Why is safety important?

Safety is important for many reasons. The obvious reason is to keep you healthy. Another important reason we work on safety skills is because a person who is not safe in the community must be escorted by someone else anytime he or she goes into the community to shop, socialize, or work.

Why is safety harder to maintain after a brain injury?

Safety is harder to maintain after a brain injury because a person's ability to understand and react to the environment has been changed. Some of these changes may be due to physical problems with walking, coordination, balance, or speed. Other changes may be from problems with vision, perception, hearing, or concentration. To be safe we must be able to notice and respond to everything in our environment.

What are some examples of community safety?

1. Stopping on the curb before crossing the street.

2. Looking in all directions for traffic before crossing the street.

3. Using crosswalks whenever they are available.

4. Keeping one's head up to notice things in the environment.

5. Choosing the safest route between two places.

6. Obeying traffic signs and "WALK/DON'T WALK" signals.

7. Wearing warm clothing and proper shoes for being outdoors.

8. Being especially careful around puddles, ice, stairs, etc.

Are there any problems you have that make it harder for you to be safe in the community? Write them here:

NOTE: This is a list of baseline criteria, others may be added on an individual basis.

References

Brooks, D. N. (1990). Cognitive deficits. In M. Rosenthal, E. R. Griffith, M. R. Bond, and J. D. Miller (Eds.), *Rehabilitation of the adult and child with traumatic brain injury* (2nd ed.). Philadelphia: F. A. Davis Co.

Brooks, N., Campsie, L., Symington, C., Beattie, A., & McKinlay, W. (1987). The effects of severe head injury on patient and relative within seven years of injury. *Journal of Head Trauma Rehabilitation*, *2*(3), 1-13.

Cervelli, L. (1990). Re-entry into the community and systems of post-hospital care. In M. Rosenthal, E. R. Griffith, M. R. Bond, and J. D. Miller (Eds.), *Rehabilitation of the adult and child with traumatic brain injury* (2nd ed.). Philadelphia: F. A. Davis Co.

Condeluci, A., & Gretz-Lasky, S. (1987). Social role valorization: A model for community reentry. *Journal of Head Trauma Rehabilitation*, *2*(1), 49-56.

Corthell, D. W., & Tooman, M. (1985). *Rehabilitation of traumatic brain injury* (Twelfth Institute on Rehabilitation Issues). Menomonie, WI: University of Wisconsin-Stout, Stout Vocational Rehabilitation Institute, School of Education and Human Services.

Dinardo, Q. (1971). *Psychological adjustment to spinal cord injury*. Doctoral dissertation. University of Houston.

Eames, P. (1989). Head injury rehabilitation: Towards a "model" service. In R. Ll. Wood & P. Eames (Eds.), *Models of brain injury rehabilitation*. Baltimore: Johns Hopkins University Press.

Fraser, R. T., Clemmons, D. C., & McMahon, B. T. (1990). Vocational rehabilitation counseling. In J. S. Kreutzer & P. Wehman (Eds.), *Community integration following traumatic brain injury*. Baltimore: Paul H. Brookes.

Fraser, R. T., McMahon, B. T., & Vogenthaler, D. (1988). Specific considerations for vocational rehabilitation with the head-injured. In S. Rubin & N. Rubin (Eds.), *Contemporary challenges to the rehabilitation profession*. Baltimore: Paul H. Brookes.

Gordon, W. A., Hibbard, M. R., & Kreutzer, J. S. (1989). Cognitive remediation: Issues in research and practice. *Journal of Head Trauma Rehabilitation*, *4*(3), 76-84.

Howard, M. E. (1988). Behavior management in the acute care rehabilitation setting. *Journal of Head Trauma Rehabilitation*, *3*(3), 14-22

Leland, M., Lewis, F. D., Hinman, S., & Carillo, R. (1988). Functional retraining of traumatically brain injured adults in a transdisciplinary environment. *Rehabilitation Counseling Bulletin*, *31*(4), 289-297.

McKinlay, W. W., & Hickox, A. (1988). How can families help in the rehabilitation of the head-injured? *Journal of Head Trauma Rehabilitation*, *3*(4), 64-72.

McMahon, B. T., Shaw, L. R., & Mahaffey, D. P. (1988). Career opportunities and professional preparation in head injury rehabilitation. *Rehabilitation Counseling Bulletin*, *31*(4), 344-354.

Neistadt, M. E., & Marques, K. (1984). An independent living skills training program. *The American Journal of Occupational Therapy*, *38*(10), 671-676.

Patrick, P. D. (1990). *The evolution of community re-entry programs*. Presented at the Post-graduate Course on Rehabilitation of the Brain-Injured Adult and Child, 14th Annual Conference, June 8, 1990, Williamsburg, VA.

Parente, R., & Anderson-Parente, J. K. (1990). Vocational memory training. In J. S. Kreutzer & P. Wehman (Eds.), *Community integration following traumatic brain injury*. Baltimore: Paul H. Brookes.

Shaw, L. R., & McMahon, B. T. (1990). Family-staff conflict in the rehabilitation setting: Causes, consequences, and implications. *Brain Injury*, *4*(1), 87-93.

Swenson, E. (1976). *The relationship between locus of control expectancy and successful rehabilitation of the spinal cord injured*. Doctoral dissertation, Arizona State University.

Wood, R. Ll. (1987). *Brain injury rehabilitation: A neurobehavioral approach*. Rockville, MD: Aspen.

13

Programming for Skill Maintenance And Generalization

Charles J. Durgin
Lynn P. Cullity
Patrick M. Devine

13

Programming for Skill Maintenance And Generalization

Charles J. Durgin
Lynn P. Cullity
Patrick M. Devine

Advances in emergency medical care and evacuation procedures have greatly increased the number of people surviving severe brain injury (Mullins, 1989). This increased medical success, advocacy movements, and healthcare economic incentives have led to a drastic increase in the number of rehabilitation programs designed to service people who have sustained a brain injury (Uomoto & McLean, 1989). Along with these changes there has been an increased interest in and need for greater clinical knowledge in identifying the most effective approaches to assisting these individuals and their families.

Although the field of brain injury rehabilitation is still in the early phases of evolution, there has been a great deal of progress in identifying effective clinical interventions. As our clinical knowledge increases, it is critical to identify practical and efficacious methods of addressing the often life-long problems that face the individual and family. One area of concern that requires additional attention by researchers and clinicians alike is the issue of skill generalization.

The purpose of this chapter is to discuss a variety of program obstacles that can impact on service delivery which, if not addressed, will likely compromise the long-term benefits of rehabilitation. Included in this discussion is an analysis of the many clinical, staff, program, and discharge variables that influence the transfer of skills. A number of recommendations covering conceptual approaches to service delivery and practical suggestions to support the individual's transition to home are offered.

The Challenge of Skill Generalization in Rehabilitation

STRIVING TO PROVIDE EFFECTIVE REHABILITATION SERVICES

One of the most challenging and important goals of rehabilitation is to provide services that will allow each person to generalize the gains made during treatment to the discharge environment (Wilson, 1987). This is frequently difficult to attain given that many individuals who have sustained a brain injury have difficulty transferring the skills acquired in one environment to the next (Olson & Henig, 1983). For this reason, service providers must make an aggressive effort to address the problem of skill generalization. Unless this occurs, the individual may lose many of the critical gains that were achieved during active treatment (Hogan, 1988). Many experienced professionals in the field of rehabilitation recognize that it is not unusual to see persons with brain injury appear to succeed at rehabilitation only to fail at meeting the demands of everyday living (Ben-Yishay, 1985).

In this regard, evaluating the individual's level of success in the discharge environment is a more realistic reflection of outcome than performance in the rehabilitation setting (Hart & Hayden, 1986). From the standpoint of benefits to the person with brain injury and to society, a rehabilitation program that improves functioning in the facility but not in the discharge environment is indistinguishable from a maintenance program (Haffey & Johnston, 1988). Due to the seriousness of these problems, rehabilitation professionals must systematically program for generalization rather than passively expecting it to occur as an outcome of the training procedures utilized (Stokes & Baer, 1977).

WORKING TO PREVENT A "SECOND TRAUMA" TO THE INDIVIDUAL AND FAMILY

Any discussion of skill generalization must take into consideration the needs and strengths of the family, as well as the general capabilities of those in the discharge environment. The serious impact of traumatic brain injury on the family (Livingston & Brooks, 1988; Brooks, Campsie, Symington, Beattie, & McKinlay, 1987; Brooks, Campsie, Symington, & Beattie, 1986) requires that professionals take active and sensitive measures to help the family recognize the problems that they will likely face (Lezak, 1987).

Although it is hard, if not impossible, to predict all of the problems the family system will face following discharge, in many cases the rehabilitation team has knowledge of how family members can intervene to help the individual achieve optimal success (behaviorally, vocationally, physically, cognitively, etc.). Unless this information is provided in a manner which family members can understand and use, they (as well as the injured person) are at risk of experiencing a "secondary traumatic experience" that may set the tone for all future efforts to restore family stability.

An example of this was graphically illustrated at a conference recently when, during a family panel presentation, the husband of a woman with a brain injury discussed his experience. His wife was hit by a car during one of their routine evening walks and sustained a serious brain injury. After an extensive period of acute inpatient rehabilitation, his wife was discharged to the family home. Upon her return, the husband found himself shocked and totally unprepared for the volume and intensity of her daily needs for care. To compound this, in a period of only a few weeks, his wife attempted suicide on a number of occasions. The "trauma of discharge" had left the husband confused, emotionally distraught, and without hope. From his account it was clear that his wife found her predicament equally disturbing. In the midst of these problems the husband elected to move out of the house. He indicated that his departure had, in effect, split him with his two grown daughters, one who understood his actions and one who could not.

As the audience asked him to elaborate, he expressed the desire to have had more specific information regarding what he and his wife might have potentially faced following discharge. Based on this presentation alone, it was not possible to clearly determine the type of support that this family had received, or if the outcome would have been different if additional methods of support had been offered. What was strikingly evident, however, is how quickly the family system fell apart once his wife returned home. While this may be an extreme example, similar problems face many people when they return home from structured rehabilitation settings without appropriate preparation.

It is important to note that this situation occurred following discharge from an acute care setting where evaluating the individual's emotional reaction to returning home can be difficult since acquired problems often become more evident in unstructured environments. To address situations like this, and other clinical problems with their own unique complications, the three-phase model outlined at the end of this chapter describes a procedure that can help staff and family members evaluate and discuss the specific needs of the individual prior to and following discharge.

ADDRESSING THE TRAINING NEEDS OF STAFF WITH DIVERSE PROFESSIONAL BACKGROUNDS

Many staff hired to provide rehabilitation services have not had any formal training in treating the many complex and often subtle aspects of brain injury (Lezak, 1978). Unless these issues are addressed through facility-based staff training there is a strong likelihood that the clinical treatment offered will not produce the desired outcome. There are a number of intervention principles that staff must understand if they are to provide services that will assist persons with brain injury both during rehabilitation and following discharge. Outlined below are a variety of fundamental yet critical training issues that can have a direct impact on the staff's ability to deliver services that will have a lasting benefit.

Understanding the Goals and Purpose of Rehabilitation

It is important for all staff to have a clear philosophical foundation that can serve to guide their approach to treatment. This will keep staff focused on what they are striving to accomplish clinically, as well as to help them to set realistic goals for themselves and their peers. All program staff must have a clear working definition of rehabilitation.

In the broadest of terms, rehabilitation aims both to assist the individual to achieve a better quality of life and to prevent serious problems. Understandably, persons with brain injury are at increased risk in a number of critical areas compared to the general population. These include developing psychiatric problems (Brown, Chadwick, Shaffer, Rutter, & Traub, 1981), losing valuable social supports (Wesolowski, 1987), becoming more dependent on others, developing drug and alcohol problems (Sparadeo & Gill, 1989), coming into conflict with the legal system (McMahon & Satz, 1981), sustaining a second or third brain injury, and/or developing serious long-term health-related complications (Trieschmann, 1990). Additionally, these individuals are generally more vulnerable to being taken advantage of by others (Lezak, 1988). Staff members need to clearly recognize these implications and should work to reduce the likelihood of having any of these scenarios from becoming a reality.

The Commission on Accreditation of Rehabilitation Facilities (CARF, 1990) defines rehabilitation as:

> *The process of providing, in a coordinated manner, those comprehensive services deemed appropriate to the needs of a person with a disability, in a program designed to achieve objectives of improved health, welfare, and the realization of one's maximum physical, social, psychological, and vocational potential for useful and productive activity. (p. 125)*

Although this is an excellent global definition, it is critical that rehabilitation professionals look more closely at the specific ways in which treatment should aim to enhance and support the areas mentioned above, particularly when the person cannot independently perform important skills at discharge. In this regard, the goal of rehabilitation must be to clearly define the conditions under which the individual and his or her family will achieve success in all critical areas of life after intensive rehabilitation services have discontinued. This should include a careful analysis of the potential risks associated with a lack of support in all critical areas of need (e.g., community safety, behavioral problems, medical issues). Obtaining this knowledge will not only improve facility-based treatment but will allow the rehabilitation team to better assist all parties in the discharge setting. This may include teaching family members to reinforce specific behaviors, set limits, prompt the use of compensatory strategies, prevent anticipated problems, and to structure the physical environment. Unless staff can understand, apply, document, and effectively teach specific interventions known to be effective they will be of little value addressing the long-term needs of the individual and family.

Recognizing the Impact of Cognitive Problems in All Areas of Social and Independent Living

Understanding the impact of cognitive deficits on functional behaviors can be completely understood only if staff to know how to perform real-life functional assessments (Diller & Ben-Yishay, 1989). Additionally, it is critical that treatment goals are structured to reflect the unique cognitive abilities of each individual served. This is particularly important in that it is the cognitive problems that often present the greatest obstacles to individuals as they work to achieve a higher level of independent functioning (Brooks, 1984).

Until staff directly observe and experience the difficulties that many persons with brain injury have outside of structured clinical treatment settings, they are likely to misjudge the individual's abilities. Placing the individual in real-life performance situations that are similar to the demands in the discharge environment will help to increase the accuracy of the clinical assessment. Furthermore, staff should recognize that memory and self-regulation problems often result in a slow learning curve requiring staff to persist at interventions even though there may be no initial signs of improvement.

Understanding Specific Teaching Strategies that can be Developed to Facilitate the Transfer of Skills

Problems in addressing this topic often occurs due to confusion associated with the terminology used. Generalization can imply both the full-strength maintenance of skills, as well as the broadening or expansion of skills learned in treatment (Scott, Himadi, & Keane, 1983). In either event it is important for staff to understand the outcome that they are programming for and to be able to structure interventions to maximize the individual's potential to transfer the use of their skills outside the treatment setting.

Scott, Himadi, & Keane (1983) made several recommendations for successfully training generalization. They recommend training with multiple and/or relevant persons, training significant others to deliver reinforcement, training in multiple settings, scheduling regular booster sessions post-treatment, and training in multiple scenes (i.e., role-playing using a variety of problem solving situations). They also suggest discrimination training to help the person identify when they need to initiate a strategy, training cognitive self-monitoring strategies to mediate performance, and the use of thorough assessment techniques to evaluate the transfer of skills. All of these teaching principles should be incorporated into the service delivery model and should be addressed by treatment team members when working on individual outcome goals. The case example below illustrates how Scott, Himadi, and Keane's (1983) intervention recommendations have been applied to day-to-day clinical intervention in a post-acute setting.

CASE EXAMPLE

At the age of 17, Lisa received a severe closed head injury secondary to a motor vehicle accident. She was in a coma for five months, received a total of 10 months of acute rehabilitation, and had returned home for 18 months before entering a residential post-acute program. Upon admission Lisa demonstrated severe problems with impulse control, social judgement, and egocentric thinking. She was highly demanding of others' attention. Although her memory skills were also impaired she was able to retain information with repetition. One of her greatest social problems was her inability to delay receiving attention. Socially, her intense, obtrusive, and chronic interruptions were so disruptive that she not only frustrated staff, but she received frequent reprimands from other clients. Upon entering any social situation she would immediately interrupt everyone present to have one of her questions or concerns addressed. These disruptions occurred irrespective of whether or not there were environmental cues that clearly suggested waiting.

Since Lisa did not have the cognitive ability to ascertain when to enter an ongoing conversation she was taught to strategically position herself and wait to be acknowledged by others. Given these cognitive problems discrimination training focused on positioning and waiting rather than deciding when and how to interject. Because she was motivated to be accepted by others and had a high need for attention, natural reinforcers (e.g., praise) were given each time she demonstrated improved self-control.

Outlined in Table 1 is a description of the training procedures employed to teach Lisa to both control her interrupting and to learn a more adaptive strategy to successfully initiate social contact. The systematic use of the teaching techniques described in Table 1 resulted in Lisa being able to control her behavior and to independently use the compensatory strategies outlined. These gains resulted in allowing her the opportunity to successfully provide secretarial assistance in a busy office, and to develop more positive social relationships in all settings.

Table 1
Case Example of Employing Training Techniques that Facilitate Generalization

Training Techniques	**Implementation Procedures**
Discrimination training/ cognitive self-monitoring strategy	Given the inability to discriminate when to enter a conversation, the individual was taught how to position herself and wait to be acknowledged by others (concrete rules to get attention)
	The "self-talk" strategy "STOP-LOOK-LISTEN-WAIT" was trained in all settings
	Treatment sessions included role-playing correct and incorrect performance to help the individual anticipate and correct problems
	Reinforcement of successive approximations of success in all situations was provided
	Videotaping and structured peer feedback was used to highlight behavioral successes and problems that need attention
	Self-charting (staff-supported) was implemented in all social situations to both measure performance and to facilitate improved self-regulation
Multiple/relevant persons and significant others to deliver reinforcement	All program staff were taught how to intervene (administrative, clinical, residential, etc.)
	Family members were taught to utilize the intervention
Multiple settings and multiple scenes	Practice trials were implemented during 1:1 sessions, in small groups, during planned encounters in the rehabilitation program, and throughout numerous community contacts
	Training was implemented in these various settings using a coaching model to ensure successful use of strategies, and to monitor the effectiveness of staff in adhering to the intervention
	A wide variety of social scenarios were simulated throughout training to provide the individual with practice in making appropriate social contact

(Continued at the top of the next page)

Training Techniques	Implementation Procedures
Booster sessions post-treatment/thorough assessment to evaluate generalization	Staff in the discharge environment were taught to reinforce these strategies to support skill maintenance
	Frequent follow-up consultation was provided by an assigned case manager to address problems
	Post-discharge treatment sessions were provided to assist the individual to use the strategies in the new setting
	Documentation in the discharge environment was structured to monitor generalization

Providing Treatment that is Integrated, Outcome-Focused, and Functionally Based

Providing highly integrated rehabilitation services is important to foster a stable, consistent, and potent therapeutic environment for people who are often confused and in need of structure (Leland, Lewis, Hinman, & Carrillo, 1988). This requires staff to be able to effectively communicate their goals to others, be comfortable with implementing therapeutic interventions that they have not been formally trained in, and work effectively with support staff (nursing aides, residential staff, etc.). For example, the use of applied behavioral analysis techniques are known to be effective in assisting people with brain injury (Horton & Miller, 1984). However, many staff need ongoing training to be competent in this area. Unless staff receive direction in this and other important specialty areas for which they have not been adequately trained, the effectiveness of the treatment offered will be significantly compromised (Wood & Burgess, 1988).

The rehabilitation plan should be designed to achieve an outcome that will provide the greatest improvement in the individual's ability to function in the discharge environment (Haffey & Lewis, 1989; Haffey & Fryer, 1988). This requires that the team set clear priorities so that the individual and family alike are not overwhelmed. Furthermore, all programming must be grounded in delivering services that improve the individual's ability to succeed in the demands of day-to-day living (Fussey & Giles, 1988; Frey, 1984). This requires staff, particularly in the later stages of recovery, to shift the emphasis of their interventions from the remediation of specific impairments to lessening the degree of disability caused by the underlying problems (Ylvisaker, Szekeres, Henry, Sullivan, & Wheeler, 1987; Wood, 1989). This involves employing the use of a compensatory model of intervention (Prigatano, Fordyce, & Zeiner, 1986) as opposed to addressing the underlying impairment to correct the functional breakdowns. An example would be training the individual to use a journal to compensate for memory loss as opposed to expending extensive resources to restore memory function when it is unlikely to improve significantly.

Effectively Including Family Members in the Rehabilitation Process

The fundamental importance of the family involvement in rehabilitation has been strongly emphasized (McKinlay & Hickox, 1988; Williams & Kay, 1991; Durgin, 1989). Including family members in the rehabilitation process, however, can be a difficult adjustment for many staff (Shaw & McMahon, 1990). To truly understand how facility-based intervention relates to life following discharge, it is critical that staff understand the realities of having a disabled family member living at home (Seligman & Darling, 1989; Seligman & Seligman, 1980). This requires that all staff members understand the trauma, role disruption, losses, and financial consequences of having a loved one sustain a brain injury. By being sensitive to individual family issues, the team can better evaluate how the family can provide the greatest level of support and can determine what kinds of expectations are realistic. Staff should not make global assumptions about what families can contribute or manage, but should base their recommendations on an individualized family assessment (Brown & McCormick, 1988; Bishop & Miller, 1988) and their own interactions with the family during the rehabilitation process.

Developing a responsive treatment model, training, and providing strong leadership to drive clinical treatment will help to enhance the quality of services provided by staff new to the field of brain injury rehabilitation.

THE POWER OF THE THERAPEUTIC ENVIRONMENT AND GENERALIZATION

Many of our efforts in rehabilitation are designed to define and create a positive therapeutic environment that is uniquely responsive to the needs of people who have sustained a brain injury. Through these efforts many programs have been successful in bringing individuals to their highest post-injury level of functioning. Much of this success is the result of creating a carefully structured environment that utilizes well-developed procedures and approaches which maximize the probability of success. This includes many program characteristics ranging from the clinical techniques of professionals to the physical layout of the treatment setting.

The ideal rehabilitation program is flexible, supports the individual's needs in many life areas, and responds to problems and crises quickly and rationally. The ideal program has the capacity to mobilize a variety of resources when necessary and can distribute the responsibility of treating the individual over many staff. In short, the ideal program anticipates how to prevent problems, provides a "safety net," and generally creates an environment that can significantly reduce the individual's stress level in important areas of daily life.

All of these variables set the context in which persons with brain injury demonstrate their abilities. Therefore, staff need to clearly identify the specific program components that have led each individual to their current level of functioning. Staff must also be able to convey how to intervene (feedback strategies, specifying how to prevent problems, etc.). One method of systematically evaluating environmental influences on behavior that has been widely adopted in many post-acute programs has been the development of separate residences that gradually offer reduced levels of supervision as the individual progresses. These range from highly supervised and structured behavioral residences to community-based apartments that offer a more normalized living environment. This is one effective strategy to evaluate the individual's ability to generalize the use of compensatory strategies into settings with less support and structure. Although this is a helpful model to train and evaluate generalization, the program variables discussed above still need to be carefully considered.

The authors experienced an example of underestimating the potency of the therapeutic environment after discharging an individual who had successfully completed all phases of a post-acute rehabilitation program. At the point of discharge the individual had been living for a few months in the independent living apartments on facility grounds. Although he had a history of alcohol abuse, he was able to refrain from drinking throughout all phases of treatment. The rehabilitation team had concerns about his use of alcohol following discharge but did not expect the rapid decline that occurred (particularly since he moved to an apartment less than a half-mile from the facility). Within three days he began excessive drinking and was at risk of losing both his job and his apartment. Apparently the rule of "no alcohol on facility grounds" and his close proximity to social and therapeutic contacts provided enough structure to help this individual control the problem. Discharge follow-up resulted in his return to the facility for a one month extension to further address these issues. Following additional intervention and subsequent discharge with external case management support, he has successfully worked and lived on his own for two consecutive years. This example illustrates the importance of seemingly subtle program components that provide very strong support to individuals which, if underestimated, can mislead the team in determining the level of support needed following discharge.

Providing the Type of Support Needed in the Discharge Environment

Rosenthal & Young (1988) suggested that the PLISST Model (Annon, 1974) has many positive characteristics that can be helpful in guiding staff when intervening to help families. This model has four stages that recommend: 1) giving the family permission to express their hopes and fears to a supportive staff member, 2) initially offering limited information about the consequences of traumatic brain injury from one consistent source, 3) providing specific information about the problems and interventions being employed, and 4) offering intensive psychological counseling to help the family cope with the problems caused by the injury.

There are a number of aspects of this approach relating to generalization that merit further emphasis. Of particular importance is establishing an effective pace in conveying information to the family. This enables the family to process information better and can help to prevent family members from becoming overwhelmed. Another important element is the provision of specific information resulting in family members acquiring the technical knowledge and insights to help them better understand the problems at hand. Both of these factors must be taken into consideration when preparing the family to carry on the supports needed following discharge. Listed below are several areas of support that are important to provide to individuals within the discharge environment.

- CLARIFYING PROBLEMS THAT ARE EXPECTED TO CONTINUE - This will minimize surprises surrounding the individual's limitations and problems.

- SPECIFYING THE SKILLS THAT THE INDIVIDUAL CAN BE EXPECTED TO PERFORM INDEPENDENTLY - This will reduce the evolution of increased dependency in the discharge setting and minimize the burden that family may experience unnecessarily.

- DIRECTION AND TRAINING RELATIVE TO THE ANTICIPATED ASSISTANCE AND/OR SUPPORT NEEDED BY THE INDIVIDUAL - Ideally this training should involve more than sharing verbal information. Directly observing the family members' abilities to support the individual, collaborating on treatment programs, and evaluating interventions as a team can facilitate the carry-over of effective environmental support.

- SPECIFIC WRITTEN RESOURCES THAT CLEARLY DESCRIBE THE TYPES OF SUPPORT NEEDED TO FACILITATE AN OPTIMAL LEVEL OF INDEPENDENCE - This information will help to establish and maintain a balance between the individual's abilities and family expectations. Families may not be able to extract this information from standard reports. Furthermore, many clinical reports do not explicitly describe the specific types of support needed to maintain the skills learned during rehabilitation.

- ASSISTANCE IN IDENTIFYING AND EVALUATING RESOURCES IN THE LOCAL COMMUNITY - Families may benefit from professional guidance in evaluating the effectiveness of home community resources in meeting the individual's post-discharge needs.

- FOLLOW-UP CONTACTS TO MONITOR THE TRANSITION AND TO TROUBLESHOOT ANY ONGOING PROBLEMS - Home visits, additional conferences, phone calls, planning a brief return to programming to reevaluate specific concerns, and coordination with an external case manager are helpful strategies to evaluate generalization.

The extent to which this information and support is effectively provided to the people in the discharge setting will, to a large degree, influence the potential for the individual to maintain his or her level of functioning. Furthermore, if the outcome goals are maintained post-discharge, the individual will be in a good position to continue to make further progress over time as is common with many people who have sustained brain injury.

Moving from a Model of Intervention to a Model of Long-term Support

Gross & Schultz (1986) developed a conceptual approach to intervention following traumatic brain injury. Their model represents a continuum of intervention that is designed to address a wide range of cognitive abilities. Each of the five models outlined assumes a different relationship between the individual and therapist, depending on the learning and performance capabilities of the individual. For example, individuals who are severely compromised in their ability to learn new skills may require intensive environmental structure to improve task performance. In this case the Environmental Control Model would be appropriate to use. The next level of intervention is the S-R Conditioning

Model. The emphasis of this model is to reinforce specific behaviors with the expectation that individuals will be able to modify their behavior and that they may potentially be able to maintain the gains even after the reinforcement is withdrawn. Intervention in both the Environmental Control Model and S-R Conditioning Model is directed at modifying the way that the environment influences behavior. Although some degree of learning and generalization may take place, it is the manipulation of the environment by staff that facilitates improved performance.

The other three models of intervention – Skill Training, Strategy Substitution, and Cognitive Cycle Models – are different in that the intervention is directed at helping individuals modify the way that they act on the environment. These models assume that the individual can transfer learning, compensate for problems across multiple situations, and demonstrate the ability to solve increasingly complex problems. It is important to note that all intervention models are designed to be used in an integrated fashion to address the unique learning needs of each individual. For example, the authors used the Environmental Control Model (intensive supervision) to protect a sexually disinhibited woman from being taken advantage of, until a behavioral program could be established (i.e., S-R Conditioning Model), which in time gave her the support to regulate her own behavior (Skills Training Model). Individuals can pass through the different levels of support for a given skill, or, in some cases, may require the use of different intervention strategies for a variety of problems. Gross and Schultz (1986) recommend that staff consider the use of these models when establishing a plan to address each of the presenting problems.

The value of this conceptual approach is that it explicitly delineates a continuum of support, accounting for the various social and environmental factors that facilitate performance. Although these models are designed to guide intervention, they can be used to project the type and level of assistance that the individual will need in the discharge setting. As the individual's ability levels are determined, staff will be able to specify the environmental supports that need to be provided, and define the areas that individuals are able to manage and regulate on their own. This is essentially a process of identifying the critical events that must occur in the person with a brain injury and in the environment if the projected outcome goals are to become a reality (Haffey & Lewis, 1989). The development of the supported employment model of vocational rehabilitation (Wehman, Kreutzer, Wood, Morton, & Sherron, 1988) is an excellent example of aggressively engineering environmental supports to maximize an individual's potential. This type of approach needs to be replicated for persons of all ability levels across all life areas if rehabilitation is to deliver positive long-term outcomes. Described below are recommendations for effectively documenting these findings so that the appropriate supports can be provided by those in the discharge environment. Included in this description are recommendations specific to programming for skill generalization.

DEVELOPING MEANINGFUL DOCUMENTATION THAT CAN BE UTILIZED IN THE DISCHARGE SETTING: THE CLIENT RESOURCE BOOK

The content development of the individualized Client Resource Book (CRB) follows Gross and Schultz's (1986) continuum of intervention. It provides clearly written guidelines, using nontechnical language, that precisely describe the environmental supports and/or self-initiated strategies known to enhance performance in the specific areas of concern (memory compensation, safe use of transportation, etc.). Depending on the needs and abilities of the individual, the CRB can be written by individuals for their own use or developed primarily by the staff to help the individual access support from others.

In many cases the content is designed to allow the person with a brain injury to forward the materials to others who can use the information in a supportive capacity. An example would be guidelines for future employers that specify strengths and particular needs in the workplace. All of the information is designed to provide a greater level of understanding to the parties in the discharge environment who are in a position to help.

CRB development is an ongoing process that involves all members of the rehabilitation team. The three-phase procedure for developing the CRB is described in Table 2. Included in this description are recommendations for enhancing skill generalization. Table 3 provides an overview of the various content areas that are considered for inclusion in the CRB. All of the material in the CRB is strictly based on the unique needs of each individual and the capabilities of the support system in the discharge environment.

Table 2

Procedure for Developing the Client Resource Book while Programming for Generalization

Programming Phase	Procedure
PHASE I - Assessment/ Treatment Planning	Evaluate the individual's strengths, acquired impairments, functional problems, pre-injury interests/ abilities, level of awareness of presenting problems, and current goals. Review family goals and assess in detail the options for discharge. The assessment should include a comprehensive analysis of potential resources available in the discharge setting (transportation, outpatient services, support groups, recreational options, etc.). Write measurable goals reflecting the anticipated skills that need to be acquired for a successful outcome (taking into consideration the feasibility of accessing community and/or family resources). In other words, the rehabilitation plan should be designed to help the individual function more independently in the discharge environment and should not simply focus on increasing skills equally in all areas. This information will help clinicians to set clear treatment priorities so that their efforts will address the areas of greatest need for each individual and family. Structure the treatment plan to determine: 1) if the individual is going to be able to independently perform compensatory strategies and 2) the type of support needed for skills the individual cannot perform independently. This process is outlined in PHASE II. Focus on teaching the priority skills that present the greatest obstacles for the individual to return to a more safe, independent, and productive lifestyle. Document the treatment priorities in a manner that clearly specifies the goal, the strategies for the individual to learn, the teaching guidelines for others to follow, and the environmental supports that need to be in place. This information is then distributed to the family members and all rehabilitation staff and will serve as a foundation for the evolution of the resource book. The content can include anything from simple food shopping guidelines to a more technical behavioral plan depending on the presenting problems. This information is then evaluated and updated in the next phase.

(Continued)

Programming Phase	Procedure
PHASE II - Intervention/ Evaluation	Structure treatment in such a manner that the individual will be presented with the same types of demands that he or she will be facing in the discharge environment (community mobility, social contacts, work responsibilities, independent living, school pressures, etc.). Direct training in these situations will decrease the number of variables that impact on generalization. If direct intervention in the environment in which these activities naturally occur is not possible, the simulation of the anticipated demands during treatment can increase the potential that the skills learned will be transferred. Teach the various strategies that have been targeted to determine the individual's ability to call upon and perform the skills as planned. To reliably evaluate the person's ability to generalize these skills, the person should be asked to perform the tasks under a wide variety of conditions (e.g., different settings, different social supports, varied use of materials and any other forms of variability that might be expected). It is critical to remember that measures must be taken to systematically teach generalization before staff can confidently predict how the individual is likely to perform after discharge. Collect information through direct observation across setting, solicit input from staff, and structure home visits to evaluate performance specific to the goals established. Data should be collected specific to the rate of learning as well as the level of problem solving that the individual is able to perform in various settings. This information will help the team reevaluate initial discharge goals and provide a framework to update the initial rehabilitation plan. Staff should be able to clearly define the conditions under which clients are able to perform at their highest level (behaviorally, academically, ADLs, etc.). This information is then used to update the original guidelines/strategies that were outlined for staff/ families to follow and for the individual to learn. Modifications may include increasing expectations, fading the current environmental supports, and/or providing other forms of assistance that have not been attempted. As the date of discharge draws nearer, this information is again reviewed and modified as is routine with any ongoing clinical intervention.

(Continued)

Programming Phase	Procedure
PHASE II (Continued)	If the initial assessment was on target, only minor programming changes are generally required. In the event that more significant changes need to be introduced, such as when the individual makes particularly rapid progress, the initial information outlined should be adjusted accordingly. Whenever possible, it is recommended that the individual be directly involved in the process as a part of ongoing treatment, to promote his or her explicit awareness of the strategies being taught, and the need for external support when necessary.
PHASE III - Discharge Preparation/Discharge Follow-up	The rehabilitation team should be in agreement as to the level of assistance the individual needs specific to the demands in the discharge setting. This should include issues of supervision and concerns relating to risk management. Meet with the family and future support staff to finalize any changes that have been made in the type of assistance that the individual requires. Document changes in a clear fashion to be used as a long-term resource. This has typically included a written contribution from each specialist describing what needs to occur to maintain the skills of concern. At this time it is important to stress the importance of using the written resources as it conveys the techniques that can be called upon to compensate for acquired problems (including both environmental supports and self-initiated strategies). When there is a strong need for environmental structure, a staff member should accompany the individual to the discharge setting to ensure that the proper supports are put in place (e.g., structuring the living space to fit with the abilities/needs of the individual). Follow-up through home visits, phone calls, or any other necessary contacts to evaluate the transition. The rehabilitation program should retain one copy of the resource book to use as a guide in reviewing the individual's adjustment and general use of strategies that were used during treatment.

Table 3
Content Typically Included in the Client Resource Book

Skill Area	Content Examples
Cognition/Communication	Memory aids/cueing devices Journal strategies Communication guidelines Planning/problem solving checklists
Psychosocial/Behavioral	Behavioral programs/contracts Relaxation strategies Conflict resolution guidelines Adjustment/transition supports Self-regulation strategies
Daily Living Skills	Self-care strategies Safety/community mobility guidelines Financial mangement supports Consumer activity guidelines Cooking task sheets
Physical	Endurance-related limitations/stategies Transferring/ambulation guidelines Use of adaptive equipment
Medical	Medication guidelines Dietary recommendations Specific medical restrictions
Vocational	Employer guidelines Personal resumé/references Profile of vocational strengths and limitations Task-specific vocational strategies
Educational	Strategies for teachers Learning strategies/supports for the student to utilize Testing and evaluation recommendations
Recreational/Leisure	Recreational interests/options Adaptations for participation Strategies for accessing recreational activities

It is important to recognize that the resource book itself is only one component of the comprehensive approach to treatment emphasized throughout this chapter. One of the great benefits of this tool is that written material can be used as a post-discharge reference to evaluate skill generalization in addition to providing clear guidelines specifying the strategies that have improved the individual's emotional adjustment and level of independence. The resource book can also be used by future support staff as a practical foundation, developed by an interdisciplinary team, to ensure the continuity of treatment.

Conclusion

Providing truly effective rehabilitation services to people that have sustained a traumatic brain injury is a challenging endeavor. Neuropsychological, family, staff, organizational, and economic dynamics present tremendous complexities that need to be managed in the pursuit of offering individualized services. While confronting these and other matters it is essential that rehabilitation professionals remain focused on the most critical therapeutic priorities and take systematic measures to aggressively program for skill maintenance and generalization.

Furthermore, service providers need to develop a clear vision of how they can more effectively impact on the long-term needs of each individual and family. Central to this process is developing treatment and discharge plans that make the best use of the individual's financial resources. These issues not only have a direct bearing on how we design our treatment programs, but challenge us to find creative ways to extend our support into the real world.

If providers fail to attend to the life-long needs of persons with brain injury and their families during rehabilitation, they will not only compromise the treatment offered to those that they currently service, but they also risk having the broader medical and human service community develop a perception that underestimates how rehabilitation can have a favorable impact. The priorities that providers set today will clearly impact on the long-term opportunities that people with brain injury will have in the future. Fortunately, there are known techniques and approaches that can be employed that can help enhance the quality of rehabilitation services presently offered.

References

Annon, J. S. (1974). *The behavioral treatment of sexual problems. Vol. I.* Honolulu: Enabling Systems.

Ben-Yishay, Y. (1985). *Holistic neuropsychological rehabilitation program for chronic, traumatically head injured individuals.* Workshop presented at meeting of The National Academy of Neuropsychologists, Philadelphia.

Bishop, D. S., & Miller, I. W. (1988). Traumatic brain injury: Empirical family assessment techniques. *Journal of Head Trauma Rehabilitation, 3*(4), 16-30.

Brooks, D. N. (Ed.) (1984). *Closed head injury: Psychological, social and family consequences.* New York: Oxford University Press.

Brooks, D. N., Campsie, L., Symington, C., & Beattie, A. (1986). The five-year outcome of severe blunt head injury: A relative's view. *Journal of Neurology, Neurosurgery, and Psychiatry, 49*, 764-770.

Brooks, N., Campsie, L., Symington, C., Beattie, A., & McKinlay, W. (1987). The effects of severe brain injury on patient and relative within seven years of injury. *Journal of Head Trauma Rehabilitation, 2*(3), 1-13.

Brown, B. W., & McCormick, T. M. (1988). Family coping following traumatic head injury: An exploratory analysis with recommendations for treatment. *Family Relations, 37*, 12-16.

Brown, G., Chadwick, O., Shaffer, D., Rutter, M., & Traub, M. (1981). A prospective study of children with head injuries, III; Psychiatric sequelae. *Psychological Medicine, II*, 63-78.

Commission on Accreditation of Rehabilitation Facilities. (1990). *Standards manual for organizations serving people with disabilities.* Tucson, AZ: CARF.

Diller, L., & Ben-Yishay, Y. (1989). Assessment in traumatic brain injury. In P. Bach-y-Rita (Ed.), *Comprehensive neurologic rehabilitation*, (Vol. 2, pp. 161-174). New York: Demos.

Durgin, C. (1989). Techniques for families to increase their involvement in the rehabilitation process. *Cognitive Rehabilitation, 7*(3), 22-25.

Frey, W. (1984). Functional assessment in the 80s: A conceptual enigma, a technological challenge. In A. Halpern & M. Fuhrer (Eds.), *Functional assessment in rehabilitation* (pp. 11-43). Baltimore: Paul H. Brookes.

Fussey, I., & Giles, G. M. (Eds.) (1988). *Rehabilitation of the severely brain injured adult: A practical approach.* London: Brooks.

Gross, Y., & Schultz, L. E. (1986). Intervention models in neuropsychology. In B. Uzell & Y. Gross (Eds.), *Clinical neuropsychology of intervention* (pp. 179-214). Boston: Martinus Nijhoff.

Haffey, W. J., & Fryer, L. J. (1988). *Head injury: Functional outcomes and community re-entry.* Presented at the conference by American Rehabilitation Educational Network, Pittsburgh.

Haffey, W. J., & Lewis, F. D. (1989). Programming for occupational outcomes following traumatic brain injury. *Rehabilitation Psychology, 34*(2), 147-158.

Haffey, W. J., & Johnston, M. V. (1988). An information system to assess the effectiveness of brain injury rehabilitation. In R. Wood & P. Eames (Eds.), *Models of brain injury rehabilitation* (pp. 205-233). London: Chapman & Hall.

Hart, T., & Hayden, M. (1986). Issues in the evaluation of rehabilitation effects. In M. Miner & K. Wagner (Eds.), *Neurotrauma: Treatment, rehabilitation and related issues* (pp. 197-212). Boston: Butterworths.

Hogan, R. T. (1988). Behavior management for community re-integration. *Journal of Head Trauma Rehabilitation, 3*(3), 62-71.

Horton, A. M., & Miller, W. G. (1984). Brain damage and rehabilitation. In C. J. Golden (Ed.), *Current topics in rehabilitation psychology* (pp. 77-105). Orlando, FL: Grune and Stratton.

Leland, M., Lewis, F. D., Hinman, S., & Carrillo, R. (1988). Functional retraining of traumatically brain injured adults in a transdisciplinary environment. *Rehabilitation Counseling Bulletin, 31*, 289-297.

Lezak, M. D. (1987). Living with the characterologically altered brain injured patient. *Journal of Clinical Psychiatry, 39*, 592-598.

Lezak, M. D. (1978). Subtle sequelae of brain damage: Perplexity, distractibility, and fatigue. *American Journal of Physical Medicine, 57*, 9-15.

Lezak, M. D. (1988). *Psychosocial repercussions of emotional disturbances in head injury.* Presented at the conference: Head Injury: An integrated approach to behavioral rehabilitation, Boston.

Livingston, M. G., & Brooks, D. N. (1988). The burden on families of the brain injured: A review. *Journal of Head Trauma Rehabilitation, 3*(4), 6-15.

McKinlay, W. W., & Hickox, A. (1988). How can families help in the rehabilitation of the head injured? *Journal of Head Trauma Rehabilitation, 3*(4), 64-72.

McMahon, E. A., & Satz, P. (1981). Clinical neuropsychology: Some forensic applications. In S. Filskov & T. Boll (Eds.), *Handbook of clinical neuropsychology* (pp. 686-701). New York: Wiley.

Mullins, L. L. (1989). Hate revisited: Power, envy, and greed in the rehabilitation setting. *Archives of Physical Medicine and Rehabilitation, 70*, 740-744.

Olson, D. A., & Henig, E. (1983). *A manual of behavior management strategies for traumatically brain-injured adults.* Chicago: Rehabilitation Institute of Chicago.

Prigatano, G. P., Fordyce, D. J., & Zeiner, H. K. (1986). *Neuropsychological rehabilitation after brain injury.* Baltimore: Johns Hopkins University Press.

Rosenthal, M., & Young, T. (1988). Effective family interventions after traumatic brain injury: Theory and practice. *Journal of Head Trauma Rehabilitation, 3*(4), 42-50.

Scott, R. R., Himadi, W., & Keane, T. M. (1983). A review of generalization in social skills training: Suggestions for future research. *Progress in Behavior Modification, 15*, 114-167.

Seligman, M., & Darling, R. B. (1989). *Ordinary families, special children: A systems approach to childhood disability.* New York: Guilford Press.

Seligman, M., & Seligman, P. A. (1980). The professional's dilemma: Learning to work with parents. *The Exceptional Parent, 10*, 511-513.

Shaw, L. R., & McMahon, B. T. (1990). Family-staff conflict in the rehabilitation setting: Causes, consequences, and implications. *Brain Injury, 4*(1), 87-93.

Sparadeo, F. R., & Gill, D. (1989). Effects of prior alcohol use in head injury recovery. *Journal of Head Trauma Rehabilitation, 4*(1), 75-82.

Stokes, T. F., & Baer, D. M. (1977). An implicit technology of generalization. *Journal of Applied Behavior Analysis, 10*, 344-367.

Trieschmann, R. B. (1990). Sickness treatment or health care: Implications for head injury. *Journal of Head Trauma Rehabilitation, 5*(1), 57-64.

Uomoto, J. M., & McLean, A. (1989). Care continuum in traumatic brain injury rehabilitation. *Rehabilitation Psychology, 34*(2), 71-79.

Wehman, P., Kreutzer, J., Wood, W., Morton, M. V., & Sherron, P. (1988). Supported work model for persons with traumatic brain injury: Toward job placement and retention. *Rehabilitation Counseling Bulletin, 31*(4), 298-312.

Wesolowski, M. D. (1987). Differences in sizes of social networks of rehabilitation clients versus nonclients. *Rehabilitation Counseling Bulletin, 31*(1), 17-27.

Williams, J., & Kay, T. (1991). *Head injury: A family matter.* Baltimore: Paul H. Brookes.

Wilson, B. A. (1987). *Rehabilitation of memory.* New York: The Guilford Press.

Wood, R., & Burgess, P. (1988). The psychological management of behavior disorders following head injury. In J. Fussey & G. Giles (Eds.), *Rehabilitation of the severely brain-injured adult: A practical approach* (pp. 43-68). London: Brooks.

Wood, R. (1989). *Behavior management in outpatient and community programs.* Presented at the conference: Head injury: An integrated approach to behavioral rehabilitation, Boston.

Ylvisaker, M., Szekeres, S., Henry, K., Sullivan, D., & Wheeler, P. (1987). Topics in cognitive rehabilitation therapy. In M. Ylvisaker and E. Gobble (Eds.), *Community re-entry for head injured adults* (pp. 137-215). Boston: College-Hill Press.

14

Sequencing Family Services in Response to Changing Needs

Linda R. Shaw

14

Sequencing Family Services in Response to Changing Needs

Linda R. Shaw

The dramatic impact of a traumatic brain injury (TBI) has been well-documented (Camplair, Kreutzer, & Doherty, 1990; Shaw & McMahon, 1990; Brooks, 1984; Rosenthal & Young, 1988). The head injury rehabilitation literature is replete with theories about why families experience difficulties in coping, with many focusing upon psychodynamic explanations (Shaw, 1990). Families and professionals alike have acknowledged the stressors confronted by families, often accompanied by calls for provision of such services as information sharing, counseling, family therapy, and support groups (Shaw & McMahon, 1990). Unfortunately, many of these recommendations lack specificity and are more often related to service providers' perceptions of family needs than to the actual expressed needs of family members. For example, Shaw (1990) found that rehabilitation professionals tend to perceive the provision of family counseling services as being of paramount importance in addressing family needs. Consequently, rehabilitation professionals tend to focus their efforts in this area, failing to recognize that many families simply do not consider counseling to be a high priority need.

The lack of attention to designing family interventions to meet the specific expressed needs of family members is further evidenced by a failure to adapt interventions to the changing needs of family members over time (Camplair, Kreutzer, & Doherty, 1990). Family members are confronted with a multitude of stressors throughout and beyond the rehabilitation process. There is ample evidence to suggest that the intensity of family stress, and even the nature of the stressors themselves, tend to vary over time.

Limitations of Needs Assessment Studies

Numerous studies have been conducted to determine the nature of the stressors confronted by families at various points along the continuum of recovery. The majority of these studies examine families' perceived "burden" or stressors at various temporal intervals post-injury. While this approach has resulted in much useful information, it is not able to control for the widely varying rates of recovery among persons with TBI. For example, a single measure taken at three months post-injury might find one client having made substantial gains and functioning independently in many areas while a second client may have made only minimal progress and/or experienced significant setbacks. The varying rates of recovery might be expected to affect the nature and degree of stressors upon family members at any given interval post-injury.

A second group of studies assesses family needs at different stages of treatment (e.g., intensive care unit, acute rehabilitation). While these studies may be assumed to more effectively reflect the needs of family members of persons functioning at similar levels, they do not necessarily account for the varying lengths of time post-injury that the families have had to adapt to their altered life circumstances. Again, this factor might be expected to affect family needs. Few such studies assess the needs of family members while clients are in the latter stages of treatment (e.g., outpatient or post-discharge). This is understandable given the relative scarcity of categorical outpatient programming for TBI clients and given the problems of accessing subject pools post-discharge. Additional methodological problems hamper the utilization of such studies in understanding the ways in which family needs vary over time. These include the following:

1. Variations in sample selection criteria resulting in limited comparative utility. Such variations include inconsistencies in severity of injury, rehabilitation services received, cultural and geographical factors, and relationship to the client.

2. Variations in methodology result in limited comparative utility. Research on family needs has been conducted by telephone interview, structured personal interview, mailed questionnaires and other approaches. Often reports of research utilizing such methods fail to report any information regarding the reliability and validity of the instrumentation.

3. Sample sizes are frequently small and tend to shrink over repeated measures, especially in longitudinal studies.

4. Little information is available regarding the influence of demographic and other variables (e.g., family coping styles).

In spite of these methodological issues, some studies have provided useful information about family stressors and needs. These studies may provide clues regarding the uniformity and/or variations in family stressors and needs over time and at various levels of client treatment. Consequently, several studies and their relevant findings are summarized below.

Temporal Interval Studies

Several studies have assessed family needs at various temporal intervals post-injury (Panting & Merry, 1972; Thomsen, 1974; Romano, 1974; Rosenbaum & Najenson, 1976). Unfortunately, such studies tend to be difficult to utilize for comparative purposes for the reasons cited above. Two groups of researchers, however, have undertaken longitudinal studies of issues related to family needs which reduce (although they do not eliminate) many of these problems. They will be referred to here as the "British Studies" and the "Scottish Studies."

BRITISH STUDIES

Oddy, Humphrey, and Uttley (1978a, 1978b) evaluated the family members of 54 head-injured adults at one, six, and 12 months post-injury. At one month, 39% of the family members exhibited significant depressive symptomatology. At this interval, depression was positively correlated with length of post-traumatic amnesia (PTA) and the length of hospital stay, rough indicators of severity of injury. The proportion of family members with high levels of depression had decreased substantially by the six-month evaluation to 20% and remained relatively constant at the one-year measurement interval (23%). Surprisingly, neither length of PTA nor duration of hospital stay were associated with depression at six and 12 months, suggesting that the nature of the stressors had changed. Rather, at both six and 12 months, confusion and verbal expansiveness and number of symptoms reported by families were significantly associated with depression. In addition, failure to return to work by 12 months post-injury was also correlated with depression.

When asked to describe the main source of stress, relatives at both the six- and 12- month intervals most frequently reported some aspect of the client's current condition such as poorly controlled behavior, fear of epilepsy, and the physical demands of coping with the client. The second most common source of stress mentioned at both six and 12 months was anxiety over the client's future. Families also mentioned fear of another accident almost as frequently. Relatives were also asked about their own health at the six- and 12- month intervals. At both intervals about 25% reported having had an illness, usually stress-related, during the preceding six months.

In a related study, Oddy and Humphrey (1980) reported that at 12 months there was clear evidence of a trend toward increased friction between the injured individual and family members, most notably with siblings. Poorer family relationships tended to be associated with the existence of behavioral problems, but only if the patient had at least one sibling in the home. Poor family relationships were also associated with a high number of subjective complaints. At a two-year follow-up, however, family relationships were not significantly poorer than those of a control group (Oddy & Humphrey, 1980). The authors concluded that "family relationships, despite signs of disruption after 12 months, appeared to have settled again by the two-year assessment" (p. 801).

In their report of the two-year follow-up to the above studies, Weddell, Oddy, and Jenkins (1980) report that "after two years most parents and spouses had a reasonably realistic view of the situation and were behaving in a constructive fashion" (p. 262). Relatives were concerned with the client's lack of friends and social contacts and tended to include their relative in their own social activities. They note that many families at this point had picked up where rehabilitation professionals had left off and many had designed their own at-home rehabilitation programs using "common sense and past experience" (p. 262).

The authors note that these endeavors might be facilitated by increased family and professional cooperation.

A seven-year follow-up (Oddy, Coughlan, Tyerman, & Jenkins, 1985) found few changes in either client symptomatology or family stressors. Families were still struggling to find ways to address the employment and social needs of their TBI relative, often with minimal success.

SCOTTISH STUDIES

McKinlay, Brooks, Bond, Martinage, and Marshall (1981) investigated relatives' "subjective burden," which was defined as the amount of psychological strain attributable to patient changes. Relatives were surveyed at three, six, and 12 months post-injury. While the mean subjective burden rating remained constant at each interval, the degree of subjective burden was associated with different patient characteristics at different measurement intervals. Consistent with the Oddy, Humphrey, and Uttley (1978a) study, subjective burden was significantly associated with length of PTA at three months. However, by 12 months that association no longer existed. At three and six months post-injury, memory problems were related to subjective burden, but were not significant at 12 months. Conversely, while level of dependency was not a significant factor at three months, it became significant at six and 12 months. Several patient characteristics (i.e., emotional problems, subjective complaints, and disturbed behavior) were significantly related to subjective burden at all three evaluation intervals.

Based upon the results of the McKinlay et al. (1981) study, it seems reasonable to assume that during the first year post-injury the nature of the stressors confronted by a family changes, possibly due to changes in the patient. However, the change in stressors may also be related to changes in the family's ability to adapt over time.

Brooks and McKinlay (1983) reported additional findings on the same sample. Focusing on the issue of behavior and personality change, they found that although the relatives did not perceive that patients' personality changes had become more troublesome over the first year post-injury, their own subjective burden associated with personality changes increased substantially, again suggesting an increasing difficulty on the caregivers' part to tolerate personality changes. At three months a high degree of subjective burden was associated with a high degree of dependency on the part of the client. At six and 12 months this association was no longer significant. At six months the presence of a group of eight symptoms describing various types of behavioral or personality change had become significantly associated with high burden, although they had not been significant at three months. These symptoms included: quick-tempered, cold, dislikes company, unhappy, lifeless, cruel, mean, and unreasonable. These characteristics continued to be significantly associated with high subjective burden at 12 months and, in addition, several other characteristics became significant including irritable, listless, childish, insensitive, and changeable. Brooks and McKinlay (1983) note that personality change in and of itself may not be sufficient to cause high burden since other factors (such as personal resources) may also contribute to the relatives' sense of burden. However, when the relative does report a high degree of burden the chances are very great (92% in this study) that the patient will have been judged to have exhibited personality change. Conversely, the relationship between subjective burden and physical change is very weak. They conclude that "after the first six months of injury during which physical recovery is at its maximum one of the main thrusts of rehabilitation effort should be directed toward the family at least as much as toward the patient. Attempts should be made to classify, to understand, to predict, and importantly, to modify the changes in personality and behavior in the patient which may have such an impact upon the family. Teaching the family members to recognize and to manage personality and behavior change may be a crucial aspect of rehabilitation for this group of patients" (p. 343).

In a related study, Livingston, Brooks, and Bond (1985) noted that while relatives' social functioning is good in the first few months following the brain injury, problems have begun to develop by three months and these remain constant throughout the first year. Many relatives experience psychiatric symptoms and high anxiety. This may be associated with a perception that their relative does not appear to be improving, lack of understanding about cognitive and social deficits, and lack of information about prognosis and outcome. Relatives' degree of burden was not predicted by severity of injury, but rather by the level of subjective complaints which the patient voiced.

A follow-up study was conducted at five years post-injury (Brooks, Campsie, Symington, Beattie, & McKinlay, 1986). The researchers found that the level of subjective burden upon the relatives of TBI patients had increased from 24% with high burden levels at one year to 56% at five years. The proportion of families reporting low burden levels decreased from 43% at one year to 10% at five years. At the five-year assessment, high subjective burden was significantly associated with disturbed behavior and injury severity as indicated by length of PTA.

A notable finding at five years was that the frequency of aggressive behavior had increased markedly. Many relatives reported being afraid of their TBI relatives and constant anxiety about provoking violent outbursts. The authors note that this finding differs from that of Weddell et al. (1980) and may be accounted for by the fact that all of the clients in the latter study had received rehabilitation services, whereas the Brooks et al. sample had not. The authors speculate that the increase of reported negative behaviors among clients in their study may stem from frustrations associated with repeated failure to resume vocational, social, and leisure activities as well as decreased tolerance on the part of the relative and a tendency to mistakenly attribute routinely occurring negative behaviors to the head injury. Relatives continued to report high levels of dependency on the part of the client, mostly related to concern over the clients' impaired judgement and inability to be left alone at home.

In a study by Brooks, Campsie, Symington, Beattie, and McKinlay (1987), individuals with head injuries and their families were assessed at varying intervals post-injury. This allowed the authors to use a cross-sectional approach in examining the varying factors associated with family burden at various intervals post-injury. This study confirmed earlier findings of increasing levels of behavioral disturbance and moderate or high degrees of subjective burden as "the patient...begins to understand the full impact and chronicity of his or her injury and its effects on his or her social and occupational life" (p. 10). Longer periods of PTA were associated with higher degrees of subjective burden on families. However, the presence of behavioral, cognitive, affective, and dependency deficits were even more potent predictors of relative burden.

In addition to severity and the presence of specific symptomatology, the authors found that other factors may mediate the existence of severe burden. First, several characteristics of the relative him/herself appear to play a role. This finding is consistent with that of Livingston, Brooks, and Bond (1985) who examined the influence of several family characteristics on anxiety and impaired social functioning, including social class, age, prior psychiatric and medical status, and work history. They found the relatives' prior psychiatric and medical status, to be significantly associated with these problems. Interestingly, subjective burden was related to the relatives' perceived availability of help even though half of the "high burden" relatives did not perceive that they needed help.

Though additional longitudinal research would unquestionably be very useful in forming a clearer understanding of the ways in which relatives' needs change over time, it appears that the needs of relatives do, in fact, vary over the course of rehabilitation and beyond. Consequently the kinds of interventions needed should vary as well.

Needs Assessment Studies: Levels of Care

While the available information on the critical factors influencing the shift in needs is limited, it seems reasonable to assume that one of these critical factors might be changes in the level of care. For many TBI individuals the recovery process is characterized by movement to several different facilities specializing in various levels of care (McMahon & Fraser, 1988). As Pancsofar and Blackwell (1986) have observed, the experience of moving leaves one with a feeling of ambivalence, feelings of joy-sadness, hope-dejection, and excitement-indifference (p. 57).

They rightly note that even though the move may be perceived as a positive step toward community re-entry, the "displaced person" tends to experience considerable anxiety about the demands of the new living environment and his or her ability to adapt to those demands. Such anxiety is often shared by others close to the TBI individual (i.e., family members). As the patient moves closer and closer to discharge, families begin to anticipate the burden of care shifting to them and the implications of fitting the presence of the TBI individual into the fabric of their daily lives.

There have been some attempts to identify the needs of family members of TBI individuals within particular treatment settings.

ACUTE CARE

Mathis (1984) assessed the needs of families of patients with severe TBI who were hospitalized on an intensive care unit (ICU). Using a structured interview design adapted from an earlier study by Molter (1979), she found the 10 most important need statements of family members to be:

1. To feel that hospital personnel cared about my relative
2. To know I would be called at home if there were any changes in my relative's condition
3. To know exactly what was being done for my relative
4. To be reassured that the best care possible was being given my relative
5. To have my questions answered honestly
6. To be told about how my relative was going to be treated medically
7. To receive information about my relative's condition at least once a day
8. To feel accepted by hospital personnel
9. To feel there was hope
10. To have specific facts concerning my relative's progress

The priority needs listed above seem to echo an urgent need for information on current condition, patient care issues, and prognosis. At this critical juncture, families may not be concerned so much with understanding the long-term consequences of the TBI as they are with more urgent prognostic issues (e.g., Will the injured family member survive?). It would appear that while the patient is being treated in the ICU, families' most critical needs are for information, reassurance, and acceptance.

Of interest in the Mathis study was the finding that while families generally agreed about whether a need statement was important or not, there was considerable variability in the degree of importance they ascribed to each need statement. Mathis observed that "these findings emphasized the need to individualize planned nursing care for family members" (p. 43).

Mauss-Clum and Ryan (1981) asked 40 family members of patients who were on a TBI rehabilitation unit to identify their most critical needs at the time of the injury versus the help actually given. They found that almost unanimously, families' first priority was the need for a kind and clear explanation of the patient's condition. Almost as important was families' need for a discussion of realistic expectations for the patients' recovery. Emotional support, financial counseling, and advice about accessing community resources were seen as important, but not critical. The researchers observed that the families tended to strongly object to early pessimistic prognoses. While the families wanted to receive accurate prognostic information, they reported that hope was an important support to them and they wished to be assured that everything possible was being done to promote the best possible outcome. They realized, only in retrospect, that they had a critical need for assistance with accessing financial resources. The families felt that they badly needed professionals to bring the need for financial planning to their attention, as they were too preoccupied with their family member's survival to focus on financial matters.

When asked what kind of help families actually received, slightly over one-half said they received emotional support and a kind and clear explanation of the patient's condition. Only 23% felt they had received a realistic prognosis. Ten percent received financial counseling, three percent received resource counseling, and a full 20% denied that they had received any information or counseling at all.

The majority of families said they would have attended a family support group, but only because they were desperate to get their questions answered. They were so focused on the patient's physical recovery that they were not interested in taking time out to address their own emotional support needs at that stage. Mauss-Clum and Ryan (1981) speculated that meeting the intense need for information is of immense value in helping families make decisions and gain control of a confusing and frightening situation, a view mirrored by others (Lloen & Snyder, 1979).

INPATIENT REHABILITATION

There is a serious lack of attention in the literature to an empirical identification of the needs of family members during the inpatient rehabilitation stage. Shaw (1990) examined family and professional perceptions regarding family involvement in the rehabilitation process within a post-acute rehabilitation facility setting. Although the author was not specifically attempting to identify family needs, families were asked to rate the importance of their inclusion in various aspects of the rehabilitation process. Speculations about the needs of these family members may be inferred from their responses. The most notable finding was that, in general, family members strongly desired the opportunity to participate in virtually all aspects of the rehabilitation process. Items concerning availability of information and education were considered to be very important to families with 10 of the top 15-ranked items reflecting this need.

Families expressed the desire for concrete written information about their relatives' status as well as the opportunity to meet and converse with staff about their relatives' progress and prognosis, both informally and in formal staffings and educational meetings. Families desired the opportunity to have input into decisions regarding the family member and to assist in discharge planning. They appeared to demonstrate an acute awareness of the fact that they would be a primary support to the client after discharge and wanted involvement in making decisions and arrangements in planning for discharge. Families also expressed a strong desire to be notified immediately about changes in health and/or behavioral incidents.

Shaw (1990) noted that "having lived with uncertainty about their loved one's very survival, most families are understandably adamant about receiving any information that might threaten their family member's hard-won health status" (p. 169). Shaw also noted that given the well-documented deleterious effect of behavioral problems on families, it is not surprising to find families so concerned with behavioral dysfunction. Families strongly desired access to instruction on how they should interact with clients, reflecting probable anxiety over their uncertainty about how to respond to clients' fears, personality changes, and communication and cognitive changes.

The need for training on how to deal with injured family members was also identified as a strong family need in a study by Otsby, Sakata, and Leung (1988). Families expressed the desire to be able to act in the role of advocate for their injured family member, as they deem necessary (Shaw, 1990). It is interesting to note that while families and rehabilitation facility staff generally tended to agree on the appropriateness of family involvement in most areas, there were some notable differences in the two groups' priorities. The difference in opinion about the need for family counseling mentioned earlier was probably the most interesting example. Other areas where families and professionals differed substantially included families' desire for frequent and unrestricted contact with the client, many issues related to sexuality, the degree of active family involvement in treatment and decision making, receipt of written documentation of client activities/progress, and notification regarding schedule changes and minor health/behavioral problems. Often the differences between staff and families on these issues were a matter of degree, with families much more adamant about their need for inclusion in these activities/areas than were professionals.

Shaw (1990) theorized that family complaints about lack of inclusion in the rehabilitation process, lack of information, etc. may stem more from differing perceptions about the relative importance of various issues than from staff deliberately disregarding family needs. Shaw offered several recommendations for clinicians, facility management, and researchers based upon her findings.

OUTPATIENT/POST-DISCHARGE

The number of studies identifying family needs during outpatient treatment and after discharge from treatment facilities is very small, probably for the reasons discussed earlier. Studies conducted in this setting have primarily been undertaken by public service agencies or advocacy groups. They attempt to document unmet needs as a precursor to stimulating the development of more appropriate services and service delivery systems.

The Illinois Department of Rehabilitative Services (DORS) (1986) conducted a needs survey of persons with TBI (primarily severe) and their families. Ninety-five percent of the head-injured subjects lived at home, either independently or with others. Average length of time post-injury was seven years. The top four-ranked unmet needs were:

1. Public awareness/understanding
2. Employment
3. Recreation
4. Financial assistance

The report highlighted the need for independent or supervised living centers, respite care, recreational programs, day care, support groups and counseling for spouses, and appropriate vocational rehabilitation services.

A comprehensive needs assessment was conducted by the Wisconsin Department of Health and Social Services (DHSS) Brain Injury Task Force and the University of Wisconsin-Stout Research and Training Center (DHSS, 1988). This assessment was much broader in scope and was based on the responses of 715 family members of persons with head injuries. The TBI individuals' injuries had occurred an average of six and one-half years prior to the survey. DHSS reports that "of services not received, vocational training and job placement were identified as the most needed services, followed by supported employment, work adjustment, vocational rehabilitation, education, financial assistance, behavior management programs and social skills training" (p. iii). They note that "all of these services are directly related to the person's ability to seek, hold, or train for appropriate jobs" (p. iii). The final report describes the status of the families represented in this survey as follows:

> *Families in this group found themselves having severe financial difficulties, unable to purchase some basic services. Family members tried to fill all roles, particularly that of case managers. Those already working in the health care professions were found to be providing, on their own, therapies to the head injured person because they were not readily available in the community. Oftentimes, medical professionals provided little understanding of the injury or support for families. Families did not know what to expect or how to deal with what was happening and families were left to find their own services. They often found no support groups in any setting. Some were now forced to live with much of their own pain and suffering and with violence and destruction from the head injured person, characteristics which did not exist before the injury. Families as well as the person with the head injury became socially isolated. (p. 33)*

Discussion

The preceding review of the literature leads to some tentative conclusions regarding the needs of family members of persons with TBI. There appears to be convincing evidence that families have:

1. Significant needs which represent challenges to professionals, throughout and beyond the rehabilitation process;
2. Some needs which remain relatively constant but vary somewhat in intensity and focus; and
3. Needs which change over time as some needs are met and new ones arise. Such needs commonly arise in response to changes in treatment settings or environments, changes in the availability of emotional support and resources, changes in the demands placed upon both the TBI individual and family members, and/or changes in the family's gradual recognition of the permanence, extent of deficits, and challenges presented by TBI.

Despite methodological problems in making comparisons between the needs identified at various points in the different studies cited, some tentative observations may be possible. These observations will, however, need to be confirmed by additional research before they may be considered conclusive. Such tentative observations are summarized here under four broad headings: Information Needs, Involvement Needs, Direct Assistance Needs, and Counseling/Support Needs.

INFORMATION NEEDS

One of the most critically important needs identified by family members in virtually every needs assessment is the need for information. The intensity of families' need for information beyond the acute stage may be partially due to the possibility that only when survival is assured does the stress level of family members recede enough for them to process the information they are being given (DePompei, Zarski, & Hall, 1987). While this need seems to remain constant throughout the process, the type and amount of information appears to vary. Immediately after the TBI the information most critically needed is prognostic including not only predictions about the patient's survival, but regular, frequent updates on health status. Although families do desire information to help them understand TBI at this early stage, the desire for information which feeds hope is probably more acute at this time.

As the patient's condition stabilizes, the family begins to perceive that the brain is not going to mend like a broken bone and that, indeed, this injury is quite unlike anything in their experience. The needs for information about TBI, rehabilitation procedures, and what to expect in the future become more critically important. As specific problems/ issues arise, information targeted toward those issues becomes critical. As noted earlier, families desire specific information on how to react/ respond to the patient's cognitive, behavioral, and communicative issues. The need to receive written reports in addition to verbal updates becomes more important upon admission to the rehabilitation center where families may not have the opportunity to access staff personally due to geographic remoteness. The need for information regarding health status remains high at this stage and the concern for information regarding behavioral problems/incidents becomes extremely important as well. Prognostic information remains important but shifts from a focus on the question of survival to questions about what families should expect at discharge and predictions about the degree of recovery ultimately expected by treatment professionals.

After discharge, the need for information remains but again, shifts somewhat in focus. Confronted with the problems of social, vocational, and financial difficulties, families are suddenly in the position of having to seek assistance and solutions on their own. At this juncture, families need information about how to access and utilize resources in the community. They need to know how to effectively advocate for their TBI relative and how to obtain respite and support for themselves as they assume the responsibility of becoming "case managers," as well as primary caregivers.

In some instances families tolerance for the client's behavioral symptomatology may begin to wear thin at this point. Given limited access to professional assistance, families especially need to know how to manage behavioral dysfunction, particularly in those cases where the client is physically aggressive/abusive. Families need information about the needs of siblings. They need to understand both the dynamics of interactions between the TBI and siblings and how to assist family members in adjusting to the presence of the TBI individual in the home.

After discharge, families need help in understanding the common problem of vocational dysfunction, both in terms of understanding the role of the cognitive and behavioral dysfunction in clients' failure to secure and/or maintain employment, and in terms of learning the role they may play in obtaining appropriate vocational services. All too often, vocational rehabilitation has been inadequately addressed in the rehabilitation setting and families have little information to rely upon in their efforts to understand and address this issue.

Families also require information to assist them in addressing clients' lack of social outlets and interpersonal relationships. While rehabilitation facilities often address "social skills problems," few families feel equipped to deal with the loneliness and social isolation which result from clients' ongoing deficits in this area.

INVOLVEMENT NEEDS

Another broad category of family needs which remains constant but changes in focus concerns issues related to direct involvement in treatment or care. Throughout the recovery process, the majority of families remain concerned and wish to be actively involved in efforts directed toward facilitating the client's recovery. The intensity of these needs appear to vary, however, given the specific circumstances and the availability of professional intervention.

Immediately following the TBI there tends to be an intense need for action on the part of the family. DeBosky and Morin (1985) noted that families tend to experience high degrees of anxiety and panic which they are unable to relieve by activity designed to assist their family member due to their lack of expertise in medical/health care. Shaw (1990) notes that "...at the very time that family members feel most in need of intervening to assist and protect their injured family member, they must turn him/her over to the care of strangers" (p. 74). Similarly, Marlatt (1988) comments that immediately following the onset of a major crisis, families feel an urgent need to resume parental/caregiving roles. During acute care and rehabilitation, families confront this dilemma of the need to be involved coupled with the need to rely on professionals' expertise. Consequently, families may have strong needs to be included in treatment in every possible way short of actual medical/surgical intervention. Barin and Leger (1985) noted that "...a parent's anxiety can take many forms. Sometimes it takes the form of 'doing.' One mother may insist that her child receive several hours of physical therapy daily (on the theory that if some therapy is good, more is better), whereas another may persist in preparing special 'health food' for her child despite dietary and medical contraindications" (p. 105).

The need for active involvement remains strong throughout the period of residential rehabilitation (Shaw, 1990) but undergoes several changes when the client is discharged home. At that point, the family often becomes solely responsible for every aspect of the client's care and adjustment, often while feeling ill-prepared to do so. Families who may have repeatedly asked for an increased role in the rehabilitation of their loved one during rehabilitation may feel that the entire responsibility has suddenly been dumped in their laps. The need for involvement remains, but is now accompanied by an increase in the need for some ongoing assistance from the professional community. Families often begin to feel burdened by the heavy responsibilities they are forced to assume and feel the need for relief in the form of assistance from community service providers, appropriate supervised living and day treatment programs, and respite programs.

DIRECT ASSISTANCE NEEDS

Early after the TBI, families tend to function in a state of shock. As noted earlier, several studies of the needs of family members at the time immediately following the injury found that families were so focused upon the needs of the injured family member that their own needs paled by comparison. Yet, in retrospect, they realized that they had needs they wished had been addressed. Help with such practical matters as financial assistance, childcare, and resource identification would have been very helpful (Mauss-Clum & Ryan, 1981). It is important to note, however, that initially families may not be able to articulate these needs.

During rehabilitation, after the immediate crisis has passed, families may become more aware of the need to attend to practical matters and to their other responsibilities. At this stage families may seek out help with dealing with insurance coverage issues, transportation, and childcare needs (Shaw, 1990). During rehabilitation, however, the family's focus remains very much on the patient. During acute care and rehabilitation, the majority of the client's needs are being addressed by professional staff, minimizing the family's need for additional direct assistance.

After discharge, another major shift in emphasis occurs. As noted in the preceding chapter, assistance from professionals is withdrawn at the very point at which new needs are manifested. Families may attempt to utilize community resources for social and recreational outlets and vocational assistance for their TBI family member only to find them nonexistent, inaccessible, or inadequate. Limited insurance coverage may severely restrict the availability of needed therapies. Noble, Conley, Laski, and Noble (1990) make the following observation:

> *Coverage is more likely to be available for acute medical service and convalescence than for long term rehabilitation and social services. The value placed on human life and cognitive functioning means that, in most cases, every possible resource that a family can command will be expended on initial medical care and treatment. (p. 31)*

The study conducted by the Wisconsin DHSS (DHSS, 1988) identified assistance with vocational rehabilitation as a critical need. The need for assistance in securing appropriate vocational rehabilitation services is further punctuated by the findings of Oddy, Humphrey, and Uttley (1978) that the client's failure to return to work by 12 months post-injury was correlated with depression in family members. The time-interval studies discussed earlier clearly document families' needs for assistance with meeting the social and recreational needs of persons with brain injury up to seven years after the TBI (Oddy et al., 1985; Brooks et al., 1987).

COUNSELING/SUPPORT NEEDS

The need for counseling and support persists for years beyond the injury, however, there are substantial variations in the ways in which such needs are experienced at different points in the rehabilitation process. Early on, families rather firmly reject professionals' attempts to provide them with counseling. In Molter's (1979) study, emotional support was assigned a very low priority by family members. Mauss-Clum and Ryan's (1981) families felt that while emotional support was important, it "was not of immediate concern" (p. 166). However, in the study by Mathis (1984), families ranked the need statement "to feel accepted by hospital personnel" as eighth in importance out of 45 need statements.

In none of these studies were relatives enthusiastic about attending a support group for the purpose of receiving emotional support. In attempting to explain this phenomenon Mauss-Clum and Ryan (1981) observed that "...it seemed that families might be so involved in grieving at the patient's bedside that they would be reluctant to take time out for a group session" (p. 167). In the initial crisis period families appear to focus on their own emotional needs only to the extent that they hope that staff will understand and accept them enough to ensure that their other patient-directed needs are met (e.g., the needs for information regarding condition and prognosis, reassurance that the patient is receiving the best possible care). Related to the need for support is the fact that families also express strong needs to be able to feel hopeful and tend to have strong negative reactions to early pessimistic prognoses on the part of medical personnel (Mauss-Clum & Ryan, 1981).

As the client stabilizes and enters the rehabilitation phase, the need for emotional support becomes more apparent to family members, with the majority expressing a desire to be afforded the opportunity for emotional support and to attend support groups (Shaw, 1990). However, as mentioned earlier, Shaw found that while families felt they should have the opportunity to participate in such activities as marital, sexual, family, and adjustment counseling, they did not see this as a high priority need. Shaw theorized that "...families tend to view the source of their problems as external to themselves and are [still] primarily focused upon information and other needs associated with the client's recovery" (p. 176). For these reasons several researchers have recommended that rehabilitation professionals should offer practical, information-oriented support groups as opposed to groups emphasizing in-depth counseling or psychotherapy (Cole, 1985; Longo & Bond, 1984; Mathis, 1984).

The previously mentioned need for information about behavioral issues manifested at this point may be addressed through training in behavioral management techniques. Such instruction necessarily involves the provision of supportive counseling as the application of such techniques and the behaviors themselves tend to be extremely upsetting to families. In general, previous studies lead to the natural conclusion that the greater the amount and intensity of personality change and behavioral symptomatology present, the greater will be the family's need for counseling and support.

At the point of discharge when families are faced with the day-to day reality of coping alone with behavioral issues, dependency issues, vocational and social concerns, the need for support and/or counseling may become more intense. Interfamilial relationships may become disrupted, especially when there are siblings present in the home, resulting in needs for family counseling. In addition, discharge improves clients' access to alcohol and illegal substances and frequently substance abuse becomes an extremely disruptive problem at this time (Langley, Lindsay, Lam, & Priddy, 1990). Families frequently find themselves in need of assistance in coping with the effects of substance use and abuse by their TBI relative, assistance which is often not readily available (see Chapter 10).

The Problem of Meeting Family Needs Post-discharge

In this chapter the author has endeavored to demonstrate the ways in which the needs of families of persons with TBI are ever-present, yet may change in focus and intensity over time and circumstances.

Recognition of the varied needs of families at different points post-injury should help professionals to become more flexible, creative, and responsive to specific family needs. Unfortunately, this is possible only to the extent that professionals have ongoing contact with families. The scarcity and adequacy of community resources seriously restricts access to professionals by family members after discharge from rehabilitation facilities. Kreutzer, Zasler, Camplair, and Leininger (1990) observe that:

> *...many communities lack transitional living, outpatient rehabilitation, day rehabilitation and vocational rehabilitation services.... Following discharge insurance coverage for rehabilitation may be exhausted or may not include outpatient services. Families may have to devote considerable time to seeking, visiting and evaluating treatment facilities. In some cases services may be too far away or simply unavailable within a day's traveling distance. In other cases, lengthy daily travel may be required to allow the person with traumatic brain injury to participate in outpatient rehabilitation on a regular basis. Family members providing transportation may need to give up their jobs or reduce work hours, which exacerbates financial stresses. (p. 249)*

These authors and others (Cervelli, 1990) have proposed methods for meeting the needs of individuals with TBI and their families post-discharge. However, all acknowledge that until significant improvement occurs in the availability and accessibility of appropriate services and resources, families will continue to struggle alone. It is incumbent on professionals to continue to advocate for recognition of the gravity of the situation and to promote positive change through education, political action, and support of like-minded groups and individuals.

References

Barin, J. J., & Leger, D. (1985). Working with the family: The rehabilitation phase. In M. Ylvisaker (Ed.), *Head injury rehabilitation: Children and adolescents* (pp. 101-115). San Diego: College Hill Press.

Brooks, N. (1984). Head injury and the family. In N. Brooks (Ed.), *Closed head injury: Psychological, social and family consequences*. Oxford: Oxford University Press.

Brooks, N., Campsie, L., Symington, C., Beattie, A., & McKinlay, W. (1986). The five-year outcome of severe blunt head injury: A relative's view. *Journal of Neurology, Neurosurgery & Psychiatry, 49*, 764-770.

Brooks, N., Campsie, L., Symington, C., Beattie, A., & McKinlay, W. (1987). The effects of severe head injury on patient and relative within seven years of injury. *Journal of Head Trauma Rehabilitation, 2*(3), 1-13.

Brooks, N., & McKinlay, W. (1983). Personality and behavioral changes after severe blunt head injury: A relative's view. *Journal of Neurology, Neurosurgery & Psychiatry, 46*, 336-344.

Burke, W. H., Weselowski, M. D., & Guth, W. L. (1988). Comprehensive head injury rehabilitation: An outcome evaluation. *Brain Injury, 2*(4), 313-322.

Camplair, P. S., Kreutzer, J. S., & Doherty, K. R. (1990). Family outcome following adult traumatic brain injury: A critical review of the literature. In J. S. Kreutzer & P. Wehman (Eds.), *Community integration following traumatic brain injury* (pp. 207-224). Baltimore: Paul H. Brookes.

Cervelli, L. (1990). Re-entry into the community and systems of post-hospital care. In M. Rosenthal, E. R. Griffith, M. R. Bond, & J. D. Miller (Eds.), *Rehabilitation of the adult and child with traumatic brain injury* (pp. 463-475). Philadelphia: F. A. Davis.

Cole, T. M. (1985). *Intimacy: A healing influence after brain injury*. Presented at Post-graduate Course on Rehabilitation of the Brain-injured Adult and Child: 9th Annual Conference. Williamsburg, VA.

Department of Health and Social Services Brain Injury Task Force (DHSS). (1988). *Final report to the secretary*. April 6, 1988.

DeBosky, D. S., & Morin, K. (1985). *A "how to handle" manual for families of the brain injured*. Tampa, FL: Hillsborough County Hospital Authority Printing and Graphic Services.

DePompei, R., Zarski, J. J., & Hall, D. E. (1987). A systems approach to understanding CHI family functioning. *Cognitive Rehabilitation, 5*(2), 6-11.

Illinois Department of Rehabilitative Services (1986). *The head injured: Their unmet needs*. July, 1986.

Kreutzer, J. S., Zasler, N. D., Camplair, P. S., & Leininger, B. E. (1990). A practical guide to family intervention following adult traumatic brain injury. In J. S. Kreutzer & P. Wehman (Eds.), *Community integration following traumatic brain injury* (pp. 249-273). Baltimore: Paul H. Brookes.

Langley, M. J., Lindsay, W. P., Lam, C. S., & Priddy, D. A. (1990). A comprehensive alcohol abuse treatment programme for persons with traumatic brain injury. *Brain Injury*, *4*(1), 77-86.

Livingston, M. G., Brooks, D. N., & Bond, M. R. (1985). Patient outcome in the year following severe head injury and relatives' psychiatric and social functioning. *Journal of Neurology, Neurosurgery & Psychiatry*, *48*, 876-881.

Lloen, M., & Snyder, M. (1979). Psychosocial aspects of care of the long-term comatose patient. *Journal of Neurosurgical Nursing*, *11*(4), 235-237.

Longo, D. C., & Bond, L. (1984). Families of the handicapped child: Research and practice. *Family Relations*, *33*(1), 57-65.

Marlatt, J. (1988). The role of the family in rehabilitation. *Journal of Rehabilitation*, *54*(1), 7-8, 77.

Mathis, M. (1984). Personal needs of family members of critically ill patients with and without acute brain injury. *Journal of Neurosurgical Nursing*, *16*, 36-44.

Mauss-Clum, N., & Ryan, N. (1981). Brain injury and the family. *Journal of Neurosurgical Nursing*, *13*, 165-169.

McKinlay, W. W., Brooks, D. N., Bond, M. R., Martinage, D. P., & Marshall M. M. (1981). The short-term outcome of severe blunt head injury as reported by relatives of the injured persons. *Journal of Neurology, Neurosurgery & Psychiatry*, *44*, 527-533.

McMahon, B. T., & Fraser, R. T. (1988). Basic issues and trends in head injury rehabilitation. In S. Rubin & N. Rubin (Eds.), *Contemporary challenges to the rehabilitation counseling profession* (pp. 197-216). Baltimore: Paul H. Brookes.

Molter, N. (1979). Needs of relatives of critically ill patients: A descriptive study. *Heart and Lung*, *8*, 332-339.

Noble, J. H., Jr., Conley, R. W., Laski, F., & Noble, M. A. (1990). Issues and problems in the treatment of traumatic brain injury. *Journal of Disability Policy Studies*, *1*(2), 19-45.

Oddy, M., Coughlan, T., Tyerman, A., & Jenkins, D. (1985). Social adjustment after closed head injury: A further follow-up seven years after injury. *Journal of Neurology, Neurosurgery & Psychiatry*, *48*, 564-568.

Oddy, M., & Humphrey, M. (1980). Social recovery during the year following severe head injury. *Journal of Neurology, Neurosurgery & Psychiatry*, *43*, 798-802.

Oddy, M., Humphrey, M., & Uttley, D. (1978a). Stresses upon the relatives of head injured patients. *British Journal of Psychiatry*, *133*, 507-513.

Oddy, M., Humphrey, M., & Uttley, D. (1978b). Subjective impairment and social recovery after closed head injury. *Journal of Neurology, Neurosurgery & Psychiatry*, *41*, 611-616.

Otsby, S., Sakata, R., & Leung, P. (1988). *Head injury rehabilitation: Persistence of problems and perceived needs within the two years post-treatment.* Paper presented at the 12th Annual Post-graduate course on Rehabilitation of the Brain-injured Adult and Child. Williamsburg, VA, June, 1988.

Pancsofar, E., & Blackwell, R. (1986). *A user's guide to community re-entry for the severely handicapped*. Albany, NY: State University of New York Press.

Panting, A., & Merry, P. H. (1972). The long-term rehabilitation of severe head injuries with particular reference to the need for social and medical support for the patient's family. *Rehabilitation, 38*, 33-37.

Romano, M. D. (1974). Family response to traumatic brain injury. *Scandinavian Journal of Rehabilitation Medicine, 6*, 1-4.

Rosenbaum, M., & Najenson, T. (1976). Changes in life patterns and symptoms of low mood as reported by wives of brain-injured soldiers. *Journal of Consulting and Clinical Psychology, 44*, 881-889.

Rosenthal, M., & Young, T. (1988). Effective family intervention after traumatic brain injury: Theory and practice. *Journal of Head Trauma Rehabilitation, 3*(4), 42-50.

Shaw, L. R. (in press). Family and professional perceptions of the appropriateness of family involvement in the head injury rehabilitation process (Doctoral dissertation, Florida State University, 1990). *Dissertation Abstracts International.*

Shaw, L. R., & McMahon, B. T. (1990). Family-staff conflict in the rehabilitation setting: Causes, consequences and implications. *Brain Injury, 4*(1), 87-93.

Thomsen, I. V. (1974). The patient with severe head injury and his family. *Scandinavian Journal of Rehabilitation Medicine, 6*, 180-183.

Weddell, R., Oddy, M., & Jenkins, D. (1980). Social adjustment after rehabilitation: A two-year follow-up of patients with severe head injury. *Psychological Medicine, 10*, 257-263.

Index

Index

A

B

C

D

E

F

G

H

I

J

L

M

N

O

P

Q

R

S

T

V

W